Current Surgical Practice Volume 5

Invited contributions mostly based on lectures given at the Royal College of Surgeons of England

Current Surgical Practice Volume 5

Edited on behalf of the Royal College of Surgeons of England by
John Hadfield, CBE, TD, MS, FRCS
Formerly Surgeon, Stoke Mandeville Hospital, Aylesbury; Vice-President and Chairman of the Court of Examiners, Royal College of Surgeons of England

Michael Hobsley, TD, DSc, PhD, MChir, FRCS
David Patey Professor of Surgery, University College and Middlesex School of Medicine, London

and
Tom Treasure, MD, MS, FRCS
Thoracic and Cardiac Surgeon, St. George's Hospital, London

with a Foreword by
Sir Ian P. Todd, KBE, MD, MS, PRCS
President of the Royal College of Surgeons of England; Consulting Surgeon to St Bartholomew's and St Mark's Hospitals, London

Edward Arnold
A division of Hodder & Stoughton
LONDON   AUCKLAND   MELBOURNE

© 1990 Edward Arnold

First published in Great Britain 1990

British Library Cataloguing in Publication Data
Current surgical practice.
  Vol. 5–
  1. Medicine. Surgery
  I. Title
  617

ISBN 0–340–52850–8

All rights reserved. No part of this publication may be reproduced or transmitted in any form or by any means, electronically or mechanically, including photocopying, recording or any information storage or retrieval system, without either prior permission in writing from the publisher or a licence permitting restricted copying. In the United Kingdom such licences are issued by the Copyright Licensing Agency: 33–34 Alfred Place, London WC1E 7DP.

Whilst the advice and information in this book is believed to be true and accurate at the date of going to press, neither the author nor the publisher can accept any legal responsibility or liability for any errors or omissions that may be made. In particular (but without limiting the generality of the preceding disclaimer) every effort has been made to check drug dosages; however, it is still possible that errors have been missed. Furthermore, dosage schedules are being continually revised and new side-effects recognized. For these reasons the reader is strongly urged to consult the drug companies' printed instructions before administering any of the drugs recommended in this book.

Typeset in Baskerville by Anneset, Weston-super-Mare, Avon
Printed and bound in Great Britain for Edward Arnold,
of Hodder and Stoughton Limited, Mill Road, Dunton Green,
Sevenoaks, Kent TN13 2YA by Butler and Tanner Ltd., Frome and London.

Contributors

H. Barr, FRCS, FRCS(Ed)
    Senior Surgical Registrar, University College Hospital

J. P. Blandy, DM, MCh, FRCS
    Professor of Urology, The London Hospital Medical College; Surgeon, The London Hospital; Urologist, St Peter's Hospital, London

P. B. Boulos, MS, FRCS
    Senior Lecturer, University College and Middlesex School of Medicine; Honorary Surgeon, University College Hospital

J. W. Brooke Barnett, MB, BS
    Secretary, The Medical Defence Union

L. Delbridge, MD, BSc (Med), FRACS
    Senior Lecturer in Surgery, University of Sydney

R. K. Ghandhi, MS, FRCS(Ed), FACS, FAMS, FCPS
    Honorary Paediatric Surgeon, Sir H. N. Hospital; Chairman of Board of Surgical Studies, University of Bombay; formerly Professor of Paediatric Surgery and Dean of Faculty of Medicine, University of Bombay

S. Griffin, FRCS
    Research Fellow and Honorary Registrar, The Middlesex Hospital

G. J. Hadfield, CBE, TD, MS, FRCS
    Formerly Vice President and Chairman of the Court of Examiners, Royal College of Surgeons of England; Surgeon, Stoke Mandeville Hospital, Aylesbury, Bucks

M. Hobsley, TD, DSc, PhD, MChir, FRCS
    David Patey Professor of Surgery, Head of Department of Surgery, University College and Middlesex School of Medicine, London

Contributors

J. D. Hardcastle, MA, MChir, FRCS, FRCP
Professor of Surgery, University of Nottingham; Surgeon, University General and City Hospitals, Nottingham

G. Jantet, MB, FRCS
Surgeon, The Ealing Hospital, London; Honorary Vascular Surgeon and Senior Lecturer in Surgery, Hammersmith Hospital and Royal Postgraduate Medical School, London

G. Keen, MS, FRCS
Cardiothoracic Surgeon, Bristol Royal Infirmary; Clinical Lecturer in Surgery, University of Bristol; Formerly Hunterian Professor of Surgery, Royal College of Surgeons of England

D. Kirk, MA, DM, FRCS
Urologist, Western Infirmary, Glasgow; Honorary Clinical Lecturer, University of Glasgow

J. Kirkham, MA, MChir, FRCS
Honorary Senior Lecturer and Surgeon, St George's Hospital and Medical School; Surgeon, St James' Hospital, London

J. M. Little, MD, MS, FRACS, FACS
Professor of Surgery, Westmead Hospital, The University of Sydney; Chairman, Department of Surgery, Westmead Hospital; Honorary Professor, Sun Yat-Sen University Guangzhou, People's Republic of China

M. C. Mace, MB, BS, FDS RCS (Eng), MRCS (Eng), LRCP (Lond)
Oral and Maxillo-facial Surgeon, Stoke Mandeville Hospital and Milton Keynes Hospital; Honorary Clinical Lecturer, United Medical and Dental Schools of Guy's and St Thomas' Hospitals

M. Mercadier, MD, FRCS
Professor of Surgery, The American Hospital, Paris, France

A. R. Mehta, MS, FICS
President, Indian Society of Head and Neck Oncology; Past President, Association of Surgeons of India; Surgeon and Chief of Head and Neck Service 'C', Tata Memorial Hospital, Bombay; Head of Department of Oncology, Dr Balabhai Nanavata Hospital, Bombay; Consultant in Oncology, Jaslok Hospital, Bombay

S. A. Mehta, MS
Research Fellow, Department of Surgery, Tata Memorial Hospital, Bombay, India

N. Mortensen, MD, FRCS
Surgeon, Departments of Surgery and Gastroenterology, John Radcliffe Hospital, Oxford

Foreword

CME—Continuing Medical Education—is the catch-phrase of the moment. Undoubtedly it becomes increasingly necessary and increasingly difficult to keep abreast of progress in whatever branch of surgery one specializes. At the same time, there is an ever-escalating need for surgeons to be conscious of their limitations and to be responsible for their own actions and those of their juniors. Unfortunate though it may be, there is a greater tendency for patients to sue—largely due to the greater expectations which advances in surgery have made possible.

This book—a very welcome and worthy successor to the four volumes which have preceded it—addresses the two subjects mentioned above: (i) specific advances, and (ii) what to do in unforeseen circumstances.

The editors have, once again, selected subjects, introduced by acknowledged experts, which challenge most of us at some stage in our careers. However, before you delve into your specific chapter, please read the Preface and Introduction; everyone can learn from the wisdom expounded in this brief entr'acte. From time to time, iatrogenic problems will occur. With the increased emphasis on audit and quality control, our mistakes and unforeseen outcomes will be discussed by our colleagues, peers and juniors. There is no doubt that much may be learned from those who have experienced the problem already.

My Council congratulates the editors on a further outstanding volume and thanks them most sincerely for bringing together so much information in so few pages. John Hadfield has edited, with colleagues, all the previous volumes and is now laying down his pen. We wish him a long and happy retirement, and thank him for all he has done, not only for Current Surgical Practice, but also for the Royal College of Surgeons.

Sir Ian Todd, KBE PRCS
June 1989

R. J. Nicholls, MChir, FRCS
   Surgeon, St Mark's and St Thomas' Hospitals

T. C. Northfield, MD, FRCP
   Physician, St James' Hospital, London; Reader in Medicine, St George's Hospital Medical School, London

J. P. Pryor, MS, FRCS
   Urological Surgeon, King's College and St Peter's Hospitals; Formerly Dean, Institute of Urology

T. S. Reeve, CBE, MB, BS, FRACS, DDU, FRACR (Hon)
   Professor of Surgery, Royal North Shore Hospital, University of Sydney, Australia

S. H. Richards, FRCS
   ENT Surgeon, University Hospital of Wales, Cardiff; Member of the Court of Examiners, Royal College of Surgeons of England

P. G. Stableforth, MB, FRCS
   Orthopaedic and Trauma Surgeon, United Bristol Hospitals

J. P. S. Thomson, MS, FRCS
   Surgeon, St Mark's Hospital for Diseases of the Rectum and Colon and Homerton Hospital, London; Honorary Lecturer in Surgery, St Bartholomew's Hospital Medical College, London

T. Treasure, MD, MS, FRCS
   Thoracic and Cardiac Surgeon, St. George's Hospital, London

M. H. Wheeler, MD, FRCS
   Surgeon, University Hospital of Wales

R. A. Williams, MA, FRCS, FRCS(Ed)
   ENT Surgeon, The Middlesex Hospital; Queen Elizabeth II Hospital, Welwyn Garden City; King Edward VII Hospital for Officers, London; Honorary Consultant Otolaryngologist to the Army

Preface

This is the fifth volume of *Current Surgical Practice*. Volumes 1 and 2, published in 1976 and 1978 respectively, have passed their tenth birthdays—the half-life period of medical knowledge—and have now gone out of print. It is not our policy to rewrite earlier chapters; we only persist with them when they give the reader something new and different.

We still retain our original intention of recording lectures given at the Royal College by authorities expressing their opinions rather than presenting standard review articles. An effort is made with each book to present 'the growing edge of surgery': broad-based in the generality of the subject and seeking contributions from leaders in all disciplines, outside as well as within surgery, whose work adds to surgical knowledge and progress. In Volume 3 we widened our field of choice further to Fellows of the College who, by virtue only of distance, were normally unable to come to the College and give a lecture. The late Professor A. K. Basu of Calcutta writing on surgery in tropical countries, and Professor A. G. R. Sheil of Sydney writing on renal transplantation, started this new approach, and the tradition was continued in Volume 4 by Professor T. E. Udwadia of Bombay writing on peritoneoscopy. In Volume 5 there are two chapters from Australia, by Professor Tom Reeves on cancer of the thyroid, and by Professor Miles Little on abdominal hydatid disease; and two from Bombay, by Professor R. K. Gandi on children's surgery in the tropics, and by Professor A. R. Mehta and S. A. Mehta of the Tata Memorial Hospital on cancer of the oral cavity.

The chapter by Tim Northfield and John Kirkham, detailing the joint approach by the therapeutic team of physician and surgeon to acute gastrointestinal haemorrhage, demonstrates that surgery is no longer an island in the sea of medicine.

The other contributions from our colleagues in the UK cover a cross-section of the generality of surgery, embodying new work and ideas on a variety of subjects. The chapter by Martin Mace on facial fractures, which are clearly the province of a facio-maxillary expert, is included as the patient first presents in the Accident and Emergency Department and the injury may in any case be part of a multiple injuries complex.

The section on iatrogenic surgical disease presents a broad canvas of the circumstances, problems, decisions, treatment and medico-legal aspects of this important subject. The intention is to view the general problem by studying examples of the particular. Each chapter, written by an authority, tells the reader how to tackle the acute situation. This time we have sought help from Europe and are grateful to Professor Maurice Mercardier of Paris for his chapter on bile duct injuries.

This book is the work of many hands. The editors have therefore left each chapter as a single entity rather than producing uniformity, which might mask all the variations in approach and might obliterate the authors' personal styles.

We are grateful to our friends who, as contributors, have again made this venture possible. The President, Members of the Council, specialist associations, the Penrose May Tutor and the Regional Advisers and Tutors have all, in many ways, contributed to surgical teaching and training and hence to this book: to them we offer our thanks.

The generality of surgery remains the sheet-anchor of basic surgical knowledge. It is our intention and hope that this book and its companion volumes represent this concept in fact.

A great deal of organization is needed to bring any book to presentation and we have received help from many sources. Special thanks in this respect must be recorded to Mr Paul Price and his staff at Edward Arnold and to Miss Sue Allen of the Department of Surgery at the Middlesex Hospital.

This is the last volume that John Hadfield will be editing, and he is especially grateful to the many friends who have helped with this enterprise.

London John Hadfield
1989 Michael Hobsley
  Tom Treasure

Contents

Contributors

Foreword

Preface

1	**Specialism and generalism in surgery** Michael Hobsley	1
2	**Towards endoscopic therapy for bleeding peptic ulcers: targets and weapons, trials and costs** Tim Northfield and John Kirkham	8
3	**Lasers and their application to surgery** P. B. Boulos and H. Barr	21
4	**Postoperative thromboembolic disease: a tantalizing enigma** Tom Treasure and Steven Griffin	38
5	**Facial fractures** Martin Mace	52
6	**Cancer of the oral cavity: cheek, tongue and alveolar margins** Ashok R. Mehta and Sahir A. Mehta	66
7	**Cancer of the thyroid** Tom S. Reeve and Leigh Delbridge	85
8	**Avoiding bowel ostomies** R. J. R. Nicholls	100
9	**New thoughts and methods in colorectal cancer** Neil Mortensen	113
10	**Familial adenomatous polyposis** James P. S. Thomson	128

11	**Hydatid disease of the liver** J. Miles Little	146
12	**Prostatic carcinoma** David Kirk	162
13	**Male infertility** John P. Pryor	179
14	**The practice of children's surgery in India** R. K. Gandhi	194
15	**Benign diseases of the breast** John Hadfield	208

IATROGENIC SURGICAL DISEASE

	Introduction John Hadfield, Michael Hobsley and Tom Treasure	221
16	**The philosophy of medical defence** J. W. Brooke Barnett	223
17	**Facial palsy** R. A. Williams and M. Hobsley	231
18	**The laryngeal nerves** Malcolm H. Wheeler and Stephen H. Richards	237
19	**Bile duct injuries** Maurice Mercardier	251
20	**Spinal cord damage associated with surgery of the descending aorta** G. Keen	260
21	**The ureter** John P. Blandy	270
22	**Injuries from bandages, splints, plasters and tourniquets** P. G. Stableforth	278
23	**The saphenofemoral junction: damage and bleeding** Georges Jantet	286
24	**Anorectal stenosis** J. D. Hardcastle	296
	Index	301

1

Specialism and generalism in surgery

Michael Hobsley, TD, DSc, PhD, MChir, FRCS

There is at present considerable debate about whether the balance between specialism and generalism in surgery is ideal, or needs shifting in the direction of specialization. It is interesting that no-one seems to favour the view that the balance needs adjusting towards generalism, and *a priori* this suggests that there should be some degree of movement towards the specialist side. Nevertheless, the object of this article is to examine the 'pros' and 'cons' of changes in either direction, without (one hopes) any prejudice.

A natural trend

The first point to make is that the trend towards specialization is entirely natural. Put three human beings together on a desert island, and it is as certain as anything can be in this world that one will be put in charge (or assume command) of cooking, one of house-building and one of food provision. Give the band a fourth person, and some new role will be invented for him, perhaps the organization of transport for escape. It is an interesting feature, however, that the demarcation between the specialities will only extend to the organizing and controlling strata of the occupation—the cook will expect help from the house-builder with peeling the potatoes, the house-builder will need help to erect a heavy corner pole, and so on. Perhaps the inferences to draw are that no man is an island and that no speciality can thrive on its own, without support from other specialities; and also perhaps that all specialities are likely to contain zones that do not require the attention of the specialist himself (zones of general interest).

The second point is that certain prerequisites are essential if specialization is to flourish. The first is stability and freedom from outside attack. It may be that our band of intrepid castaways have to spend some time at the beginning in repelling attacks from hostile savages, whether man, beast or both. In such circumstances, each man will probably have to snatch a bite to eat as best he can, whenever he can spare a moment from the fray. The second prerequisite is time. It may take some time for members of the band to recognize that there might be advantages in specialization, and for each member to opt for the particular speciality of his choice. The process of making this choice depends upon more than the individual's preference, past history of experience, or even demonstration of present skills: there is the factor of perceived seniority which will decide between conflicting claims of two (or more) individuals to a single speciality. All these features have relevance to our discussion of the place of specialization in surgery, and will be recalled later.

Advantages of specialization

One does not need to labour the advantages of specialization because they are obvious. The specialist accumulates experience of the speciality more rapidly than he would were it diluted with material from other fields. In a discipline like surgery in which manipulative skills are essential, the specialist is likely to be much more expert in the performance of an operation which he does frequently than is the non-specialist who only has an occasional opportunity to perform the procedure. The rapid accumulation of data facilitates research in the field, and as our knowledge increases so our decision-making becomes sharper and more refined. All these advantages summate to produce a quicker route towards the object of the exercise—better treatment for our patients.

Disadvantages of specialization

Nevertheless, there is another side to the coin, perhaps best summarized in the hackneyed definition of a specialist as a man who knows more and more about less and less: the limiting situation is that he knows everything about nothing. He may be the world expert on an esoteric condition, but what is his value as a clinician if he has to wait a year to see his next case? Of course that is an exaggeration, but there is no doubt that the compartmentation of hospital medicine into smaller subspecialties makes it more difficult to steer the patient in the right direction. In countries like the UK with a strong system of primary care, the onus is on the general practitioner to find the right expert for his patient, but he cannot be expected to be completely efficient in this regard. In default, it becomes the responsibility of the local consultant to whom the patient is originally referred to pass him on to the best expert. That second referral implies the willing agreement of the first surgeon to the policy of specialization. It also implies that the patient is willing to travel. A final disadvantage is that the stricter the compartmentation, the more difficult cross-fertilization. It is noteworthy how often the most dramatic advances come from the application of experience or expertise from another specialist field to a particular problem. The spectacular advances in plastic surgery achieved with full-thickness free vascularized grafts owe everything to advances in the technique of grafting small blood vessels, made by the vascular surgeons. Ideally there must be more than one forum in which experts can talk to each other across the boundaries of the special fields.

In other words, unbridled specialization has its dangers: the shift towards increased specialization should not go too far.

The present situation

It is salutary to review the present state of affairs in the light of the above conclusion, paying attention to three different aspects.

The medical student

First and foremost, the undergraduate curriculum must continue to be firmly based on the development of clinical skills—history-taking and physical examination. If the student can take a precise history and make an accurate examination, he is as well equipped as possible for dealing with unusual situations. No matter what his area of practice in his later medical life, he will be best able to deal with situations outside his immediate zone of familiarity.

Secondly, coverage on the course must be as wide as possible: there should be no substantial lacunae that might lead to a lack of awareness of potential treatments. Specialization by exclusion must not be allowed to occur in our undergraduate medical schools although the acquisition of extra knowledge in depth in a particular field should continue to be encouraged. The suggestion sometimes made that surgery itself could be excluded from the medical curriculum as being a discipline more suited to postgraduate studies would be farcical were it not for the seriousness of some of its protagonists.

Thirdly, the medical course must develop and emphasize the natural innate curiosity of all of us, and combine it with resolution and patience, so that the qualified doctor is trained to test received wisdom, to look below the surface of the obvious, to demand the best rather than the usual for his patient.

Of course, specialization is sometimes mainly in the eye of the beholder. I shall never forget the shock of realizing, on the first day of my first house-job, that I was considered to be the local expert on the removal of a plaster cast!

The general practitioner

It seems reasonable to assign to the general practitioner the responsibility for discovering the interests of the general surgeons at his local district general hospital: referral to the 'wrong' consultant is time-wasting, inefficient and therefore costly. For most of the time, this is not too onerous a task for the general practitioner: the decision usually lies between gastroenterology, vascular and breast and metabolic problems. Occasionally the clinical situation has a much more esoteric flavour, and it is in these cases that the practitioner's knowledge is much less likely to be comprehensive. Can every family doctor in the country be expected to know those very few surgeons who have special experience of the dumping syndrome and the operation of the reversal of pyloroplasty?

The 'general' surgeon

From the outset it is important to differentiate between the district general hospital and the university hospital. The analysis can be developed more clearly by considering the latter first.

All hospitals have a responsibility towards medical education and research as well as to the care of patients, and in the university hospital the care of the patients is the supreme consideration, just as it is in the district general hospital. However, in the university hospital the commitment to teaching and research forms a greater proportion of the whole effort than it does elsewhere and this extra commitment is recognized in extra funding. It is therefore usually in university hospitals that the process of differentiation of a new specialist interest takes place. How exactly does this process occur?

There are many possible routes, but I would like to suggest that all of them are variants of one of two different groups: rare conditions and common conditions.

In the case of rare conditions, the role of the university hospital is to act as a focal point to which patients with the condition can be referred from general practitioners, or from surgeons of first referral, from far and wide—indeed, for the rarest conditions, from perhaps the whole country. The concentration of many patients with the condition, or group of conditions, under the care of a single surgical team permits advances in management to arise from the simple process of audit of outcome, quite apart from the application of complicated techniques of investigation. Furthermore, if the operative procedures required in management are demanding and difficult to learn, then the fact that they can be practised often in the special centre results in the rapid development of the necessary skill, at first in the head of the team and later in the juniors who pass through the firm as part of their training. The trainees are then able to go out and start new centres elsewhere, thereby reducing the distance that patients with the condition need in future to travel. It must, however, be clearly understood that there is a logical limit to which this process of diffusion should be confined if the advantages of the specialization are not to be lost.

An example may be quoted to support the statement of the previous sentence. The incidence of salivary gland tumours in the UK is 1 per 100,000 (i.e. about 500 per annum). Most of these are parotid tumours. Groups of surgeons who might deal with these problems include not only 'general' but also facio-maxillary, plastic, otolaryngological and perhaps neurosurgeons. If the process of diffusion were allowed to be complete, it would follow that each surgeon would perform parotidectomy at most about once a year. My own experience with this operation leads to the view that, no matter how well-trained the surgeon in the performance of parotidectomy, he would soon lose the fine edge of his expertise at this rate of strike. Indeed, I think the number performed each year should not be allowed to fall below 20 and preferably should be in the range of 25–30. In other words, there is really only room in the UK for about 20 centres specializing in diseases of the salivary glands.

The situation with common clinical problems is very different. If all the patients requiring attention for varicose veins and similar problems were averaged out among the whole cadre of general surgeons, there would still be a sufficiently large number of patients for each surgeon to maintain his expertise at treating such problems. The raison d'être of a varicose vein clinic at a university hospital is not primarily to attract a larger than average share of the patient pool (although its presence will inevitably tend to do just that); rather it is to bring to bear on the problems of venous disease a greater weight of attention and research than can be deployed in the average district general hospital. The armamentarium required for the purpose consists of complicated investigation techniques and the ultimate luxury of extra pairs of hands over and above the service need, both these items being too expensive to provide at every district general hospital. One hopes for an immediate return as a result of this outlay—the definition of techniques of management that are relatively simple and which can be communicated to district general hospitals where they can then be used without the necessity for expensive investigations or extra personnel. Of course one cannot expect that such immediate benefits will always accrue, but there is nearly always some less direct benefit in terms of an increase in knowledge which may ultimately find application in some other field.

The example I wish to offer of this phenomenon is the group of operations contained under the heading of mammaplasty. These operations were rightly developed mostly by plastic surgeons; but now that the principles underlying them have been carefully established, and because the technical skill needed is not excessive, it is possible to hand the procedure back to the general surgeons. This is just as well, because the patient load is so large (as a result of the previous vogue for mastectomy) that the plastic surgeons would not be able to carry the whole responsibility with their relatively small numbers unless some of them were prepared to specialize more or less exclusively in this field.

The differences outlined between district general and teaching hospitals are generalizations, and as with all generalizations there are many exceptions to them. While to give examples would be invidious, we all recognize that many important advances have been made by laborious, dedicated and inspired work at district general hospitals in many fields such as hernia, carcinoma of the breast and gastroduodenal diseases. However, one can make no progress in this discussion without some generalizations. One such is that there is no further useful generalization that can be made about specialization in university hospitals. What happens in such a hospital depends on a variety of factors including finance, the interests of persons and departments (including particularly those of the medical school) and the demands of medical students for their education.

At the district general hospitals, however, it is possible to proceed to further generalizations, based on some very simple but ineluctable mathematics. The number and size of such hospitals has to be a compromise of factors tugging in opposite directions. On the one hand it is inhumane and costly to expect patients and their visitors to have to travel too far. On the other hand, small hospitals are expensive to run and it is more difficult to conduct a good medical practice in them because of difficulties with the coverage of all the specialist services that could prove to be necessary in the management of any individual patient. In the UK official thinking on the optimal size of a hospital has varied over the years, but at present seems to suggest an order of 600–1000 beds, the exact size depending on such factors as the density of population, the ease and frequency of methods of public transport, and the location of neighbouring hospitals.

In such a hospital the general surgical workload at present seems to be undertaken by three or four general surgeons. The definition of a general surgeon in this context is any surgeon who is prepared to accept the responsibility for emergency admissions that do not fall clearly and distinctly into specialist fields such as orthopaedics, otolaryngology, eyes and (with some exceptions) urology. Principles of continuity of medical care demand that the surgeon should have his own junior staff on emergency call with him, and since the juniors cannot be on duty more often than one-in-three then a trio of surgeons can neatly cover the emergency take every third day. There seems at present to be some demand that the rota of junior staff should become one-in-four, and it will then be essential that there are four general surgeons—otherwise a surgeon would only be on call with his own junior staff on one day in twelve.

Keeping for the moment to the idea of three general surgeons, how might they undertake a greater degree of specialization? At present the answer seems to be that one becomes a gastroenterologist, one a peripheral vascular surgeon, and one a breast and endocrine surgeon—but they still remain general enough to accept their one-third share of the emergency admissions, and to accept the responsibility of looking after the patients of their two colleagues when the latter are away on leave. This basic competency in the field of their colleagues' expertise is assured by their period of higher surgical training which at present has a strong emphasis on a period of about two years (at least) in district general hospitals.

Suppose now that we decide to introduce a greater degree of specialization. The gastroenterological surgeon becomes one oesophago-gastroduodenal (probably plus hepatobiliary) and one coloproctological surgeon, and so on so that there are now six general surgeons. Will they still take part in a rota for emergencies? Will the elderly patient admitted with a profuse haematemesis be under the immediate care of the surgeon who during his working day deals solely with large bowel problems or with the thyroid and parathyroid glands? Alternatively, will every specialist general surgeon be on the whole time for emergencies in his field? In the latter event there is no longer such a discipline as general surgery and therefore no longer any training ground for general surgeons. This brings us back to the questions, who shall decide which specialist shall be called to deal with any individual emergency admission? and how will that person be trained? The other problem with replacing the three general surgeons with six specialist surgeons is that the hospital must be doubled in size and catchment area in order to ensure that each surgeon has an adequate workload.

My own feeling is that the process of specialization at district general hospital level has probably gone about as far as it can safely go, given the geographical and demographic constraints of the UK. As the three general surgeons at a hospital grow older, more experienced, and one hopes wiser, they will naturally tend to develop special interests and special expertise. Colleagues will begin to recognize the availability of an opinion better than their own, perhaps a technical skill greater than they can offer, and a system of internal referrals, or even of prior sorting of general practitioner referrals, will grow up. However, this process will take time, and it will probably not be until any one surgeon is within sight of retirement that his practice will have become very specialized. The care of emergency admissions will not be jeopardized. This rather fluid process of evolution also allows for an elasticity in the process of specialization rather than the rigid compartmentation of *a priori* definitions of subspecialties. My own surgical career has been founded on an interest in the salivary glands and gastroduodenal diseases, and these certainly do not conform to any one of the traditional specialist compartments.

Finally there is the question of how a vacancy shall be filled. There are two major possibilities: that one of the remaining surgeons will wish, with the agreement of his colleagues, to take over the vacant position with something approximating to the degree of specialization of the previous incumbent; or that a new appointment will be made to take up that position. Whichever solution is implemented, there will be the problem of finding someone with the right qualifications in terms of special experience. At present there is little difficulty experienced: with our present plethora of junior hospital doctors aiming at a general surgical career, few become appointed as consultants until they have completed five or six years of higher surgical training, and this means that in any efficient rotation most senior registrars have been exposed to two years of at least two of the three major subspecialties. If, however, Achieving a Balance works, we should within a few years be expecting our senior registrars to be in post only three or four years, and the question of subspecialty orientation assumes greater importance. Probably the best way to deal with this is to define firms, departments or other clinical units which have been adjudged by peer review, in the light of well-defined criteria, to be recognized as providing special experience in one of the subspecialties. Recognition that the individual senior registrar is well qualified to apply for a post as a consultant surgeon with special experience in gastroenterology will be self-evident in the case of someone who has spent a total of two years in one (or two) specialist gastroenterology units. In the interests of elasticity, I would suggest that this criterion need not be the only one employed, but it should make easier the work of referees and appointment committees. Any greater degree of specialization might be a bonus for a particular appointment which might benefit from that particular set of skills, but to aim at such super-specialization would be counterproductive in terms of ensuring a smooth transition between senior registrar and consultant grades—the number of jobs a senior registrar would become eligible to apply for would be potentially so much smaller that the vagaries of chance would produce long gaps of time with no such suitable jobs becoming vacant.

2

Towards endoscopic therapy for bleeding peptic ulcers: targets and weapons, trials and costs†

Tim Northfield, MA, MD, FRCP, and
John Kirkham, MChir, FRCS

Objectives

'The ultimate objective of treatment is to ensure that the largest possible number of patients who enter bleeding leave hospital alive.'—Norman Tanner, 1950

While Norman Tanner succinctly defined the ultimate objective of treatment for acute upper gastrointestinal haemorrhage,[1] Avery Jones played a major role in defining the important risk factors for continuing medical treatment of these patients.[2] He showed that rebleeding (continued or recurrent haemorrhage following hospital admission) is associated with a ten-fold increase in the mortality rate; and that the presence of a chronic peptic ulcer and an age of over 60 are also associated with an increased mortality rate. In the light of these findings, a policy of emergency surgery was introduced in those groups having an adverse prognosis with continued medical treatment, in the hope that this would reduce the mortality rate. This certainly prevents rebleeding, but convincing evidence that it reduces the mortality rate is lacking. Several studies suggest that the overall mortality rate has not changed over the last few decades, despite initiation of this policy.[3-5] The problem is that emergency surgery involves a general anaesthetic and an abdominal incision in an ill patient; and that patients are at risk of dying of the complications of emergency surgery, including pneumonia and pulmonary embolism.

---

†This chapter is based on the Hopkins Endoscopy Prize Lecture at the Jubilee meeting of the British Society of Gastroenterology in September 1987. It was delivered by Professor Northfield on behalf of colleagues collaborating in a seven-year research programme based on the Norman Tanner Gastroenterology Unit, St James' Hospital (now transferred to St George's Hospital on closure of St James') and the Department of Gastroenterology, University College Hospital. The programme involved Mr Kirkham and Drs Northfield and O'Sullivan at St James' Hospital, and Drs Salmon and Bown at University College Hospital. Three successive research senior registrars, Drs Storey, Swain and Matthewson, were responsible for the day-to-day running of the programme at both hospitals; and Mr Rees, Health Economist, was responsible for a costing exercise carried out at St James' Hospital. The programme was funded by research grants to Dr Northfield from the Office of the Chief Scientist, DHSS, who provided financial support for the research senior registrars and the Health Economist, and also provided equipment including lasers.

The objective of our research programme into this subject, which we initiated a decade ago, is to determine whether endoscopic therapy for bleeding peptic ulcers reduces the mortality rate, by reducing the risk of rebleeding without the need for a general anaesthetic and an abdominal incision. In assessing the success of ourselves and of others in achieving this objective, we aim to address four questions:

1. What is the best *target* for endoscopic therapy?
2. What is the best *weapon*?
3. Do controlled *trials* show convincing benefit?
4. Do the ends justify the *cost*?

Targets

> 'The ulcer is cicatrised over its whole extent with the single exception of a point in the centre, which is occupied by the eroded artery.'—Brinton, 1857

This description of a visible vessel in the base of an ulcer is based on autopsy studies over a century ago by Brinton,[6] who felt that this phenomenon 'quite explains the intermittent, though repeated, character of these haemorrhages'. The endoscopic observation of a visible vessel was emphasized by Schindler in the late 1930s and by Tanner in the late 1940s. More recently, Foster and colleagues[7] have published a retrospective analysis of 89 patients with peptic ulcer. They found an incidence of 67 per cent for stigmata of recent haemorrhage (SRH), defined as visible vessels, adherent clot, and red or black spots in the base of an ulcer. They reported that this finding carried a 42 per cent risk of rebleeding in their series, compared with 3 per cent in those having no SRH. The mortality rate was 13 per cent, versus 3 per cent in the control group. Griffiths and colleagues[8] focused on the finding of a visible vessel in their 157 peptic ulcer patients. They reported an incidence of 18 per cent. This was associated with a rebleeding rate of 100 per cent, compared with 22 per cent in the control group having no visible vessel. The mortality rate was 18 per cent, compared with 3 per cent in the control group. These two retrospective analyses appeared at the same time as we were planning our research programme, and the finding of SRH appeared to provide potential targets for endoscopic therapy as well as indicating high-risk patients.

We decided to study the incidence and prognosis of these SRHs prospectively in the patients entering our clinical trials.[9] Of the first 826 such patients, approximately half (49 per cent) were found to have a peptic ulcer on endoscopy. In those patients in whom it was possible to examine fully the ulcer endoscopically (80 per cent of the total), approximately half had a visible vessel (Fig. 2.1), whereas only one fifth had some other SRH, and the remaining third had no SRH. Of those dying, 95 per cent had endoscopic visualization of a visible vessel, 5 per cent had visualization of some other SRH, and no patient died who had had no SRH observed at endoscopy (Fig. 2.2). The prognostic significance of SRH has been further explored in those not receiving endoscopic therapy because the SRH was inaccessible to this form of therapy, or because they

10 *Towards endoscopic therapy for bleeding peptic ulcers*

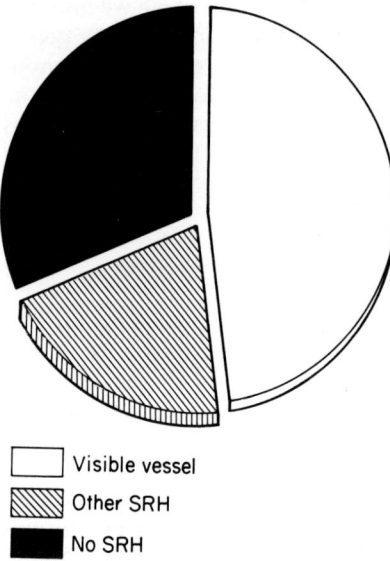

Fig. 2.1 Incidence of stigmata of recent haemorrhage (SRH).

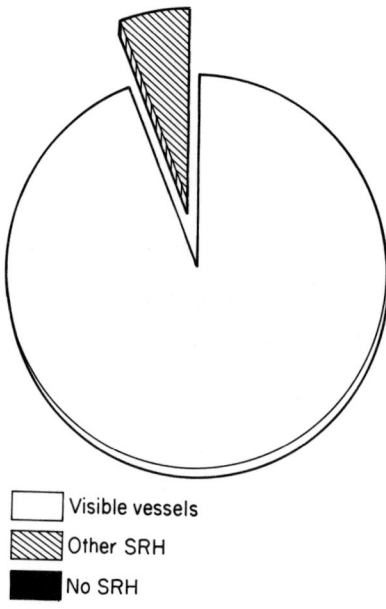

Fig. 2.2 Proportion of peptic ulcer deaths in relation to SRH.

had been randomized to the control group.[9] Fig. 2.3 shows that the endoscopic finding of a visible vessel carries a considerably increased risk of rebleeding, of emergency surgery and of death. Other SRH carry a smaller risk, but in our hands the finding of no SRH implies no risk of these three events.

The advantage of our series is that it involves a large number of patients, all of whom were studied prospectively according to a clearly defined protocol. This involved very careful examination of the ulcer crater prior to randomization, including an attempt to wash off any clot. We further validated our endoscopic finding of a visible vessel by careful histological examination of those gastric ulcers that required emergency gastrectomy in the control groups.[9] Twenty-seven such patients were available for analysis. A visible vessel had been identified endoscopically in all 27 such patients; it was identified histologically in 26 of the 27 gastric ulcers. The histological findings may have relevance to endoscopic therapy. The diameter of the visible vessel varied from 0.1 to 1.8 mm, with a mean of 0.7 mm, and it should be noted that experimentally it is difficult to stop arterial haemorrhage from a vessel more than 1 mm in diameter. The site of the vessel was submucosal in 16 of the ulcers, but subserosal in 10; this might carry an increased risk of perforation with endoscopic therapy. Pathological changes were common in the vessels, localized arteritis being found in 85 per cent, aneurysm formation in 50 per cent and recanalized thrombus in 25 per cent. The finding that these changes did not carry a risk of perforation in our clinical trials can probably be attributed to the fact that chronic penetrating ulcers are always adherent to surrounding organs such as the pancreas.

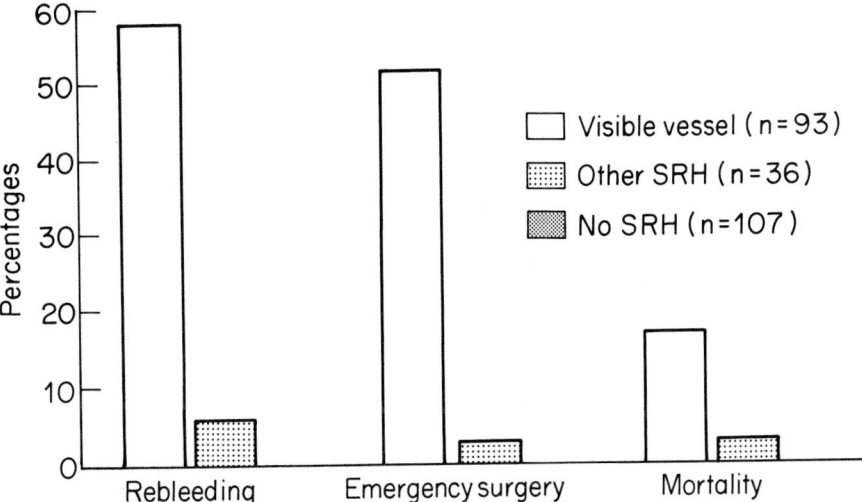

Fig. 2.3 Prognosis of patients with SRH (untreated).

Weapons

>'For arresting haemorrhage great heat is required with rigorous cauterisation, so that a firm eschar is produced which will not readily come off.'—Avicenna, 1000 AD

The weapons we have examined are *lasers* and *electrodes*, all of which act by the application of heat energy (i.e. by cauterization). We believe that the effect is analogous to that of frying a rasher of bacon, which halves in length. If an arterial vessel halves in circumference in a similar way on application of cautery, then the lumen is likely to be occluded. This is a more plausible explanation than photocoagulation of the enclosed blood. Animal experiments have been carried out comparing the Nd YAG with the argon laser, and have confirmed the theoretical prediction that the Nd YAG laser with its more penetrating beam causes more extensive damage.[10] This would be expected to make it more effective in clinical trials, although possibly carrying a greater risk of perforation.

Electrode systems are, of course, much cheaper than lasers, but they have two major disadvantages. One is that the amount of energy delivered cannot easily be controlled; and the other is the likelihood of clot adhering to the electrode itself. In animal experiments we have compared the efficacy and safety of four different electrode systems—the dry monopolar and the liquid monopolar electrode, the bipolar (or multipolar) electrode and the heater probe.[11] In the case of both monopolar electrodes, electricity passes across the patient from the electrode itself to a plate that is applied to the skin. It is thus predictable that these two methods carry the greater risk of full-thickness damage to the gastric mucosa, and this was confirmed in our animal experiments. The bipolar electrode and heater probe were both safer in this respect, and the heater probe was the more effective of the two in the sense that it required a smaller number of pulses to arrest arterial haemorrhage. This therefore became our electrode of choice for comparison with the laser in controlled trials. The heater probe applies heat energy direct to the visible vessel by means of a non-stick metal coating. A predetermined amount of heat energy is applied by means of a microchip in the tip of the heater probe, controlled by a small computer.

Trials

>'Assuredly we bring not innocence into the world,
> We bring impurity much rather:
> That which purifies is trial,
>   And trial by what is contrary.'—Milton, 17th century

The literature on endoscopic therapy for bleeding peptic ulcers is bedevilled by uncontrolled studies which report a high proportion of successes in stopping acute gastrointestinal bleeding. Often, this relates to stopping oozing from the edge of ulcers, whereas our endoscopic experience has taught us that it is spurting arterial haemorrhage from a single exposed vessel rather than oozing that causes clinically serious rebleeding. Even the observation that arterial haemorrhage is terminated by a treatment system is of limited value on an anecdotal basis, because we have often observed patients at endoscopy in whom spurting arterial haemorrhage stops and restarts spontaneously. Only randomized controlled trials can provide reliable, unbiased evidence on the subject.

We have carried out three separate controlled trials during the period 1980–86 (Fig. 2.4). The first trial compared the argon laser with control treatment,[12] the second the Nd YAG laser with control treatment,[13] and the third the heater probe (the best electrode system in our animal experiments) with the Nd YAG laser (the best laser system in our animal experiments and in our previous controlled trials) and control treatment.[14]

The criteria for inclusion and the experimental design have been carefully standardized for all three controlled trials. To qualify for inclusion, patients had to be admitted for acute gastrointestinal bleeding; they had to have a peptic ulcer identified at emergency endoscopy; this had to contain SRH accessible to endoscopic therapy; and the patient had to give written informed consent for inclusion prior to the endoscopy. Accessibility of the SRH was determined for the laser by shining the aiming beam, and for the heater probe by gently touching the SRH with the heater probe. Experimental design always included randomization at the time of endoscopy itself; stratification according to type of SRH (visible vessel, adherent clot, black or red spots, all three groups being stratified also into actively bleeding or not); and diagnosis and management

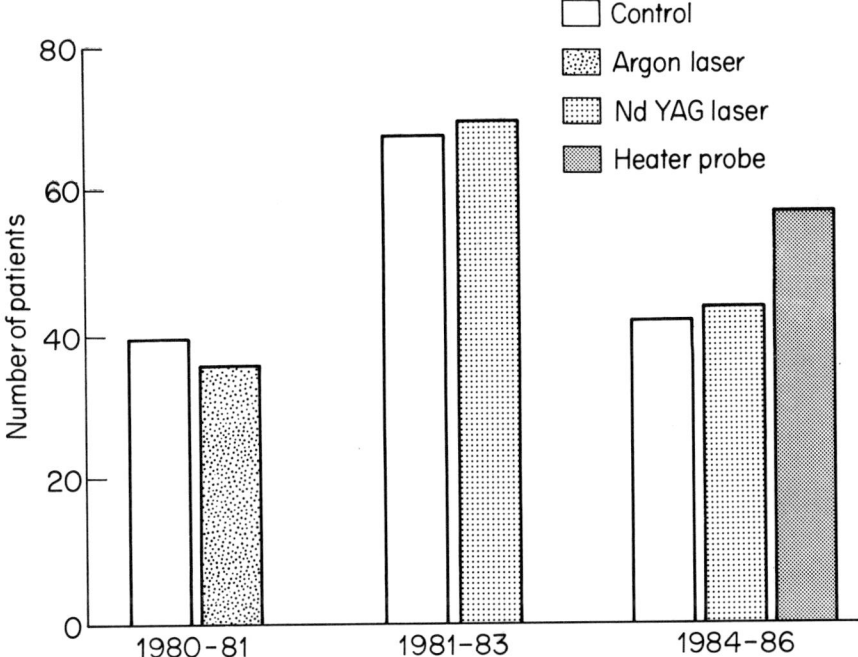

Fig. 2.4 Nature of endoscopic coagulation treatment in three controlled trials (1407 patients endoscoped, 357 randomized).

of rebleeding were carried out by a team unaware of the treatment group (the endoscopic findings themselves were reported in the notes, but the endoscopic treatment procedure was not).

As can be seen from Fig. 2.5, all treatment procedures tended to give a lower rebleeding rate than control treatment, which ran consistently at 40 per cent overall in the three trials. In the first trial, the argon laser significantly reduced the rebleeding rate only if the visible vessel group was analysed separately. The Nd YAG laser significantly reduced the overall rebleeding rate in both the second and third trials. The reduction in the heater probe group did not reach statistical significance, and was intermediate between control and Nd YAG laser treatment. With respect to emergency surgery (Fig. 2.6), all treatments used tended to reduce the rate by comparison with control treatment, and this was a significant reduction in the case of the Nd YAG laser in the second trial. It should be noted that the decision to proceed to emergency surgery was made by a team unaware of the treatment group. A significant reduction in mortality rate was achieved with the argon laser in the first trial and with the Nd YAG laser in the second trial (Fig. 2.7).

In Fig. 2.8 the results for the three trials have been combined for the first time. This can be justified on the grounds that the experimental design was identical for the three trials, and that the rebleeding rate in the control group was also identical for the three trials, suggesting that the same patient population was being studied on each occasion. With the combined results, further significant

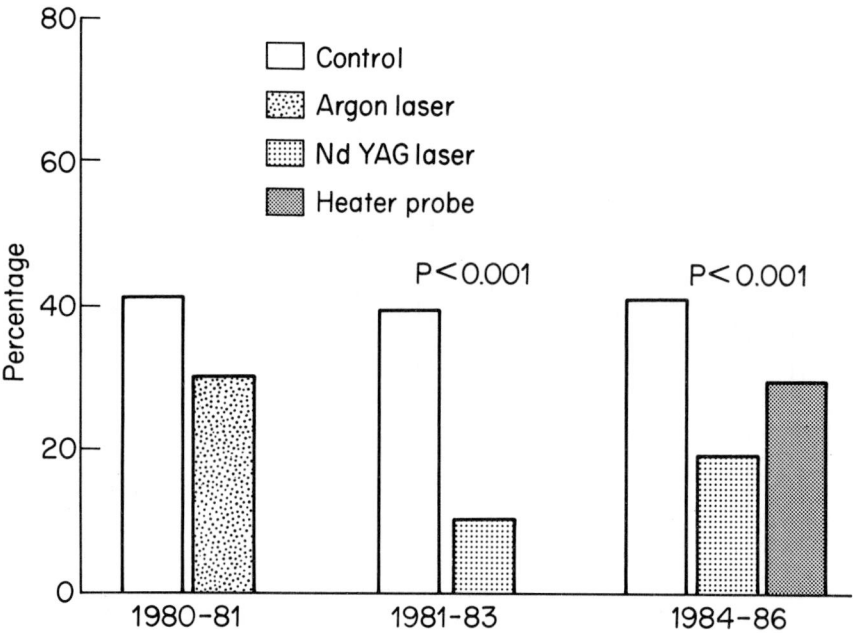

Fig. 2.5 Rebleeding rate according to method of endoscopic management.

differences emerge in addition to those already mentioned. The rebleeding rate for the Nd YAG laser was significantly lower by comparison with both the argon laser and the heater probe. The mortality rate with the Nd YAG laser was also significantly lower than for the heater probe. Thus, in our hands the Nd YAG laser was the most effective weapon, and this was not associated with any

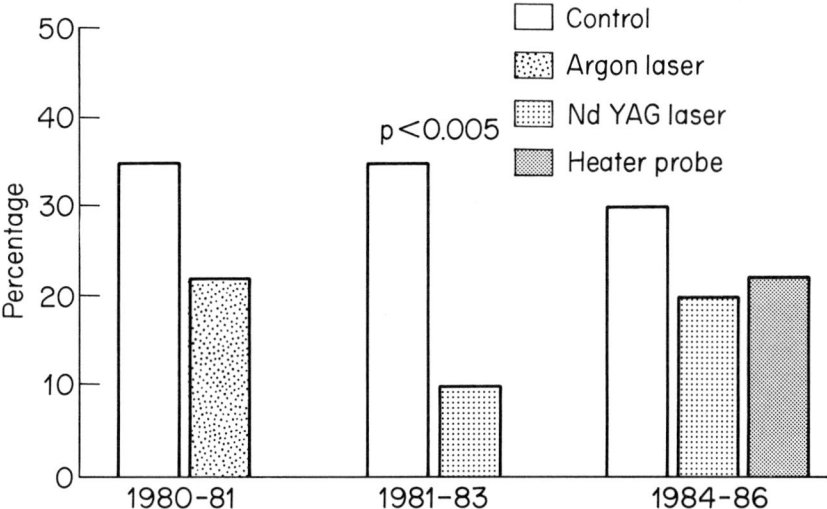

Fig. 2.6 Necessity for emergency surgery after endoscopic treatment.

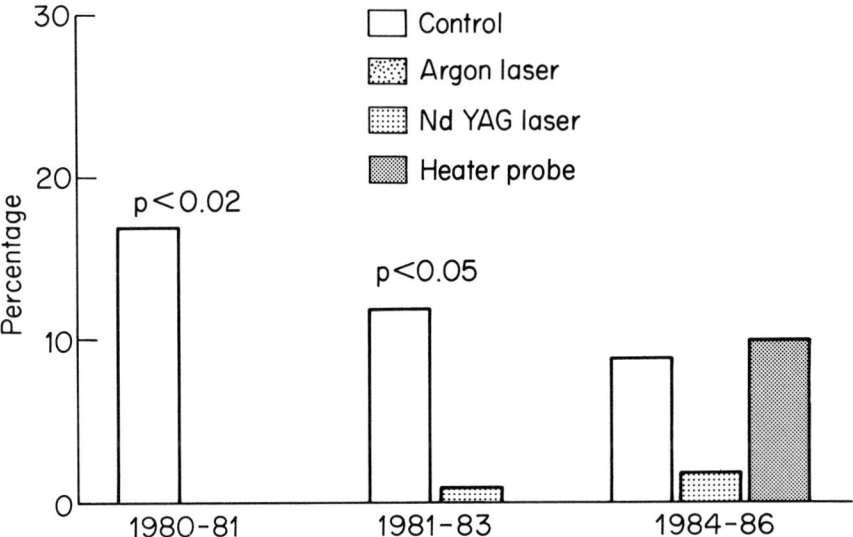

Fig. 2.7 Mortality rate subdivided according to method of endoscopic treatment.

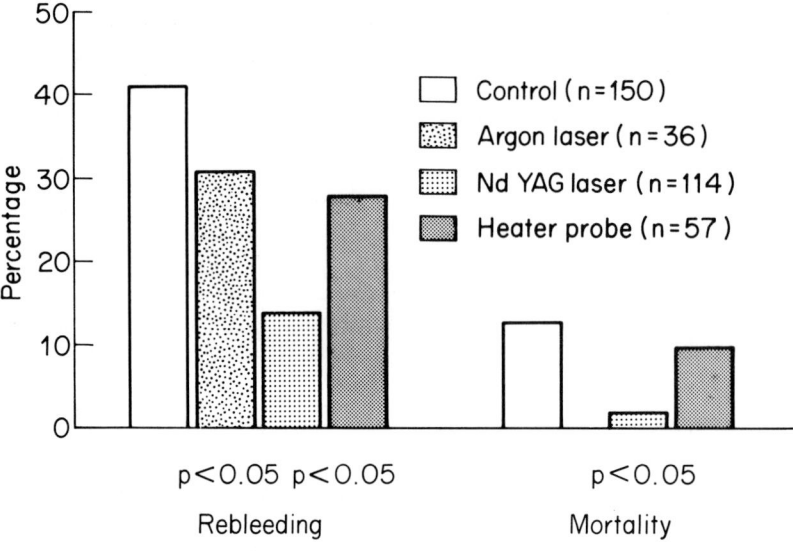

Fig. 2.8 Combined results for all methods of treatment.

increase in risk because none of the Nd YAG laser treated patients developed a perforation.

The trend observed in other controlled trials[15-19] supports our findings, although in most cases the results are not so clear-cut. Table 2.1 examines the results of other laser trials. The first four trials listed refer to the Nd YAG laser and the fifth by Vallon and colleagues[20] to the argon laser. It is noteworthy that in the trial by McLeod and colleagues[17] only 2 per cent of the total patients available were randomized into their trial. For the rebleeding rate, four of the five trials report a trend in favour of the laser (indicated by bold type in the table), and in two of the four this trend is a significant one (indicated by an asterisk). For the mortality rate, three of the trials show a trend in favour of the laser, but in none of these is it a significant trend.

With respect to other electrode trials,[20-24] the layout in Table 2.2 is the same as for Table 2.1. The first two trials listed refer to liquid monopolar electrodes,

Table 2.1 Laser trials

Study	Patients randomized	% Total	% Rebleeding L	C	% Mortality L	C
Homer et al.	42	40	*18	32	0	8
Kreis et al.	174	16	22	20	1	1
McLeod et al.	16	2	*25	100	0	25
Rutjeerts et al.	108	32	**10**	23	16	16
Vallon et al.	136	41	**29**	34	7	15

L = laser; C = control.

Table 2.2 Electrode trials

Study	Patients randomized	% Total	% Rebleeding E	C	% Mortality E	C
Freitas et al.	78	16	**31**	**53**	7	18
Moreto et al.	37	–	**56**	**71**	8	14
O'Brien et al.	204	44	***17**	**35**	13	14
Kernohan et al.	45	35	43	29	0	0
Laine	44	13	***10**	**87**	0	13

E = electrode; C = control.

and the other three to bipolar or multipolar electrodes. For the rebleeding rate, four of the five trials show a trend in favour of the electrode system and in three of the four this is a significant trend. For the mortality rate, too, four of the five trials show a trend in favour of the electrode, but in none of them is this significant.

A *new development is the use of endoscopic injection therapy for bleeding peptic ulcers*. Chung and colleagues[25] carried out a controlled trial of adrenaline injection in 68 patients with bleeding peptic ulcers (7 per cent of the total endoscoped). Repeat endoscopy was carried out at 24 hours and repeat injection given if there was further evidence of bleeding. Fifteen per cent of patients in the treatment group and 27 per cent in the control group received emergency surgery ($p < 0.02$); but although this decision was made according to predetermined criteria, one of the two surgeons involved had carried out the injection therapy. Panès and colleagues[26] studied the combined effect of injecting adrenaline plus polidocanol (a sclerosant). Fifty-five patients were randomized (13 per cent of the total). Minor rebleeds in the treatment group were treated with a second injection. Major rebleeding, diagnosed according to defined criteria by a team unaware of the treatment group, occurred in 5 per cent of the treatment group compared with 43 per cent of the control group ($p < 0.001$). There was no significant difference in mortality rate in either trial, but taken together they suggest that endoscopic injection therapy probably does have a role in the management of bleeding peptic ulcers. There is now an important need to compare this form of treatment with laser therapy.

Costs

> 'In use of equipment, insufficient attention is paid to real costs. In most cases it would be cheaper not to install the equipment, but whenever it is needed to send each student in a separate chauffeur-driven Rolls Royce to use the equipment in another institution.'—Committee of Vice Chancellors, 1968

Hospitals grasped this simple truth earlier than the universities, and have for many years been driving patients in chauffeur-driven ambulances to hospitals with more expensive equipment (e.g. for radiotherapy). There is, however, a prejudice against transferring patients in an emergency situation from one hospital to another, and this prejudice may limit the general availability of laser equipment for bleeding peptic ulcers. In fact, in the patients transferred from other centres to our unit for therapeutic endoscopy of massive upper gastrointestinal bleeding, accompanied by a nurse, a doctor and an adequate supply of blood, no problems have arisen from the transfer. This suggests that the prejudice against transfer under these circumstances is unjustified. We have examined the cost-effectiveness of lasers for treatment of bleeding peptic ulcers in the setting of a district general hospital. We have taken no account of the fact that a laser, once installed, can be used for other purposes such as symptomatic treatment of bronchial and gastrointestinal neoplasms.

The costing was performed by a professional health economist who was unaware of the endoscopic treatment received by each patient, and the costed sample consisted of the 79 patients entered into the third and last of our clinical trials at St James' Hospital.[27] Eleven major costing categories were used to cover the spectrum of hospital services directly and indirectly relevant to the patient's care, and individual patient profiles were constructed to cover all items of expenditure from the time of admission to discharge or death. Excluding capital costs, the mean costs per case were £4616 for the control group ($n = 24$), £1758 per patient for the laser treated group ($n = 25$), and £1940 per patient for the heater probe treated patients ($ = 30$). As shown in Fig. 2.9, the mean costs per day were similar for the three groups (£180, £132 and £141 respectively) and the main difference was in the mean length of stay. This was 26 days for the control group, compared with 13 and 14 days for the other two groups. As shown in Table 2.3, eight patients, five of them from the control group, each cost more than £5000. Although only representing 10 per cent of the total patients, they together accounted for 50 per cent of the total costs. These very expensive patients all required emergency surgery for rebleeding, and usually spent a period on the intensive care unit.

Assuming that the equipment has a life-span of seven years and that 35 patients per year are treated by means of the laser, the data suggest that the laser would pay for itself within five months, giving a seven-year discounted value of approximately £600 000. So long as it is used by an experienced operator, laser

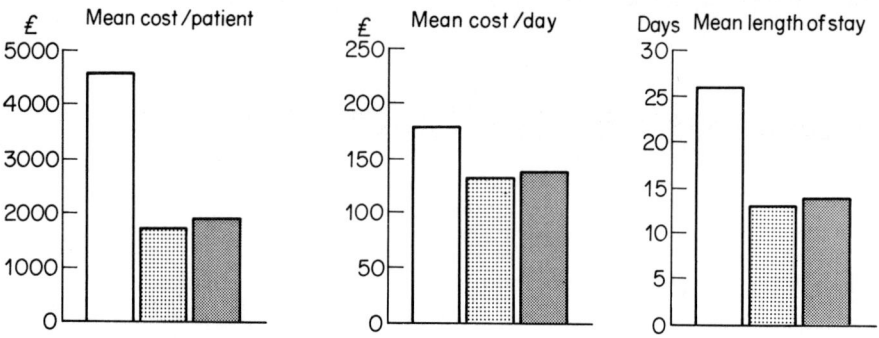

Fig. 2.9 Cost/stay analysis according to method of treatment.

Table 2.3 Very expensive patients (> £5000)

	n	Cost (£1000s)	Total cost (£1000s)
Control	5	82	110
Laser	1	5	43
Heater probe	2	17	57
Total	8	105	210

therapy would therefore appear to offer the possibility of substantial economies to the National Health Service. It should be noted, however, that in our hands there was usually a learning curve of about six months for a new laser operator to achieve an optimal reduction in rebleeding rate.

Conclusions

> 'Those disease which medicine do not cure,
>   the knife cures;
> Those which the knife cannot cure,
>   cautery cures;
> And those which cautery cannot cure,
>   are reckoned to be wholly incurable.'
> —Hippocrates, 400 BC

We conclude that the visible vessel is the appropriate target for endoscopic therapy; and that the Nd YAG laser is the best weapon in our controlled trials. These trials show a significant reduction in the rates for rebleeding, emergency surgery and mortality for the Nd YAG laser; other trials show a consistent trend towards reduced rebleeding and mortality for laser treatment. The capital cost of the laser is balanced by a reduction in hospital stay, making installation in a district general hospital potentially cost-effective.

References

1. Tanner N.C. Discussion: gastroduodenal haemorrhage as a surgical emergency. *Proc. R. Soc. Med.* 1950; **43:** 147.
2. Jones F.A. Haematemesis and melaena: with special reference to correction and to the factors influencing the mortality from bleeding peptic ulcers. *Gastroenterology.* 1956; **30:** 166.
3. Schiller K.R.F., Truelove S.C., Gwyn Williams D. Haematemesis and melaena with special reference to factors influencing the outcome. *Brit. Med. J.* 1970; **ii:** 7–14.
4. Allen R., Dykes P. A study of the factors influencing mortality rates from gastrointestinal haemorrhage. *Quart. J. Med.* 1976; **45:** 533–50.
5. Silverstein F.E., Gilbert D.A., Tedesco F.J., et al. The national ASGE survey on upper gastrointestinal bleeding. *Gastrointest. Endosc.* 1981; **27:** 73–102.
6. Brinton W. On the pathology, symptoms and treatment of ulcer on the stomach. London: John Churchill, 1857: 43–50 and 126–35.
7. Foster D.N., Miloszewski K.J.A., Losowsky M.S. Stigmata of recent haemorrhage in diagnosis and prognosis of upper gastrointestinal bleeding. *Brit. Med. J.* 1978; **1:** 1173–7.
8. Griffiths W.J., Neumann D.A., Welsh J.D. The visible vessel as an indicator of uncontrolled or recurrent gastrointestinal haemorrhage. *N. Engl. J. Med.* 1979; **300:** 1411–13.

9. Swain C.P., Storey D.W., Bown S.G., Heath J., Mills T.N., Salmon P.R., Northfield T.C., Kirkham J.S., O'Sullivan J.P. Nature of the bleeding vessel in recurrently bleeding gastric ulcers. *Gastroenterology.* 1986; **90:** 595–608.
10. Silverstein F.E., Protell R.I., Gilbert D.A., *et al.* Argon vs neodynium YAG photocoagulation of experimental canine gastric ulcers. *Gastroenterology.* 1979; **77:** 491–6.
11. Swain C.P., Mills T.N., Shamosh E., Dark J.M., Lewin M.R., Clifton J.S., Northfield T.C., Cotton P.B., Salmon P.R. Which electrode? A comparison of four endoscopic methods of electrocoagulation in experimental bleeding ulcers. *Gut.* 1984; **25:** 1424–31.
12. Swain C.P., Bown S.G., Storey D.W., Kirkham J.S., Northfield T.C., Salmon P.R. Controlled trial of argon laser photocoagulation in bleeding peptic ulcers. *Lancet.* 1981; **ii:** 1313–16.
13. Swain C.P., Kirkham J.S., Salmon P.R., Bown S.G., Northfield T.C. Controlled trial of Nd YAG laser photocoagulation in bleeding peptic ulcers. *Lancet.* 1986; **i:** 1113–16.
14. Matthewson K.M., Swain C.P., Bown S.G., Bland M., Kirkham J.S., Northfield T.C. Randomized comparison of Nd YAG laser, heater probe and no endoscopic therapy for bleeding peptic ulcer: *Gastroenterology.* 1987; **92:** 1522.
15. Homer A.C., Powell S., Vicary F.R. Is Nd YAG laser treatment for upper gastrointestinal bleeds of benefit in a district general hospital? *Postgrad. Med. J.* 1985; **61:** 19–22.
16. Krejs G.J., Little K.H., Westergaard H., Hamilton J.K., Spady D.K., Polter D.E. Laser photocoagulation for the treatment of acute peptic ulcer bleeding. *N. Engl. J. Med.* 1987; **316:** 1618–21.
17. MacLeod I.A., Mills P.R., MacKenzie J.F., Joffe S.N., Russell R.I., Carter D.C. Neodymium yttrium aluminium garnet laser photocoagulation for major haemorrhage from peptic ulcers and single vessels: a simple blind controlled study. *Brit. Med. J.* 1983; **285:** 345–8.
18. Rutgeerts R., Vantrappen G., Broeckaart L., Janssens J., Coremans G., Geboes K., Schurmans P. Controlled trial of YAG laser treatment of upper digestive haemorrhage. *Gastroenterology.* 1982; **83:** 410–16.
19. Vallon A.G., Cotton P.B., Lawrence B.H., Armengot-Miro J.R., Sellard Ones J.C. Randomised trial of endoscopic argon laser photocoagulation in bleeding peptic ulcers. *Gut.* 1981; **22:** 228–33.
20. Freitas D., Doneto A., Monteiro J.G. Controlled trial of liquid monopolar electrocoagulation in bleeding peptic ulcers. *Gastroenterology.* 1985; **80:** 853–7.
21. Moreto M., Zabella M., Ihanez S., Setien F., Figar M. Efficacy of monopolar electrocoagulation in the treatment of bleeding gastric ulcer; a controlled trial. *Endoscopy.* 1987; **19:** 54–6.
22. O'Brien J.D., Day S.J., Burnham W.R. Controlled trial of small bipolar probe in bleeding peptic ulcers. *Lancet.* 1986; **i:** 464–7.
23. Kernohan R.M., Anderson J.R., McKelvey S.T.D., Kennedy T.L. A controlled trial of bipolar electrocoagulation in patients with upper gastrointestinal bleeding. *Brit. J. Surg.* 1984; **71:** 889–91.
24. Laine L. Multipolar electrocoagulation in the treatment of active upper gastrointestinal tract haemorrhage. *N. Engl. J. Med.* 1987; **316:** 1613–17.
25. Chung S.C.S., Leung J.W.C., Steele R.J.C., Crofts T.J., Li A.K.C. Endoscopic injection of adrenaline for actively bleeding ulcers: a randomised trial. *Brit. Med. J.* 1988; **296:** 1631–3.
26. Panès J, Viver J., Forne M., Garcia-Olivares E., Marco C., Garau J. Controlled trial of endoscopic sclerosis in bleeding peptic ulcers. *Lancet.* 1987; **ii:** 1292–4.
27. Matthewson K., Rees M., Kirkham J.S., Northfield T.C. Costing of hospital management of bleeding peptic ulcer patients treated by Nd YAG laser, heater probe or no endoscopic therapy. *Gut.* 1988; **29:** A1489.

3

Lasers and their application to surgery

P.B. Boulos, MS, FRCS, FRCSEd, and
H. Barr, FRCS, FRCSEd

The last decade has witnessed a rapid development of laser technology and of the application of lasers in a variety of scientific fields including medicine. In certain areas the laser has superseded conventional treatment with impressive results and consequently has considerably influenced surgical practice.

The purpose of this review is to describe some basic principles of lasers and to present a critical evaluation of their application in an attempt to introduce the uninitiated to a clearer and better understanding of the role of lasers and their potential value in surgery.

Fundamentals of lasers

Laser is an acronym for *light amplification* by *stimulated emission* of *radiation*. This is better understood by recapitulating the basic physics of the atom (Fig. 3.1). Electrons in orbit around the nucleus of an atom have specific energy levels; electrons away from the nucleus are in higher energy levels and electrons in the ground or lower energy states are closer to the nucleus. An incoming photon with an energy level that matches the difference between two energy levels of the atom can be absorbed, producing an excited atom in which an electron moves to a higher energy state, which can thus later spontaneously return to the original lower energy state releasing the absorbed energy as another photon—this is *spontaneous emission*. However, there is another possibility, first predicted by Einstein in 1917. When the atom in the excited state is struck by another photon, this is not absorbed, but it instead stimulates the atom to release a second photon of equal frequency and energy travelling in the same direction and in perfect spatial and temporal harmony with the stimulating photon. This phenomenon is termed *stimulated emission of radiation*.

The basic structure of a laser system is a laser medium placed in a cavity producing stimulated emission of light when excited by a power source with precisely aligned mirrors at each end of the laser tube. The laser medium determines the name of each laser and different laser materials are employed. Solid-state lasers use a solid material such as a ruby crystal and neodymium embedded in the lattice of a crystal of yttrium aluminium garnet—the Nd YAG laser. Gas lasers use a gas or a mixture of gases such as helium, argon and CO_2 or excimer (excited dimer). Dye lasers employ a complex organic dye in liquid solution or suspension such as rhodamine.

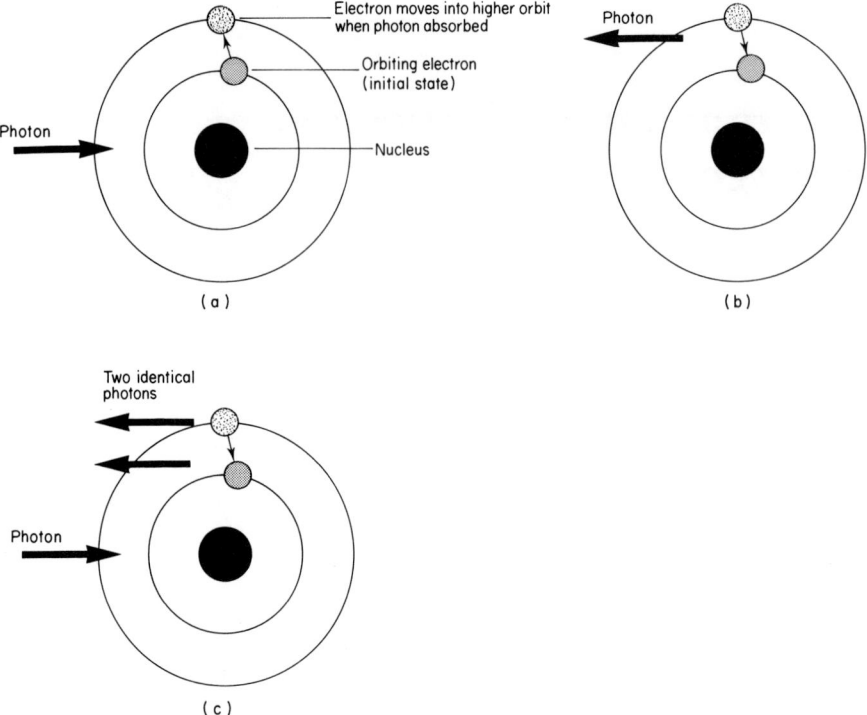

Fig. 3.1 (a) Absorption of a photon by an atom. (b) Spontaneous emission of a photon. An electron loses energy spontaneously and decays back to its initial state by emitting a photon. (c) Stimulated emission of photons. An excited atom with electrons in the higher orbit is struck by another photon. Two photons are released as the electron returns to the initial state.

An external power source stimulates the atoms in the laser medium so that the number of atoms with higher energy levels exceeds the number of atoms in a lower energy level, a condition termed *population inversion*. This 'pumping system' may be optical or electrical depending on the medium used. The excited atoms are stimulated to emit photons and, by multiple reflections between the mirrors, a cascade of stimulated emissions occurs, leading to enormous amplification (Fig. 3.2). Photons with equal energy eventually escape as the laser beam through the partially reflective mirror.

The laser light may be delivered in different forms (Tables 3.1 and 3.2). Continuous-wave lasers have a constant beam power density with time. Pulsed (long or rapid) lasers produce beams with small durations, controlled through the power source or by introducing optical switches between the mirrors.

Laser light is monochromatic (of one wavelength) and is emitted as a narrow collimated beam of high intensity. This beam for some wavelengths can be transmitted along quartz fibres, making lasers suitable for use through both rigid and flexible endoscopes. The light can be delivered with precision and at specific wavelengths, depending on the tissue effect required, and can be quantified and reproduced.

Fundamentals of lasers 23

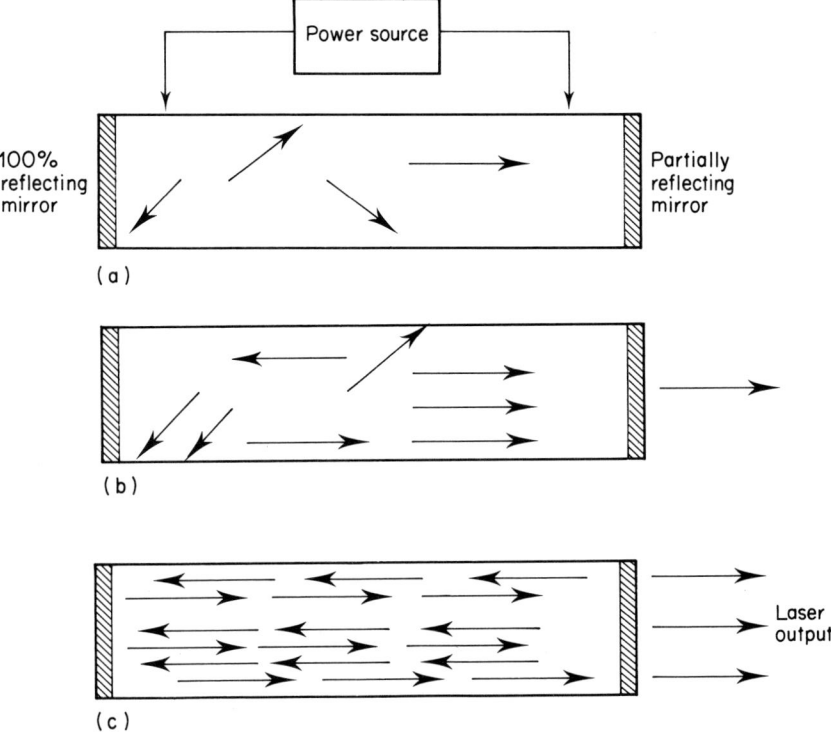

Fig. 3.2 (a) Initial spontaneous emission of photons. (b) Preferential emission along the laser (mirror) axis. (c) Laser action after several passes through the optical cavity.

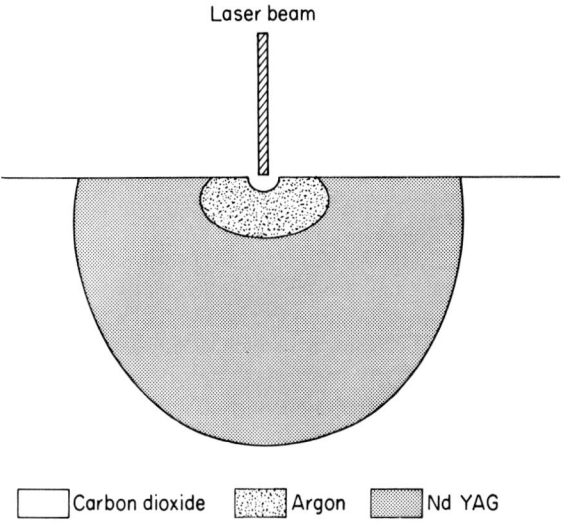

Fig. 3.3 The relative volumes of tissue affected by different lasers.

24 *Lasers and their application to surgery*

Table 3.1 Types of continuous-wave laser in surgical use

Laser	Wavelength (nm)	Power (W)	Main surgical action
CO_2	10 600	5–50	Thermal non-contact knife. Superficial tissue vaporization with little deep tissue coagulation (0.1 mm).
Nd YAG	1 064	5–100	Superficial tissue vaporization with deep tissue coagulation (5–6 mm) Haemostasis
Argon ion	488	1–10	Specific absorption in blood vessels of skin and eye Thermal coagulation but not to the depth of the Nd YAG laser (1–2 mm)
Dye	Tunable over 50 nm (usually in the red)	0.05–1	Source of light for photodynamic therapy

Table 3.2 Types of pulsed laser in surgical use

Laser	Wavelenth (nm)	Pulse Duration	Pulse Energy (J)	Main surgical action
Nd YAG Q-switched	1 064	10 ns	0.1–1	Photomechanical membrane destruction in ophthalmology Laser lithotripsy
Nd YAG	1 064	0.1 ms	0.1–1	Laser angioplasty
Dye	Tunable	0.2 ms	0.01–0.1	Laser lithotripsy
Eximer	193–355 (ultraviolet)	14–20 ns	0.01–0.1	Photoablation

Interaction of laser light with tissues

Laser light may be absorbed, reflected, transmitted or scattered when it interacts with tissue. Only absorbed light can produce a biological effect. Light that is reflected or transmitted through tissue will have no effect. Scattered light has a more diffuse effect since it is absorbed over a broader area. The resultant tissue effect is dependent on the photon energy (its wavelength), the laser power (measured in watts) and energy (power × exposure time, measured in joules).

The interaction of light with tissue depends on the tissue composition, and the wavelength of the light administered. Tissues have varying properties of light absorption and scattering depending on the rate of blood flow and concentration of pigmented material. The CO_2 laser beam is strongly absorbed in water, whereas the beams from Nd YAG and argon ion lasers are absorbed in haemoglobin and other pigments. Different wavelengths of light have different absorption characteristics in tissue. Ultraviolet wavelengths are strongly absorbed in tissue and their effects are localized to the surface. As the wavelength lengthens through the blue and green into the red, tissue becomes more transparent to allow light penetration. Nd YAG (wavelength 1064 nm in the near infrared) tissue penetration is therefore better than for the argon ion laser, which emits at two main wavelengths (at 488 and 514 nm in the blue and green regions of the visible spectrum). As the wavelength continues to lengthen into the infrared, tissue becomes opaque again, light transmission decreases and in the range of the CO_2 laser (10 600 nm) the energy is rapidly absorbed by tissue and the effects are again limited to the surface. Hence, as less light is transmitted more energy is absorbed, producing different thermal effects. The CO_2 laser beam, which is quickly absorbed, vaporizes tissue more readily than does the Nd YAG beam which, however, affects a larger tissue volume. The argon ion laser is intermediate in its transmission, absorption and thermal effect (Fig. 3.3).

Light delivered at a low intensity may not produce thermal effects, but at carefully selected wavelengths (usually red) it can activate photosensitive compounds retained in tissues, generating a toxic reaction. This forms the basis of *photodynamic therapy*.

At higher powers the same light causes *photothermal* reactions to occur. Initially, heating of soft tissue causes thermal contraction of the treated area, and higher energies kill the cells and ultimately vaporize cellular material, leaving a crater. As tissue shrinks, small vessels are sealed, with thrombosis occurring as a secondary effect. The extent of the biological effect can be selected appropriately according to the therapeutic requirement. While Nd YAG and argon ion lasers are effective in haemostasis because of the larger volume of surrounding tissue reaction, as well as for vaporizing malignant tissue, the volume heated by the CO_2 laser outside the area of vaporized tissue is too small to be of value in arresting major haemorrhage, although it can seal capillary oozing. In contrast, its highly localized effect makes it suitable as a laser *knife*—the cells immediately under the beam vaporize, with minimal damage to adjacent areas.

At very short exposure times (a few microseconds) a *photomechanical* rather than a photothermal effect can be produced, generating a shock-wave that can be used to shatter tissue or pulverize stones.

At extremely short interaction times and peak pulse power, the light energy can break intramolecular bonds and strip the electrons from the atom, producing a *photoablation* effect on the tissue.

Specific applications of lasers in surgery

Ophthalmology

Ophthalmologists were the first to treat patients with laser light. The argon ion laser beam at a wavelength of 514 nm is not absorbed by the cornea or aqueous humour, which allows safe photocoagulation of the retina in the treatment of diabetic retinopathy. Neovascularization in the diabetic eye is induced to satisfy the oxygen demands of the retina; by destroying less-needed areas of the peripheral retina the oxygen demand is reduced and the new vessels regress, reducing the risk of retinal haemorrhages and blindness. By incorporating a special electro-optical switch within the laser cavity, high-power short pulses of energy can be obtained, and with the careful use of the eye's own optics selective effects at different levels in the eye have been possible.

Nd YAG lasers have been used in the treatment of glaucoma, by creating a hole in the iris to improve drainage, and for posterior capsulotomy, without damaging the retina, by disrupting the lens capsule which may become opaque following current cataract surgery. Similarly, vitreous strands or sheets are treated. The extreme precision of the excimer is being assessed for reshaping and sculpting the cornea during keratorefractive surgery for the treatment of severe myopia.

Most of these procedures can be performed on an outpatient with a laser incorporated into a slit lamp or microscope.

Otorhinolaryngology and neurosurgery

The mouth and upper airways are accessible to CO_2 laser treatment either directly or via rigid endoscopy. Microscopic laryngeal surgery has been advanced with the use of the laser. In particular, recurrent laryngeal papillomatosis is treated more easily by this method. Although it cannot eradicate the disease, its effectiveness in preserving normal laryngeal structures and maintaining the translaryngeal airway has made it the treatment of choice.

There is controversy on the use of lasers for treatment of early carcinoma of the larynx. Radiotherapy is established to be very effective, but lasers may have a role in debulking the tumour. Of 25 patients with a T1 vocal cord carcinoma, who had initially rejected surgery or radiotherapy and were treated by CO_2 laser excision, no patient had died of tumour six years later, although three developed local recurrence that required surgery or radiotherapy.

The CO_2 laser has also been used to treat leukoplakia and similar lesions of the oral mucosa. The unique superficial vaporization of this laser allows for a precise microsurgical excision of the dysplastic tissues. It has facilitated excision of head and neck tumours, particularly lymphangiomas of the head and neck in children.

As a non-contact knife the CO_2 laser gives a clean cut in vulnerable tissue of the brain and spinal cord, without the risk of producing mechanical traction from the blade. Because of the high temperatures reached some tissues may char when a continuous-wave CO_2 beam is used in the normal way. This can be reduced by using the laser in a superpulsed mode, when the peak power is increased from 5–25 W to 250 W, but the average power remains the same. In this mode the peak power density is much higher, so that the tissue is vaporized and there is little possibility of charring.

Plastic surgery and dermatology

The real impact of lasers in plastic surgical and dermatological practice has been in the management of cutaneous vascular anomalies and port wine stains, particularly when they are grossly disfiguring on the face. The major histological abnormality in a port wine stain is an increase in vessel numbers with ectasia, which is most marked in the subepidermal region. The aim of laser therapy is to seal these abnormal vessels without damaging the overlying epidermis, thus avoiding scarring. The laser commonly used is the argon ion, since its blue/green light is absorbed more strongly in blood than in the relatively transparent epidermis. The final cosmetic result is not apparent for several months after treatment, and healing can be very variable. It is therefore essential to treat a small test patch first and observe its healing for at least four months before trying to treat the whole area. The procedure is time consuming and requires several sessions.

The results do not produce perfect skin. In 10 per cent of patients the result is classified as excellent with total lightening of the skin, 70 per cent have marked lightening without scarring, 15 per cent report little change, and 5 per cent have significant scarring.[1] If patients are given a realistic presentation of the outcome most regard treatment as worthwhile. The best results have been obtained in patients over the age of 35 with mature skin, and with purple coloured lesions on the face.

Dermatologists have used various lasers to remove tatoos, with disappointing results, the patient often being left with a scar in the shape of the tattoo. Amateur tattoos, often self-inflicted using black ink, may respond to ruby laser treatment with minimal scarring, because they tend to be placed in the superficial part of the skin. Professional artists insert the pigments at a deeper level and these tatoos remain a major challenge.

The carbon dioxide laser has been used to excise small skin lesions, but it presents little advantage over alternative methods of treatment. More recently plastic and microvascular surgeons have experimented with the possibility of welding the two ends of severed small vessels and nerves together with a low-powered CO_2 laser attached to an operating microscope. After laser welding a haemostatic anastomosis is produced, but it appears to be weaker than a standard suture anastomosis, late anastomtic aneurysms being more common after laser arterial anastomosis.[2] This technique remains predominantly experimental with few human data available.

Thoracic surgery

Most patients with bronchial cancer are inoperable at the time of diagnosis because of the extent of the disease or poor respiratory reserve, and nearly 60 per cent of these patients will have haemoptysis or airways obstruction causing dyspnoea at some stage. Chemotherapy and radiotherapy are effective in some patients; however, they are associated with considerable morbidity and toxicity. The development of bronchoscopic treatment of obstructing airways cancer is mostly dependent on the Nd YAG laser coupled into 400–600 micron flexible optical fibres that can be passed down the instrumentation channel of a standard bronchoscope. The principle of laser therapy is to remove the intrabronchial or intratracheal tumour to relieve airways obstruction or to coagulate bleeding tumours causing haemoptysis. The laser is used to vaporize and coagulate the tumour. Necrotic tumour sloughs some time after treatment, and if inhaled may occlude a major airway; therefore all dead tissue is removed with endoscopic forceps, passed down a rigid bronchoscope, immediately after laser coagulation. This provides instant improvement in the airway and reduces the risk of temporary obstruction due to oedema or slough. Treatment is therefore more effectively carried out under general anaesthesia with a rigid bronchoscope, which also allows the passage of a flexible instrument with the laser fibre through the instrumentation channel to deliver the laser beam, and a large sucker or forceps to clear the airways.[3]

Quantitative assessment of the results showed an objective improvement in the peak flow rate of 25 per cent or more and complete cessation of haemoptysis for at least one month in 88 and 58 per cent of patients respectively. Symptomatic improvement occurred in two-thirds of the patients. Complications due to haemorrhage, pneumothorax, tracheo-oesophageal fistula and pneumonia are rare. At present laser therapy is most appropriate for intraluminal tumour. However, some 40 per cent of patients with dyspnoea are breathless because of extrinsic compression of the airway. It may be possible to treat these patients by inserting a laser fibre through the bronchial wall and destroying the tumour by localized hyperthermia. Laser therapy in the future could be curative for early tumours, and may be of some value if patients are unfit for surgery owing to poor pulmonary function.

Vascular and cardiac surgery

Since the description of balloon dilatation of vascular stenosis by Gruntzig and Hopff,[4] percutaneous transluminal balloon angioplasty (PTBA) has become widely used both for peripheral blood vessels and coronary arteries. Its application is limited because, firstly, it is necessary to pass a guide wire through the lesion before it can be dilated and in many patients it is not possible to pass the obstruction; and secondly, balloon dilatation of long segments results in an unacceptable level of early reocclusion.[5] Therefore the idea of laser angioplasty or laser-assisted balloon angioplasty is very attractive. Laser angioplasty involves the passage of a laser beam down an optical fibre inserted into the artery instead of the guide wire. When an obstruction is met the fibre is advanced, creating a channel through the atheromatous material by the application of laser energy. In general this procedure should be followed with PTBA, to ensure a widely patent vessel, since at present the laser only cores out a small channel. The combined procedure is called laser-assisted balloon angioplasty. Several lasers are suitable and have been investigated experimentally, but in clinical work the argon ion and Nd YAG lasers have been predominantly used.

The advantages of this technique are that more stenoses and occlusions can be treated than those presently suitable for PTBA, and luminal patency rates may be improved because atheroma is vaporized and removed. Three possible complications have caused concern, particularly in the treatment of the coronary arteries. These are perforation of the vessel wall with haemorrhage, embolization of material dislodged by the laser action or of clot formed on the tip of the laser fibre, and diffuse damage to the vessel wall sufficient to cause aneurysm or reocclusion. Several studies have failed to show production of particulate emboli by laser angioplasty, and aneurysm formation has not been confirmed.[6] Only perforation has proved to be a major problem, but it soon became obvious that contact of a bare laser fibre with a vessel was responsible and could be avoided by using a device on the end of the fibre.

The largest experience has been gained with a device in which a metal cap is used to cover the distal end of the optical laser fibre from a continuous-wave argon ion laser. This has the effect of heating the metal tip to temperatures above 400°C, with no direct application of laser energy to the tissue. However, the use of a hot tip to which charred tissue may stick would increase the risk of embolization and diffuse thermal damage.

Clinical results for the treatment of occluded femoral and popliteal arteries has, however, shown a low incidence of complications and a very reasonable clinical outcome.[7] Fifty-six patients underwent laser-assisted balloon angioplasty; 53 per cent were considered unsuitable for conventional PTBA. Nearly 90 per cent of the lesions were recanalized and there was one perforation caused by mechanical pressure. There was no evidence of embolism or arterial spasm. Two patients suffered an acute reocclusion, and one of these required surgery. Of 26 patients followed for up to 10 months, there were two further occlusions both within three months. These results compare favourably with the results of PTBA alone, despite the group consisting of patients with more advanced disease. Laser angioplasty to the coronary arteries has been reported in a small series but with an unacceptably high rate of subsequent myocardial infarction.[8]

Several other devices are undergoing evaluation at present. Extensive experimental and early clinical studies have been performed on a sapphire-tipped device used with the pulsed and continuous-wave Nd YAG laser. Although there is some heating of the sapphire, approximately 60 per cent of the laser beam is transmitted as light. Delivery of the laser energy in pulses prevents dissipation of heat to the surrounding tissue during exposure, and therefore minimizes unwanted thermal effects in the vessel wall. The practical importance of this has yet to be demonstrated. In an early series the primary recanalization rate was 63 per cent in 40 patients, with only one late occlusion, the maximum duration of follow-up being 18 months.[9]

In the UK over 5000 legs are amputated every year for vascular disease, so there is considerable potential for laser angioplasty in the peripheral circulation. However, its role in coronary artery disease is still fraught with unacceptable risk of perforation and myocardial infarction.

Gastrointestinal surgery

Bleeding peptic ulcer accounts for 50–60 per cent of acute hospital admissions for upper gastrointestinal haemorrhage. The mortality from this disease has changed little over the past 30 years despite advances in diagnostic endoscopy and intensive care, probably because of the surgical risk factors in an increasingly elderly population. Although most episodes of acute upper gastrointestinal haemorrhage cease spontaneously, there is a need for minimally invasive treatment to avoid surgery with its associated morbidity and mortality. High risk of rebleeding is recognized when a bleeding or non-bleeding vessel is seen at endoscopy. Lasers were the first endoscopic haemostatic devices to be used. The technique of treatment is to ring the bleeding point with 6–8 laser shots (80 W for 0.5 seconds), as close as possible to the visible vessel so as to cause thermal contraction of the feeding vessel, and not to hit the vessel directly which may precipitate bleeding. Controlled trials have confirmed the efficacy of this treatment: of 39 ulcers with a visible vessel only six rebled after laser therapy, as opposed to 23 of 43 control untreated ulcers ($p < 0.005$).[10] There was a 1 per cent mortality in the laser-treated group compared with 12 per cent in the control patients. It is now clear that the Nd YAG laser is a better haemostaic device than the argon ion laser.

Other cheaper thermal methods have been explored for endoscopic therapy. A popular device is the heater probe, which can be rapidly heated to 250°C using an internal coil covered by an aluminium Teflon non-stick coat, and the probe is applied directly to the visible vessel in the ulcer base. In a trial comparing heater probe and laser therapy for ulcers, the rebleeding rate was 20 per cent after laser therapy, 28 per cent after heater probe therapy and 42 per cent in control untreated ulcers, with no significant difference in mortality in any of the groups.[11] Although at present lasers appear as the most effective endoscopic method for haemostasis, it is likely that cheaper methods will ultimately prove as effective. Endoscopic injection of adrenaline into actively bleeding peptic ulcers arrested haemorrhage in 29 of 34 patients, this being a significant improvement over untreated patients.[12] In particular, endoscopic injection of adrenaline combined with either local thermal treatment with bipolar electrocoagulation or Nd YAG laser therapy has been shown to be equally effective.[13]

Laser therapy is also effective for angiodysplasia and hereditary haemorrhagic telangiectasia, which commonly occur in the stomach, duodenum and colon and are endoscopically accessible. It eliminates the need for surgery and reduces blood transfusion requirements. Other common lesions such as oesophagitis, gastritis and Mallory–Weiss tear mostly cease bleeding spontaneously, but the laser may be useful if this does not occur. There is no rationale for laser treatment for variceal haemorrhage.

The Nd YAG laser has also been used for the palliation of malignant dysphagia due to obstructing carcinomas of the oesophagus and gastric cardia. In patients deemed unsuitable for curative resection because of the extent of the malignancy, or because of severe coexisting medical disease, a channel can be cut by vaporizing tumour. On average 80 per cent of patients swallow a solid diet following laser treatment. Major complications occur in 4 per cent, with perforation and fistulation accounting for the majority of these, and there is a mortality of 1 per cent. Laser therapy is unsuitable if the tumour is predominantly extrinsic or if a tracheo-oesophageal fistula is present. In these circumstances endoscopic intubation is the preferred treatment. A disadvantage of laser therapy is that it must be repeated, and intubation may be required to maintain adequate swallowing because of extraluminal compression or laser-induced fibrosis.

There remain certain definite indications for laser therapy. First, insertion of a prosthesis high in the oesophagus may be uncomfortable and laser therapy is preferred for treatment of tumours in this position. Also, the laser has particular value in cutting a channel through tumours completely occluding the oesophagus (when a guide wire cannot be passed), through tumour overgrowth above a prosthetic tube, and at the site of an anastomotic recurrence after oesophageal resection.

Lasers can be used in arresting repeated bleeding from inoperable or recurrent gastric carcinoma, but conventional laser therapy can be difficult because of the large surface requiring treatment. Recently it has been possible to treat some of these lesions with interstitial laser therapy, slowly coagulating the tumour by inserting a laser fibre into its centre and using low power (1–5 W) for 100–1000 seconds.[14]

Hepatobiliary and pancreatic surgery

At present lasers are used for the fragmentation of biliary calculi that are too large to be removed by endoscopic sphincterotomy. The biliary tree is approached either by percutaneous transhepatic cholangioscopy or retrogradely following endoscopic sphincterotomy. Treatment is performed under sedation with fluoroscopic control or under direct vision using the newly developed 'mother and baby endoscopes'; a small endoscope (the laser fibre passed through the instrumentation channel) is passed through the instrumentation channel of a large duodenoscope into the common bile duct. Ell and associates reported the successful fragmentation of seven out of nine common bile duct stones using high energy pulses from a Nd YAG laser.[15] It is conceivable that gall stones could be similarly treated by percutaneous transhepatic cholecystoscopy using a flexible choledochoscope. There is the potential for laser treatment in recanalizing malignant biliary strictures which are impassable by a guide wire to allow placement of an endoprosthesis. In combination with afterloading radiotherapy with iridium wires, this technique may offer long-term palliation.

Until recently the only other application was to use the Nd YAG laser as a thermal knife for reducing the blood loss during major hepatic resection. The laser was used as a naked beam or passed through a shaped sapphire to perform contact laser surgery. It appears, however, that the present lasers may be most useful for haemostasis involving large oozing surfaces of the liver due to trauma. Standard surgical techniques will continue to be employed in liver resection to allow better control of major vascular and biliary structures.

Recently there has been an increasing interest in the use of interstitial laser hyperthermia for the treatment of solid tumours that are not easily resectable. Interstitial hyperthermia involves reducing the Nd YAG laser power from 50 to 80 W for 0.5–1 second to between 1 and 2 W delivered over a longer time (up to 1000 seconds), and inserting the fibre directly into tissue. The aim of using low power is to avoid vaporization while producing hyperthermic destruction of the tissue. This is predominantly an experimental technique that has been investigated for the possible treatment of irresectable liver and pancreatic cancers.[16] For clinical treatment, multiple fibres would be inserted into the tumour under ultrasound control or at laparotomy and left until the lesion is totally destroyed. Whether this approach would prove clinically applicable remains to be demonstrated.

Colorectal surgery

Rectosigmoid cancers are best treated by surgical resection both for cure and palliation. However, there remain some 5 per cent of patients with advanced metastatic spread or severe concomitant disease who are unsuitable for operative intervention. Palliative colostomy will relieve the obstruction but not the local symptoms of discharge, bleeding, tenesmus and incontinence. Although resection would provide better palliation, it may entail a permanent colostomy and prolonged recuperation, which would be unjustifiable in patients with a limited life expectancy. Local fulguration or cryotherapy are modalities that provide some relief for these patients, but require a general anaesthetic and are deliverable only to lower rectal cancers. Endoscopic Nd YAG laser tumour vaporization has been employed for inoperable rectosigmoid carcinoma, with symptomatic improvement in bleeding, discharge and obstruction in 85 per cent of patients, and with few complications.[17] Laser therapy is also recommended for the treatment of anastomotic recurrence when the chance of resectability is limited by local infiltration and potential cure is remote.

Colonscopic Nd YAG laser therapy is also possible for benign colonic tumours. While pendunculated polyps are very effectively treated by snare diathermy, sessile and villous adenomas require surgical excision which could be a major undertaking when large or not easily accessible by the endo-anal route. The morbidity associated with radical surgery in the elderly justifies a less invasive form of treatment even if not curative, especially since half of these lesions may not be malignant. A recent study reported complete eradication of 42 of 56 villous adenomas with the Nd YAG and argon ion laser over a mean follow-up period of 11.8 months.[18] A major criticism, which is insignificant if the treatment is aimed purely at palliation, is that the specimen is not obtainable for histological examination to assess the invasiveness and the completeness of removal. The development of endoscopic ultrasound may provide the information required to allow conventional use of laser therapy for these lesions. In patients with familial polyposis coli, treatment of recurrent rectal stump polyps has proved to be efficacious and safe.

Colonscopic laser therapy has also been employed for the treatment of angiodysplasias of the colon, and avoids colonic resection in these usually elderly patients. If the lesion can be identified it can be treated with the Nd YAG laser and completely destroyed, but in the usual case with multiple lesions the difficulty is in identifying the source of bleeding. The principle of treatment is slightly different from that for bleeding peptic ulcers. First a circumferential ring of tissue around the lesion is treated to produce thermal contraction of any feeding vessels. Finally the lesion itself is treated. Similarly, laser treatment is effective in irradiation proctitis and would eliminate the need for major surgery.

Perianal conditions are suitable for treatment with the CO_2 laser, but there appears at present to be little advantage of laser treatment over more conventional therapy. In particular, laser haemorrhoidectomy has been recommended as less traumatic and better tolerated than conventional therapy. However, the results of randomized trials are awaited.

Urology

The external genitalia are easily accessible to treatment with the CO_2 laser. Penile warts, superficial penile cancers and urethral caruncles have all been successfully treated, but there are no comparative data with conventional surgery. The endoscopic treatment of urethral strictures with CO_2, argon ion and Nd YAG lasers has not really produced any improvement in management. It was hoped that by vaporizing the fibrous tissue around the stricture, it would be possible to improve on the results of bouginage and urethrotomy. However, in a series of 41 patients treated with the argon ion laser, most patients had developed recurrent strictures within six months and the overall conclusion was that this technique offered little advantage over simple dilatation.[19] The CO_2 laser causes minimal scarring and could therefore be more suitable. There is, however, no reliable delivery system and the beam cannot be transmitted through water.

The area where lasers may have the greatest impact in urology is in the treatment of bladder cancer. Transurethral resection is an established method of treatment for superficial bladder cancer. It allows histological staging of the disease, which is not possible when the tumour is totally ablated with the laser, although endoscopic ultrasound should offer a better measurement of tumour invasion and disease staging. Although only a minority of lesions will progress to invasive carcinoma, they represent a clinical problem because of the high recurrence rate. After transurethral resection, some 50–70 per cent of lesions will be expected to recur at some point in the patient's lifetime. A possible explanation for recurrence is implantation of cells dislodged at the time of resection. Theoretically this problem may be avoided by laser treatment since there is no direct tissue contact.

Laser treatment is generally carried out with the Nd YAG laser. It is coupled into a flexible optical fibre and passed through a rigid or flexible endoscope. In some instances laser therapy can be performed through a flexible cystoscope under local anaesthesia on an outpatient, whereas transurethral resection and cystodiathermy are uncomfortable in the conscious patient. In a controlled trial, transurethral resection (TUR) has been compared with Nd YAG laser therapy.[20] Patients with T1 and T2 bladder cancers were divided into three groups. Group 1 included patients with tumours less than 6 mm in diameter (the diameter of the resectoscope snare), group 2 patients had T1 tumours greater than 6 mm in diameter, and group 3 were patients with T2 greater than 6 mm. In group 1, patients were randomized to laser or TUR and all were recurrence-free. In groups 2 and 3 all patients had TUR, but in the laser group the resection site was treated with the laser one or two weeks later. In group 2, none of 29 patients who had additional laser therapy developed recurrence, but 13 of 34 patients who did not have combined treatment developed further tumours, a highly significant difference. In group 3, recurrence developed in 3 of 15 patients treated with combination therapy, and 6 of 10 patients who were treated with TUR only. These results were for local recurrence with a follow-up of two years. Recurrence rates at other sites were similar for laser (12 of 62) and TUR (13 of 60). Although the effectiveness of laser therapy is clear in group 1, in the other groups the value is difficult to assess because patients who had TUR did not have the resection sites later further treated with laser, whereas the laser group did. Laser therapy would undoubtedly be considered in the control of local symptoms in patients with advanced disease.

Laser lithotripsy was originally developed to deal with urinary calculi impacted in the ureter that could not be removed endoscopically or shattered by extracorporeal shock-wave lithotripsy (ESWL). For stone fragmentation lasers have proved to be less traumatic to the ureter when compared with ultrasound (which requires a rigid probe and is relatively slow) and electrohydraulic lithotripsy (which can cause local tissue heating). The most effective system is a pulsed tuneable dye laser (tuned to 450–500 nm) coupled into a flexible optical fibre.[21] This fibre can be passed down a flexible or small-bore rigid ureteroscope and placed in contact with the stone. The majority of stones can be fragmented with one-microsecond pulses of 25 mJ at 10 Hz for 20 seconds. Overall, 95 per cent of stones can be completely or partially removed (with subsequent spontaneous passage) from the ureter using this method. ESWL is currently the preferred method for lithotripsy of kidney and upper ureteric calculi, but laser lithotripsy is the best method of endoscopic management for impacted stones in the rest of the ureter, where the pelvic bones act as a barrier to shock-wave therapy.

Gynaecology

The CO_2 laser has its most important application in the colposcopic treatment of cervical intraepithelial neoplasia (CIN). It has been demonstrated that 99 per cent of CIN extends no further than 4 mm from the surface into the cervical crypt at the time of diagnosis. Therefore, it can be completely eradicated by vaporizing the superficial layers with the laser. The lesion must be entirely visible to the colposcope, and lesions that disappear into the endocervical canal must not be vaporized because neoplasia in the canal may be invasive. The precision of the laser is the main advantage, and the procedure can be performed on an outpatient with little sedation or local anaesthesia. In early lesions (CIN I–II) there is a 96 per cent cure rate; similar results are being reported for CIN III (97 per cent) with little morbidity when compared with other techniques such as cryotherapy, which can produce severe vaginal discharge.[22]

Since the results of laser treatment for CIN have been so good, it is now being applied to vulvar intraepithelial neoplasia (VIN) and vaginal intraepithelial neoplasia (VAIN). The results of superficial laser vulvectomy are encouraging, with 95 per cent of patients disease-free after one year follow-up. The CO_2 lasser beam cannot be transmitted down flexible optical fibres and can only be delivered via a series of mirrors in an articulated arm, which has prevented its application to some areas inside the body, including the uterus.

Recently the Nd YAG laser has been used to treat 300 patients with menorrhagia by laser ablation of the endometrium at hysteroscopy, with complete success reported for 90 per cent. If these initial findings are confirmed then the hysterectomy rate in the UK may be drastically reduced.[23]

Photodynamic therapy

Photodynamic therapy (PDT) is an interesting new technique with the potential for selective destruction of cancers. It is based on the systemic administration of certain photosensitizing agents, generally porphyrin or phthalocyanine compounds, that are retained selectively in malignant tissue, fluoresce when exposed to specific wavelengths of light, and in the presence of oxygen produce a local cytotoxic effect.

Tumour localization of photosensitizers and destruction on exposure to light is well documented. The retention of these agents appears to be related to non-specific tumour factors rather than to the photosensitizer used. In extracranial tissues the maximum tumour-to-normal ratio that can be obtained with a variety of photosensitizing agents is 2–3 : 1. In the brain, ratios of 30 : 1 can be obtained because the blood/brain barrier around tumours is destroyed.[24] PDT may therefore be of value as an adjunct to surgical treatment of gliomas. At present the treatment of gliomas has proved dismally disappointing. Local resection fails predominantly because of local microinvasion by the tumour; and radical resections involve extensive damage to normal brain. PDT might therefore be used after local resection to treat the tumour bed and selectively destroy any remaining tumour cells with survival of normal surrounding brain.[25] Early clinical trials have not yet demonstrated any definite benefit. PDT has been employed with encouraging results for cutaneous metastases of various cancers in patients in whom conventional therapy failed, and for superficial bladder, endobronchial and oesophageal carcinoma. Treatment of recurrent pelvic cancers with PDT has been reported and is undergoing further assessment.

Haematoporphyrins are not mutagenic or carcinogenic, but they do cause skin photosensitization, and so for 4–8 weeks after injection patients must not be exposed to sunlight unless covered with clothing. Phthalocyanines cause much less skin photosensitivity but are not yet ready for clinical use.

Investigation of photodynamic therapy in experimental colorectal neoplasms has demonstrated an important biological advantage compared with thermal laser destruction. Unlike thermal damage, full-thickness colonic damage produced by photodynamic therapy does not reduce the mechanical strength of the bowel or cause perforation, because the submucosal collagen is preserved. However selective necrosis is limited to a small area,[26] which will restrict its application to small tumours only. It may provide a useful method for the treatment, before malignancy has developed, of adenomatous polyps in the upper gastrointestinal tract in patients with familial polyposis syndrome.

The concept of PDT is one of the most exciting aspects of lasers in surgery, but the true role of this form of treatment has yet to be defined. It is tempting to apply photodynamic therapy clinically before the important parameters that control the degree of damage have been clarified. The major problem appears to be that most of the present generation of photosensitizers are activated by light that will not penetrate far enough into tissue. To get maximum tissue penetration, red light, generally from a dye laser (because of its tunable monochronicity and ability to be transmitted down an optical fibre), is used.

Cost-effectiveness and safety

The individual cost of a laser is variable, with a simple CO_2 laser costing £10 000 and a full dye laser system of the order of £100 000. The most commonly used Nd YAG laser costs £40 000, with maintenance and other recurring costs of approximately £4000 per annum. It is always difficult to evaluate cost-effectiveness since this requires costing of other treatment methods. Laser treatment may require several sessions, but hospital stay of patients in certain instances is probably less than if conventional treatment is offered. There are other expenses involved in laser maintenance, and direct comparisons are difficult. It appears from the control trials of the treatment of upper gastrointestinal haemorrhage that the laser may be a cost-effective solution. With heater probes costing £6000 and local adrenaline injection being less expensive, these methods may prove to be more cost-effective. However, one laser may have applications in many specialities and need not be reserved for one specific use.

The particular hazard for the operator of a laser is the risk of retinal burn if the beam is allowed to escape into the eye. To prevent this occurrence all endoscopes are fitted with an eyepiece filter and if the beam is used in the open all personnel in the room must wear safety goggles. In addition laser rooms have to be fitted with interlocks on the door which shut down the instrument should anyone enter the room during operation. Each hospital with a laser must have a designated laser safety officer to ensure that correct safety procedures are followed for the particular use of the laser.

There are particular hazards of using the laser in the larynx and bronchus with potentially flammable anaesthetic agents or materials such as endotracheal tubes. Following PDT of large tumours there may be risk of secondary haemorrhage, if the tumour is not completely destroyed. The precise nature of this problem remains to be identified. The complication has been observed following thermal laser therapy, but the main risk of this technique is perforation.

An important consideration in the development of any new technique is the risk of inducing malignant transformation. Most lasers operating in the visible and infrared range have photon energies that are too low to break molecular bonds and liberate free radicals. However, short-wavelength excimer lasers produce free radicals that may induce changes in the tissue. At present this appears to be only a theoretical risk, but careful assessment is still required.

References

1. Carruth J.A.S., Tonquet V.L.R. Review of treatment of port wine stains with the argon laser. *Lasers Surg. Med.* 1984; **4:** 191–9.
2. Flemming A.F.S., Brough M.D., Bown S.G. Hydrostatic distension as a method of assessing strength of laser-assisted microvascular anastomoses. *Proceedings of the Fourth Annual Conference of the British Medical Laser Association* 1986, London.
3. Hetzel M.R., Nixon C., Edmonstone W.M., Mitchell D.M., *et al.* Laser therapy in 100 tracheobronchial tumours. *Thorax.* 1985; **40:** 341–5.
4. Gruntzig A.R., Hopf H. Perkutane Rekanalisation chronischer arterieller Verschlüsse mit einem neuen Dilationskatheter: Modifikation der Dotter-technik. *Dtsch. Med. Wochenschr.* **99:** 2502.
5. Murray R.R., Hewes R.C., White R.I., Mitchell S.E., Auster M., Chang R., Kadir S.,

Kinnison M.L., Kaufman M.L., Kaufman S.L. Long-segment femoropopliteal stenoses: is angioplasty a boon or a bust? *Radiology*. 1987; **162:** 473.
6. Isner J.M., Clarke R.H., Donaldson R.F., Aharon A. Identification of photoproducts liberated by *in vitro* argon laser irradiation of atherosclerotic plaque, calcified cardiac valves and myocardium. *Amer. J. Cardiol*. 1985; **55:** 1192.
7. Cumberland D.C., Tayler D.I., Procter A.E. Laser-assisted percutaneous angioplasty: initial clinical experience in peripheral arteries. *Clin. Radiol*. 1986; **37:** 423.
8. Cumberland D.C., Starkey I.R., Oakley G.D., Fleming J.S., Smith G.H., Goiti J.J., Tayler D.I., Davies J. Percutaneous laser-assisted coronary angioplasty. *Lancet*. 1986; **ii:** 214.
9. Cross F.W., Bowker T.J., Marston A., Adiseshiah M., Bown S.G. Artificial circulation assessment of sapphire fibretips for use in laser angioplasty. *Brit. J. Surg*. 1986; **74:** 329.
10. Swain C.P., Kirkham J.S., Salmon P.R., Bown S.G., Northfield T.C. Controlled trial of Nd YAG laser photocoagulation in bleeding peptic ulcers. *Lancet*. 1986, **i:** 1113–7.
11. Matthewson K., Swain C.P., Bland M., Kirkham J.S., Bown S.G., Northfield T.C. A randomised comparison of Nd YAG laser, heater probe and no endoscopic therapy for bleeding peptic ulcer. *Gut*. 1987; **10:** A1342.
12. Chung S.C.S., Leung J.W.C., Steele R.J.C., Crofts T.J., Li A.K.C. Endoscopic injection of adrenaline for actively bleeding ulcers: randomised trial. *Brit. Med. J*. 1988; **296:** 1631–3.
13. Rutgeerts P., Vantrappen G., Van Hootegem Ph., *et al*. Nd YAG laser photocoagulation versus multipolar electrocoagulation for the treatment of severely bleeding ulcers: a randomized comparison. *Gastrointest. Endosc*. 1987; **33:** 199–202.
14. Barr H., Krasner N. Is it possible to control bleeding from gastro-oesophageal cancer using endoscopic laser therapy? *Gut*. 1988; **29:** A729.
15. Ell Ch., Hochberger J., Muller D., Lux G., Demling L. Laser lithotripsy of gall stones by means of pulsed Nd: YAG lasers. *Seventh Congress of the International Society for Laser Surgery and Medicine*, Munich: A149.
16. Steger A.C., Barr H., Hawes R., Bown S.G., Clark C.G. Experimental studies on interstitial hyperthermia for treating pancreatic cancer. *Gut*. 1987; **28:** A 1382.
17. Bown S.G., Barr H., Matthewson K., Hawes R., Swain C.P., Clark C.G., Boulos P.B. Endoscopic treatment of inoperable colorectal cancers with the Nd YAG laser. *Brit. J. Surg*. 1986; **73:** 949–52.
18. Brunetaud J.M., Mosquet L., Houcke M., *et al*. Villous adenoma of the rectum. Results of endoscopic treatment with argon and Nd YAG lasers. *Gastroenterology*. 1985; **89:** 832–7.
19. Hofstetter A., Frank F. Laser use in urology. In: Dixon J.A. (ed.): *Surgical Applications of Lasers*. Chicago: Year Book Medical Publishers, 1983.
20. Beisland H.O., Seland P. A prospective randomised study on Nd YAG laser irradiation versus TUR in the treatment of urinary bladder cancer. *Scand. J. Urol. Nephrol*. 1986; **20:** 209–12.
21. Watson G.M., Wickham J.E.A. Initial experience with a pulsed dye laser for ureteric calculi. *Lancet*. 1986; **i:** 1357–8.
22. Jordan J.A., Sharp F. *Gynaecological Laser Surgery*. New York: Perinatology Press, 1986.
23. Goldrath M.H. Hysteroscopic laser ablation of the endometrium. In: Jordan J.A., Sharp F. (eds.): *Gynaecological Laser Surgery*. New York: Perinatology Press, 1986.
24. Tralau C.J., Barr H., Sandeman D.R., Barton T., Lewin M.R., Bown S.G. Aluminium sulfonated pththalocyanine distribution in tumours of the colon, brain and pancreas. *Photochem. Photobiol*. 1987; **46:** 777–81.
25. Sandeman D., Bradford R., Buxton P., Bown S.G., Thomas D.G.T. Selective necrosis of malignant gliomas in mice using photodynamic therapy. *Brit. J. Cancer*. 1987; **55:** 647–9.
26. Barr H., Tralau C.J., Lewin M., Clark C.G., Bown S.G., Boulos P.B. Selective destruction of experimental colon cancer using photodynamic therapy. *Brit. J. Surg*. 1988; **75:** 611–2.

4

Postoperative thromboembolic disease: a tantalizing enigma

Tom Treasure, MD, MS, FRCS, and
Steven Griffin, FRCS

Deep vein thrombosis and pulmonary embolism are common clinical problems which confront surgeons of all disciplines and yet there can be few subjects surrounded by such uncertainty. The symptoms and clinical signs of deep vein thrombosis are neither sensitive nor specific, so confident clinical diagnosis is difficult. The response to a suspicion of deep vein thrombosis varies widely, with some opting for prolonged anticoagulation on the basis of a clinical suspicion, while others initiate a series of invasive investigations before initiating any therapy.

Pulmonary embolism presents with various clinical pictures, and again the symptoms and signs are inconclusive and it can be difficult to know how to respond. Sometimes urgency dictates that we initiate treatment on suspicion alone; but under what circumstances and to what extent the condition should be investigated may tax clinical judgement. If we do investigate before starting treatment, how much reliance can be placed on the results? *Even when the diagnosis is made with certainty there is no uniformity about the treatment.* Some patients are managed surgically by pulmonary embolectomy, and opinions vary on the relative merits of performing the operation with the help of cardiopulmonary bypass, or performing a Trendelenberg type of operation without bypass. Medical management with streptokinase is more commonly used, but the data are simply inadequate to support any firm view and in any case the three approaches—medical management, embolectomy or operation on bypass—are not interchangeable or uniformly available.

There is an obvious logic it trying to prevent the common complication, deep vein thrombosis, and the less common but lethal manifestation, pulmonary embolism; but there is still no uniformity in practice and some debate about the evidence for the efficacy of various measures. Finally, what is it sensible to do for secondary prevention? Is there a place for obstructing the inferior vena cava in some way? If prolonged anticoagulation is to be used, for how long and at what level?

Here are a series of clinical dilemmas listed in the form of questions. For each of these the practising surgeon should have a working policy:

1. Can we do anything to prevent thromboembolic complications in the surgical patient?
2. How should we respond to clinical suspicion of deep venous thrombosis?

3. How should we manage a postoperative patient who has evidence of pulmonary infarction?
4. How should we manage acute massive pulmonary embolism?
5. In which cases should we use long-term anticoagulation, and for how long?
6. Is there a place for obstructing or filtering the flow in the IVC?

Every working surgeon is confronted with these questions, the first daily and others less commonly. There will be no notice of the question, nor, in most instances, time to read or consult. Some are life and death decisions that have to be reached in moments if they are to influence the outcome. In others the response might appear over-dramatic, and dangerous, in the short term and the surgeon must believe that the response is in proportion to the magnitude of the longer term hazard. Ideally, for each, there should be a reasonable policy which is achievable within the context of the particular practice, and which can be justified on the available evidence.

We shall discuss each of these and try to offer answers. Many will disagree and opinions will change, but at any time, in any given surgical team, it would be reasonable to ask each of these questions.

1. Can we do anything to prevent thromboembolic complications in the surgical patient?

It is probable that the only conclusive way to answer this question is with evidence from suitably designed and properly conducted prospective randomized clinical trials. This is much more easily said than done. Clinical trials, in spite of the enormous efforts that might have gone into their organization, have often proved to be inconclusive, out of date by the time they report, or at best, only answer a small part of the question that the investigators posed at the outset. Trials of prevention are particularly difficult to design if the event which we are trying to prevent occurs infrequently, as is the case with the major complications of common and routine surgical procedures.

It is instructive to digress briefly to look at some research strategies that have been used to try to overcome this problem. Examples of other serious but infrequent complications of major surgery are wound infection and, particularly in cardiac surgery, stroke, both of which occur with an incidence of under 2 per cent.[1,2] If we were to randomize 100 patients undergoing operation into two study groups we would expect to record one, two or three events in the whole series and, no matter how these were distributed between the groups, it would be patently obvious, on the grounds of common sense alone, that no conclusion could be drawn. The null hypothesis that 'there is no significant difference between the outcome in group A and group B' cannot be rejected, not because we have proved they are similar, but because we would never have been able to prove them dissimilar. Even if, owing to a freak pattern of events, we did find a significant difference we would have to reject the trial as invalid because the patients in the study could not be representative of the population at risk, where we believe there to be an incidence of 1–2 per cent. This predictable failure of a trial to produce an answer is called a beta, or type-II, error and is now familiar to all those who are involved with clinical research. It means that if we are looking for a difference in an event with low frequency in the study population, we will need large numbers in the trial to obtain an answer. In the case of prevention of pulmonary embolism, which probably kills a little under 1 per cent of patients undergoing major surgery, it has been estimated that a trial of adequate power to detect a reduction in mortality for this condition would have to include 20 000 cases.[3] It is therefore unlikely that an individual unit could run a worthwhile study of prophylaxis to reduce death from pulmonary embolism.

There are three ways around this problem. One is to regard death from pulmonary embolism as the most severe manifestation of a more common problem (that is, the formation of thrombus in the deep veins) and study the common condition. By counting the occurrence of deep vein thrombosis, we increase the number of countable events. We might even go further and grade the extent of the deep vein thrombosis; and, by including the severity as well as the frequency of DVT, we can increase the data available for analysis. In our own study of median sternotomy infection we used a similar strategy by looking at all degrees of imperfect healing rather than just severe wound infection[4] and were able to show significant differences in a trial of 517 randomized patients. Similarly, a study of deep vein thrombosis, with an incidence of 20–30 per cent,[5] is likely to provide an answer with much smaller numbers than the 20 000 cases required if we take death proven to be due to pulmonary embolism as an end-point. However, in both examples we have to question whether the more common, less severe complication is reliably related to the more serious, but much less common condition which we may originally have set out to study.

In the case of wound infection it is likely that minor and very severe infections are part of the same pathological process, the ends of a spectrum of severity, and that they will be influenced by some preventive measures. *The clinical diagnosis of deep vein thrombosis is notoriously difficult, but it is clear that the relationship between DVT and pulmonary embolism is neither a simple nor a reliable one.* We believe that the fatal pulmonary embolus may have come from clinically silent deep vein thrombosis. Anecdotally there are reasons to believe that massive pulmonary embolism and clinically diagnosable deep vein thrombosis may be negatively correlated. Perhaps the aetiological factors are different and prophylaxis that will prevent one will not influence the other. In our studies of bypass-related cerebral problems we believe that the common, apparently minor changes in neuropsychological performance are quite separate from severe stroke and have a different aetiological pattern. We must seek to reduce the incidence of both but in different ways. But which of these examples does pulmonary embolism resemble? There are cases where death is due to pulmonary embolism but post mortem examination has failed to find thrombus in the veins. Nevertheless, the thrombus which obstructs the pulmonary circulation has come from somewhere in the systemic venous system. In a retrospective analysis of 195 cases of death from pulmonary embolism[6] a pathologist reported deep vein thrombosis in 162 (83 per cent). Neither pulmonary embolism nor DVT had been suspected clinically in the majority. Although one could argue that fixed and mobile thrombi are different pathological entities, they coexist sufficiently frequently for us to believe that, if the incidence of DVT were reduced, fatal embolism would be less common.

The most reliable and applicable end-point in studies of the frequency and prevention of deep vein thrombosis has been the accumulation of radio-labelled fibrinogen in the leg veins.[5] Some studies have required the confirmation of DVT by venography. Trials of prophylactic measures have included the use of stockings, compression devices and intravenous dextran infusions, but the method of prophylaxis which has the most bearing on the main subject of this chapter is perioperative administration of heparin. *The use of subcutaneous heparin, started before surgery, reduces the incidence of DVT from about 20 per cent to about 10 per cent.* A study of above 500 patients would have the power to detect this difference and many such studies have been performed. It is of interest that the findings were similar for general, orthopaedic and urological surgery. The prolongation of treatment beyond five days seemed to confer no additional benefit, and 12-hourly treatment is as good as 8-hourly.[3] Deep vein thrombosis is a substantial problem in its own right, with serious morbidity, so we might argue, for that reason alone, that it is justifiable to give heparin while recognizing that reduction in the much more common event, DVT, is not necessarily accompanied by a reduction in the incidence of fatal massive pulmonary embolism.

A second approach is to make the trial large enough, and therefore powerful enough, to avoid a beta error. This will nearly always require a multi-centre trial. All too often problems such as a low recruitment rate, variable diligence between the centres, and differences in the approach to ethical considerations have flawed trials in other conditions, leaving the conclusions questionable and easily discounted by those who do not like the answer that emerged. The International Multicentre Trial[7] reported on 4121 patients, of whom a total of 18 patients died of pulmonary embolism. The distribution of pulmonary embolism between the groups was uneven and significantly so. The incidence of fatal pulmonary embolism was reduced from 0.7 per cent (16 cases) in the untreated group to 0.1 per cent (2 cases), a difference believed to be due to the effect of heparin. Non-fatal emboli and deep vein thrombosis were also less in the group who received heparin prophylaxis.

The third technique to overcome the problems of reaching statistical proof of the efficacy of a treatment is to pool retrospectively the results of a number of trials, so called meta-analysis.[8] A massive analysis has been performed of 74 studies of the use of prophylactic heparin, including a total of 15 598 patients.[3] The overall death rate was reduced by a quarter (from about 4 per cent to about 3 per cent) and there was no significant difference in the deaths attributable to haemorrhage. The findings in the pooled data were consistent with the findings in the individual studies. The process of performing an analysis of this type is suspect and the reasons for including and rejecting studies must be inspected carefully. Some remain unhappy with this approach, but we suspect that this is because of a received perception of scientific rigor and statistical purism. *We are convinced and are prepared to conclude that there is a reduction in fatal and non-fatal pulmonary embolism with the perioperative use of subcutaneous heparin and that this provides an overall benefit in terms of survival.*

It is interesting that pulmonary embolism is almost unknown as a cause of perioperative catastrophe in cardiac surgery in which patients are totally anticoagulated with heparin (300 units per kg, that is over 20 000 units by I.V. bolus) and the effect of the bypass is to produce a fairly profound and sustained coagulopathy. However, cardiac surgical patients who have a prolonged period of postoperative immobility may succumb to relatively late embolism at three weeks when presumably they have returned to the same hazard as any other bedridden individual. The risk is increased with age, female gender, duration of immobility before as well as after surgery, oral contraceptives, pregnancy, malignancy and surgery in the region of the pelvis and lower limbs. Stasis is the most important proximate risk factor, and the occurrence of deep vein thrombosis and pulmonary embolism is well documented in fit, young people after long air flights.[9]

We believe that 5000 units of heparin, given 8- or 12-hourly, from before surgery until the patient is mobilized, is effective prophylaxis. There is no increase in the risk of serious bleeding although there is a small increase in wound haematoma. The evidence has been collected in older patients undergoing major surgery, and many surgeons have a policy that excludes younger patients having more minor surgery, but the criteria are fairly arbitrary. Others believe that the risks of the treatment have been proven to be negligible and give this prophylaxis to all patients admitted for operation, which has the considerable advantage that it is less likely to be overlooked.

2. How should we respond to clinical suspicion of deep vein thrombosis?

In its gross form, deep vein thrombosis can be diagnosed clinically with reasonable confidence. The sudden onset of severe, unilateral, leg oedema in a postoperative patient strongly suggests this diagnosis and probably merits treatment in its own right because of the severity of the symptoms and the permanent damage that may result to the venous system. Loss of patency of the deep venous system, or destruction of its valves, may lead to leg ulceration which causes great distress and afflicts a large number of patients. These patients should be treated energetically, and the practice in most hospitals is to heparinize the patient on the basis of this clinical diagnosis. There is an understandable fear that heparinization is dangerous but this may be illogical. Aspirin is available to all across the chemist's counter, warfarin is given to hospital outpatients, but heparin is usually only given in high-dependency areas of the hospital. In cardiac surgery we use heparin every day, its action decays spontaneously within hours and it can be rapidly reversed with protamine. Warfarin is used regularly, its effects take some days to wear off and it can be reversed to some extent with fresh frozen plasma. The effect of aspirin on the platelets has a half-life of five days and can only be reversed with platelet transfusions. In surgery, heparin is the most manageable of the three.

Confirming the diagnosis by phlebography should follow whenever possible. We might be asked, will it alter the management in any way? The clinical diagnosis may be wrong in up to 50 per cent of cases, and then the patient can be spared further heparinization and long-term anticoagulation. If there were evidence of loose thrombus extending into the large pelvic veins and the inferior vena cava, some would advocate use of an IVC filter, although under these circumstances we would advocate medical management rather than an intervention designed to obstruct the inferior vena cava.

What is much more difficult to deal with, and is much more common, is the patient with a less clear-cut picture who is noted to have calf tenderness, or minor oedema, or a slight pyrexia without adequate explanation. Does the patient have a deep vein thrombosis, and if so is there a risk of embolism? If it were not for the risk of pulmonary embolism it would be hard to justify elaborate investigations, intravenous heparin and prolonged oral anticoagulation given in the belief that there is an important risk to life that can be reduced by treatment. There are several problems in decision making. The clinical signs correlate poorly with phlebographic proof of the diagnosis. The investigations, if undertaken, are not insubstantial and there is often debate about their interpretation. It is also widely taught that the deep vein thrombosis that causes pain and swelling is probably securely stuck and is not endangering life; it is the quiet ones you have to watch! It is even said that if a patient with a clinically manifest DVT has a pulmonary embolism, it probably came from the other side! *So what should be done when our suspicions are aroused but the diagnosis is far from certain? Await events? Initiate investigations? Treat on clinical suspicion?*

The first statement to be made is that pulmonary embolism has, by definition, always been preceded by venous thrombosis, although there may be uncertainty about the site of origin in some cases. In autopsy studies of patients dying of pulmonary emboli, over 80 per cent have thrombus in leg veins, and in 30 per cent the most proximal involvement is in the deep veins of the calf.[6,10] By no means all and perhaps only a minority originate in the pelvic veins, so DVT of the leg cannot be disregarded as a hazard for pulmonary embolism. It is likely that only one in twenty patients with DVT has a subsequent embolism, but this may be without further warning and fatal so we believe it is an important diagnosis to make and to treat energetically.

The choice of investigation includes Doppler, Doppler with ultrasound (duplex scanning), radionuclide venography, impedance plethysmography, venography and fibrinogen scanning. This last test has been of great value in prospective studies. Fibrinogen labelled with ^{125}I is administered intravenously and counts are taken over the legs daily. Accumulation of fibrinogen in thrombus can be detected providing a valuable means of documenting DVT. It is of no use in the clinical situation which we have described. Impedance plethysmography and Doppler both require the expertise of a vascular laboratory to perform and interpret the tests. This means that they are of value in the performance of trials and evaluating patients referred to a vascular unit but are of less help to the orthopaedic surgeon, gynaecologist or any other surgeon confronted with the problem and requiring help in making the diagnosis so that management can be planned. *Our policy therefore is to perform venography*. Although this remains the objective standard it is not easy to perform well and the results are often debated. In particular there is often less than total confidence in distinguishing streaming of contrast in an underfilled vein from thrombus. *Nevertheless, it is usually helpful in making a decision.*

If deep vein thrombosis is ruled out the patient is spared anticoagulation and further anxiety. Those in whom thrombus is demonstrated are given heparin intravenously with 25 000 units as a bolus and then 1000 units per hour by infusion. *The more confident the clinical diagnosis the more likely would we be to initiate heparinization before venography*, and if venography cannot be performed within hours we would proceed on clinical judgement. Local measures are applied, such as support stockings, and the leg is either used in active walking or elevated above the horizontal. Warfarin is started and maintained for a period of at least six weeks. The ideal level of anticoagulation is a matter of conjecture, but prolongation of the prothrombin time over twice but less than three times the control value (INR of 2–3) is accepted.

Obstructing the inferior vena cava, surgically or with a transvenously sited filter to prevent pulmonary embolism, is not justifiable under these circumstances.

3. How should we manage a postoperative patient who has evidence of pulmonary infarction?

In practical terms there are two patterns of presentation of pulmonary embolism, pulmonary infarction and acute massive pulmonary embolism. Both may vary in severity and the two may occur in the same patient, but they are sufficiently different in their presentation and danger to merit separate discussion. The difference depends upon the size of the embolus. Those that are small enough to pass on into the segmental branches of the pulmonary arteries have little or no haemodynamic effect. On the other hand, only thrombus which becomes wedged well out near the periphery of the lung causes infarction. Normally the arterial supply to the lung and airways is from the bronchial arteries, which are branches of intercostal arteries distributed with the bronchi. *Only at the periphery of the lung will an occlusion of the pulmonary artery compromise the viability of the lung tissue.* The coexistence of hypoxaemia, a common enough postoperative complication, or cardiovascular impairment may increase the vulnerability to infarction.

Pulmonary infarction causes pleuritic pain and haemoptysis. In a typical case, the diagnosis is obvious. However, fewer than half of angiographically proven cases of embolism to the segmental pulmonary arteries present with haemoptysis, so many must go undiagnosed. Other respiratory symptoms are non-specific in the postoperative patient, and in the absence of haemoptysis they are unlikely to lead to a diagnosis of pulmonary infarction, which is unsuspected in the majority of cases.[6]

The patient should be examined, looking in particular for evidence of right heart abnormalities such as a heave, or elevation of the jugular venous pressure. Absence of these signs does not refute the diagnosis, but their presence adds weight and suggests that the embolism is substantial and that the patient is already compromised and would be at serious risk from further events. Tachycardia and tachypnoea are likely, but are so non-specific as to be of no diagnostic help. Auscultation may reveal a rub which would confirm the pleuritic nature of the pain, but again this adds nothing to the diagnosis. The legs should be examined for evidence of deep vein thrombosis.

Investigations should include a routine chest x-ray. Relative lucency due to reduction in vascular markings in one area compared with others may be seen but this is a very subjective change. The ECG should be taken and studied for evidence of right heart strain, such as inverted T waves anteriorly.

On suspicion of the diagnosis, ventilation and perfusion lung scans should be performed. The perfusion scan is performed by injecting intravenously albumen macroaggregates labelled with ^{99}Tc and taking a series of views of the lungs, including obliques. Ventilation scans are performed using ^{133}Xe gas. The test is positive if there are perfusion defects without a matching ventilation defect. A chest x-ray should be used to exclude some other cause, and the perfusion defects are particularly suggestive if they have a recognizable lobar or segmental distribution, and if they are multiple. *A truly normal distribution of perfusion refutes the diagnosis quite effectively, but unfortunately false positive tests are quite common* and are particularly likely to occur in patients who have other abnormalities in the chest, even patchy areas of atelectesis, which are very likely to coexist in these cases.

If the clinical suspicion is high and the perfusion scan supports, or at least does not rule out, the diagnosis, these patients should be heparinized. Analgesia and increased inspired oxygen are also given. We would not perform venography because with proof of pulmonary embolism the treatment will be the same whether deep vein thrombosis can be demonstrated or not. On the other hand, if there remained considerable diagnostic uncertainty, and particularly if there were clinical reasons to fear full anticoagulation, venography would then be appropriate to help plan management. Additional local measures as described above for deep vein thrombosis would seem sensible. If there were evidence of haemodynamic effects, we would suspect that there was a relatively large embolus and would consider pulmonary angiography.

The pulmonary vasculature is very compliant, accepting the whole cardiac output at a pressure which is normally no higher than 25 mmHg and falls to capillary pressure in diastole. Abrupt occlusion of one or other pulmonary artery during pneumonectomy is tolerated without evidence of right ventricular strain and with only modest and probably non-sustained elevation of the pulmonary artery pressure. On the other hand, *obstruction of one pulmonary artery by thrombus is not well tolerated and the pulmonary artery pressure is likely to rise to 40 mmHg or more*. The right heart, unused to abnormal resistance, will not withstand this workload for long. It is possible that this is because showers of emboli have gone into the other lung and the pulmonary vascular bed is reduced to considerably less than 50 per cent. It has been suggested that the degranulated platelets in the thrombus may be responsible. If a dog is perfused with blood from another animal with pulmonary embolism, it develops right heart strain even though it does not itself have thrombus in the pulmonary artery. A causative change in vasoactive amines has not been demonstrated.

4. How should we manage acute massive pulmonary embolism?

If any examination candidate finds himself in disagreement with his examiner on this subject he might find comfort in the knowledge that there is disagreement at the highest level. At the British Cardiac Society in 1987 the outstanding surgical experience from the Brompton Hospital in the management of 139 cases with acute massive pulmonary embolism was reviewed.[11] The favourable results of the use of embolectomy on cardiopulmonary bypass were reported. It was pointed out by another leading group with experience in this field that surgery on bypass was not necessary and that a better approach was to move the surgeon to the patient to perform a pulmonary embolectomy with inflow occlusion, an operation rather loosely referred to as Trendelenberg's operation although it is not in fact what he described.[12] It is at least possible that the favourable results with cardiopulmonary bypass were due to natural selection and were seen in spite of, not because of, the surgery. To take that argument further, it is arguable that any patient who survived to be transferred to a cardiac unit had already demonstrated an ability to survive pulmonary embolism. An alternative view is that all the patients who could be saved would do at least as well with medical measures alone.[13] So who is right?

In acute massive pulmonary embolism there is sudden and severe disturbance of the cardiovascular system owing to pulmonary embolism. The degree of haemodynamic disturbance is, in general terms, in proportion to the size of the embolus, and at least 50 per cent of the pulmonary vascular tree is obstructed.

As has already been discussed, it is possible that there were previous events and that there was already obstruction to parts of the vascular tree. It is also believed that the degree of pulmonary vascular resistance is more than can be explained by the presence of the thrombus alone and that other factors may contribute to the haemodynamic changes.

Presentation is usually with severe distressing chest tightness, dyspnoea and sometimes syncope. It is associated with defaecation (or a desire to defaecate) more often than chance would dictate. This may be because straining frees the embolism owing to a sudden surge of venous return at the end of a Valsalva manoeuvre, or because the first sensation as the embolism travels is of an autonomic surge taken to be a 'call to stool'.

A history of the patient's state in the days preceding the event and of the sequence of events must be sought out carefully because action may have to be taken without investigation. *There is a tendency, particularly in the high-risk cases undergoing orthopaedic or gynaecological surgery, for any deterioration in a patient's condition to be attributed to pulmonary embolism.* The differential diagnosis includes all the causes of acute collapse and, of course, myocardial infarction is an important alternative diagnosis. It is also important to remember that there are other causes for what is perceived as a sudden deterioration in the patient's condition, but in fact the underlying cause may be sepsis, gastrointestinal haemorrhage, or a number of other possibilities that will not be helped by either streptokinase or surgical embolectomy.

On examination tachypnoea is likely to be present. Hypotension, its severity depending on the degree of obstruction, is also likely. There is evidence of poor cardiac output as judged by peripheral cooling and weak pulses. The jugular venous pressure is raised, there is usually a right ventricular heave and an increase in the pulmonary component of the second sound.

Investigations should start with the ECG, which is usually in sinus rhythm with a tachycardia. T-wave inversion is common, and the appearance of a deep S-wave in lead I and a Q and inverted-T in lead III is characteristic but not necessary for the diagnosis.

About 15 per cent of cases of symptomatic pulmonary embolism are fatal, but a much higher proportion of cases of acute massive embolism die, many within the first hour. Of those who survive the first hour, 90 per cent can be expected to leave hospital alive. In severe cases, urgent resuscitation is required to save life. The first measure is to elevate the venous pressure even further because survival depends on the amount of blood that will get beyond the pulmonary artery occlusion and through to the left heart. Oxygen will help reduce the pulmonary vasoconstriction which is believed to exacerbate the condition. Thrombolysis will occur naturally so, if the patient can be kept alive and the degree of obstruction is compatible with survival for long enough for this to happen, improvement can be expected and treatment should be aimed at encouraging lysis of the thrombus and prevention of further embolism. However, rapid resolution is the exception rather than the rule and it is likely to be 7–10 days before there is resolution of most of the thrombus. If the patient cannot maintain a circulation or is deteriorating fast, desperate measures are required and the form which they take may well depend to a large extent upon what facilities are available. Pulmonary angiography not only confirms the diagnosis but aids emergency treatment by providing an opportunity to dislodge, break up and move on clot in the pulmonary arteries.[13] It should be considered in all but those where the only hope is with a desperate attempt at immediate surgery. However, the angiographic contrast media may cause deterioration in the patient's circulation.

Pulmonary angiography

A transvenous catheter is passed through the right heart into the pulmonary artery and an injection of contrast will show any major filling defect, seen as the abrupt cut-off of a major vessel or as a missing area of perfusion. It has been advocated, and seems reasonable, to attempt to break up this thrombus if at all possible with the catheter.[13] If some is moved on it may make the difference between life and death. *If the diagnosis is confirmed and the patient is able to maintain an output, then treatment should be medical. If there are large central emboli amenable to surgical removal, obstructing more than 50 per cent of the pulmonary circulation, and the patient's condition is not supportable for long enough to await lysis, or continues to deteriorate an hour after its instigation, surgery may be considered.*

Medical treatment—thrombolysis or heparin

The choice of anticoagulation with heparin while awaiting the natural process of lysis to occur, or the use of thrombolytic agents to speed the process, has been subjected to prospective randomized trials, but the results are not absolutely clear-cut. It is likely that this remaining uncertainty is a consequence of the ethical impossibility of withholding thrombolytic therapy in a patient who is clearly dying, and might be saved by the other treatment. It is only in this very severe group that a difference might be shown.[10,14,15] *The balance of evidence is in favour of the conclusion that thrombolysis is sufficiently faster than natural lysis to improve the chance of survival by opening up the pulmonary blood flow more quickly.*[13,16] The choice of agents now includes streptokinase, urokinase, and recombinant tissue plasminogen activator (rTPA). Streptokinase is given as 250 000 units over 30 minutes, followed by 100 000 IU/hour over the next 24 hours.[16] Its disadvantage is that it causes allergic reactions, but these are rare. It will also restore patency of the veins and lyse dangerous clot sitting within them.

Thrombolytic therapy is associated with very troublesome bleeding in patients who have had surgery within the previous fortnight, so in cases which are stable enough, after resuscitation, to await the effects of heparin, this is probably the better treatment. Thrombolysis also creates considerable difficulties in patients who are subsequently operated upon, so the choice of whether or not to operate must be made before any decision to use streptokinase. In general, for patients with acute massive pulmonary embolism, who can be supported for a few hours, we would advocate treatment with thrombolytic drugs. Bleeding from venous and arterial puncture sites is to be expected with both treatments.

Surgical treatment—with or without cardiopulmonary bypass

It is clear from the description above that the majority of patients who survive to be diagnosed and have a treatment plan formulated have a reasonably good chance of survival with medical therapy. At the other extreme, if a collapsed patient cannot be restored to a state where the heart can support the circulation rarely will anything be gained by heroic surgery. So, there is a relatively small proportion of patients who are in a state sufficiently parlous to warrant operation. Typically these will be patients who are sustaining a poor and probably deteriorating cardiac output.

The choice of whether to operate with or without bypass is irrelevant for most patients. There are only 40 cardiothoracic units in the whole of the UK and these are not evenly distributed. Surgery on bypass is not an option for most surgeons and patients, and if it is employed it is very likely that these are a group of atypical patients in whom survival was long enough to make referral possible.

Pulmonary embolectomy

The best experience of embolectomy with the use of inflow occlusion is from Clarke and Abrams in Birmingham, UK.[11] For over 25 years they have run what they call a peripatetic embolectomy service. The operation as they (and we) perform it bears little resemblance to that described by Trendelenberg in 1908. The operation is performed through median sternotomy and requires few special instruments. The sternum can be split in a variety of ways. In our own theatre we use an oscillating or reciprocating saw but the most widely available equipment is a Gigli saw.

A special long pair of artery forceps is needed to pass behind the sternum. The pulmonary artery is secured with two stitches and a large side-biting clamp (Satinsky) is tried for size and position. The superior and inferior venae cavae are snared or clamped. The heart continues to beat but the left ventricle, deprived of pulmonary venous return, does not eject. The pulmonary artery is opened via a 2.5 cm longitudinal incision and clot pulled out with Desjardins forceps, helped by the sucker; more peripheral thrombus is forced out by the anaesthetist compressing the lungs. The Satinsky clamp can be applied, the snares released, and the heart allowed to beat for a while. Clarke and Abrams advocate a single period of up to 150 seconds. We prefer to use several much shorter episodes of circulatory arrest which can be achieved by the use of the Satinsky clamp.

The Birmingham series provides data on 65 patients. In seven the diagnosis was wrong (more than 10 per cent—a worrying statistic for those who would contemplate operation without prior angiography) and in another three the operation was performed on bypass. Of the 55 who had an operation for pulmonary embolism without bypass, 31 (56 per cent) survived to leave hospital (70%CL: 48–64%). The report divided the experience into 19 who had already had a cardiac arrest with only 16 per cent hospital survivors (8–30%), and a more favourable group of 36 with 78 per cent hospital survivors (68–86%).

Pulmonary embolectomy on cardiopulmonary bypass

If the patient has a massive pulmonary embolism where cardiac surgery is available, there may be an opportunity to save a life which otherwise would have been lost. Such cases are rewarding but rare. Patients referred in from outside are rarely candidates for this form of surgery because they have already defined themselves as a surviving group, although occasionally a patient is only just surviving with a large demonstrable thrombus and surgery offers the best chance. The Brompton series documents 71 cases of embolectomy on bypass over a 23-year period, 90 per cent by a single surgeon.[14]

Cardiopulmonary bypass was established through median sternotomy in the majority, and during a period of total cardiopulmonary support averaging 27 minutes the embolectomy was performed. Overall 70 per cent survived to leave hospital (70%CL: 64–76%). If the same division is made into those who required cardiac massage there is again a large difference, with only 20 per cent surviving (12–32%) in those who had arrested (25/71) and 89 per cent (82–94%) in the more favourable group.

The mean time to operation was just over five hours in the Birmingham peripatetic service and never more than 24 hours. In the Brompton series 25 per cent of the cases were operated upon more than 24 hours after the initial event.

The experience in the two series has interesting similarities. *The unanswerable question is, would these cases have done as well or better on medical therapy?* The Brompton group have a large experience with thrombolysis and believe that there is a group for whom operation is indicated.[14,15] These are patients in whom thrombolysis is contraindicated and who are dying from removable thrombus in the pulmonary artery, or in whom the haemodynamic state is so poor that the time taken for lysis is too long to wait. Our clinical experience is in line with that view.

5. In which cases should we give long-term anticoagulation and for how long?

Some patients who have survived or have been saved from massive pulmonary embolism by surgery have a further embolism. The residual thrombus in the deep veins remains a risk. This occurred in both the Birmingham and the

Brompton series. Even patients who have had thrombolytic therapy still have the predisposition to form deep vein thrombosis. What should we do to safeguard them?

We treat all of them with heparin initially and then they are maintained on oral anticoagulants for a period. We aim to keep the prothrombin ratio at 2–2.5 for up to three months, depending on the extent to which risk factors persist. A patient who makes a rapid recovery from an otherwise straightforward operation is probably at lower risk than an elderly, plump woman mobilizing slowly after hip surgery.

6. Is there any place for operations to obstruct the inferior vena cava?

The idea of operating to obstruct the venous drainage of the lower part of the body to prevent further episodes of embolization was first suggested by Trousseau in 1868 and, although various procedures to plicate or place filters in the inferior vena cava have been suggested, for the majority of patients the disadvantages far outweigh any theoretical benefit of this approach. With anticoagulation the risk of further embolism is low, probably less than 5 per cent. We would regard this as adequate and preferable to subjecting them to operations to obstruct flow in the inferior vena cava. Furthermore, if the patient has any residual pulmonary artery obstruction, restricting venous return is likely to be detrimental because the right heart relies on the high filling pressure for its output. A removable filter which can be placed transvenously has an appeal and has its proponents.[17]

Some patients who have a DVT or are treated for pulmonary infarction may subsequently have a massive embolism, although we believe that this sequence is in fact rather uncommon. If the former group are initially treated with thrombolytics and both groups are then kept anticoagulated with heparin, the risk is probably very small. We can see no evidence in favour of obstructing the inferior vena cava in these cases. Patients who have persisting recurring pulmonary embolism may be considered for treatment but should be referred for specialist advice.

Has surgery anything to offer in the management of longstanding pulmonary embolic disease?

There is a small minority of patients who suffer recurrent pulmonary emboli which are not lysed but instead become organized. They present with pulmonary hypertension. They may present acutely and be correctly diagnosed as having had a pulmonary embolism, but in the absence of other information it may not be appreciated that the majority of the problem is due to organized thrombus throughout the vascular tree which cannot be removed by embolectomy. Alternatively they may present with chronic disability and the diagnosis of chronic pulmonary hypertension is made.

There is no medical treatment which will reverse this process. There is limited experience with thromboendarterectomy for this condition.[18] Full cardiopulmonary bypass is required. Also, because the condition is associated with considerable collateral flow as a result of the chronically obstructed pulmonary arteries, it can only be performed if the flow is reduced and the pressure kept low. The risk to the central nervous system is reduced by cooling to below 18°C, which permits periods of circulatory arrest to be used. Results in some of the patients have been impressively good.

References

1. Wilson A.P.R., Gruneberg R.N., Treasure T., Sturridge M.F. Staphylococcus epidermidis as a cause of postoperative wound infection after cardiac surgery: assessment of pathogenicity by a wound-scoring method. *Brit. J. Surg.* 1988; **75:** 168–70.
2. Smith P.L.C., Treasure T., Newman S.P., Joseph P.L.A., Ell P.J., Schneidau A., Harrison M.J.G. The cerebral consequences of cardiopulmonary bypass. *Lancet*, 1968; **i:** 823–5.
3. Collins R., Scrimgeour A., Yusuf S., Peto R. Reduction in fatal pulmonary embolism and venous thrombosis by perioperative administration of subcutaneous heparin. *N. Engl. J. Med.* 1988; **318:** 1162–73.
4. Wilson A.P.R., Treasure T., Sturridge M.F., Gruneberg R.N. A scoring method (ASEPSIS) for postoperative wound infections for use in clinical trials of prophylaxis. *Lancet*, 1986; **1:** 311–12.
5. Kakkar V.V. Prevention of venous thromboembolism. *Clin. Haematol.* 1981; **10:** 543–82.
6. Sandler D.A., Martin J.F. Autopsy proven pulmonary embolism in hospital patients: are we detecting enough deep vein thrombosis? *J. R. Soc. Med.* 1989; **82:** 203–5.
7. Prevention of fatal postoperative pulmonary embolism by low doses of heparin: an International Multicentre Trial. *Lancet*, 1975; **ii:** 45–51.
8. Bailar J.C., Mosteller F. *Medical Uses of Statistics*. Waltham, Mass.: NEJM Books, 1986.
9. Cruickshank J.M., Gorlin R., Jennett B. Air travel and thrombotic episodes: the economy class syndrome. *Lancet*, 1988; **ii:** 497–8.
10. D'Alonzo G.E. Deep venous thrombosis and pulmonary embolism. In: Dantzker D.R. (ed.): *Cardiopulmonary Critical Care*. New York: Grune and Stratton.
11. Gray H.H., Morgan J.M., Paneth M., Miller G.A.H. Pulmonary embolectomy: indications and results. *Brit. Heart J.* 1987; **57:** 572.
12. Clarke D.B., Abrams L.D. Pulmonary embolectomy: a 25-year experience. *J. Thoracic Cardiovasc. Surg.* 1986; **92:** 442–5.
13. Surgery for pulmonary emboli. *Lancet* (editorial). 1989; **i:** 198.
14. Gray H.H., Morgan J.M., Paneth M., Miller G.A.H. Pulmonary embolectomy for acute massive pulmonary embolism: an analysis of 71 cases. *Brit. Heart J.* 1988; **60:** 196–200.
15. Gray H.H., Paneth M., Miller G.A.H. Pulmonary embolectomy: its place in the management of pulmonary embolism. *Lancet*, 1988; **i:** 1441–5.
16. Dieck J.A., Ferguson J.J. Indications for thrombolytic therapy in acute pulmonary embolism. *Texas Heart Inst. J.* 1989; **16:** 19–26.
17. Janssen E.W., Janssen J., Cheriex E.C., Penn O.C. Use of a removable vena cava filter for prevention of recurrent embolism after emergency pulmonary embolectomy. *Texas Heart Inst. J.* 1989; **16:** 15–17.
18. Daily P.O., Johnston G.G., Simmons C.J., Moser K.M. Surgical management of chronic pulmonary embolism. *J. Thoracic Cardiovasc. Surg.* 1980; **79:** 523–31.

5

Facial fractures

Martin Mace, MBBS, BDS, FDS, RCS, MRCS, LRCP

The young casualty officer, during his surgical training, is often required to carry out the initial assessment of the facially injured patient, sometimes in units where specialist backup is not immediately available. The importance of an understanding of the facial skeleton and its involvement in trauma cannot be over-stressed. The facial bones surround the threshold of the respiratory tract and the organs of sight and smell. Severely displaced facial fractures threaten the patency of the airway and thus the survival of the patient.

Applied anatomy of trauma

The skull is usually considered to be subdivided into three: upper, middle and lower. The upper third is the cranium; suspended from the base of the cranium is the middle third; and articulating with the temporal bone is the lower third, the mandible.

The *middle third* comprises 18 different bones arranged as a honeycombed structure constituting air-filled passages and cavities forming a supportive framework for the ocular apparatus and the nasopharyngeal tract. It provides the bony attachment for the upper teeth. It is remarkably rigid, with the main weight-bearing structures resisting the forces of mastication directed vertically. Forces directed from a frontal or lateral direction can more easily disrupt the delicate framework.

The middle third joins the inclined plane of the base of the skull of the middle and anterior cranial fossae, formed by the frontal bone and body of the sphenoid, at about 45° to the horizontal. Trauma applied anteriorly, sufficient to disrupt this attachment from the skull base, will force the middle third backwards and downwards, gagging the dental occlusion and opening the mandible (Fig. 5.1). This movement includes the soft tissues, notably the soft palate, and the nasopharynx may be obliterated with the oropharynx significantly diminished in size. Associated mandibular fractures, where the tongue support is compromised, may result in near total occlusion of the upper respiratory tract. This is, of course, compounded if there is an associated head injury with partial or total loss of consciousness.

With high-level middle-third fractures the cribriform plate of the ethmoid may be involved, often causing a tear of the dura and a leak of cerebrospinal fluid, usually seen as a persistent rhinorrhoea.

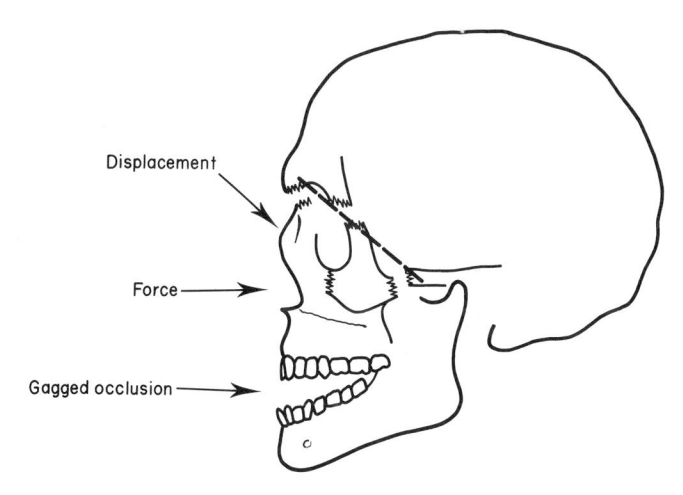

Fig. 5.1 Downward and backward displacement of the maxilla, causing nasopharayngeal obstruction and opening the mandible.

The peripheral trigeminal branches, the infraorbital and zygomatic nerves, may be crushed, giving disturbances in sensation over the facial skin in the upper lip, cheek and side of nose. The delicate structures passing through the orbital fissures, in particular the sixth cranial nerve, can also be disrupted. The superior orbital fissure syndrome—consisting of pupillary dilatation, paraesthesia of the area supplied by the ophthalmic division of the trigeminal nerve, and ophthalmoplegia—may result rarely from severe middle-third damage.

Damage to major blood vessels from a middle-third injury is unusual, despite the proximity of the maxillary artery to the posterior maxilla. Nevertheless, in displaced maxillary fractures this artery may be lacerated, causing serious nasopharyngeal haemorrhage. Facial lacerations can involve the major facial veins and artery.

The mandible constitutes the *lower third* of the facial structure occupying a prominent and exposed position. It articulates with the cranium via the condyles and glenoid fossae of the temporal bones. A large proportion of the force of a blow to the mandible could thus be transmitted to the middle cranial fossa, unless it is absorbed by the common fracture of the thin condylar neck. The horizontal rami of the mandible form a horseshoe shape, with the vertical rami passing upwards and slightly backwards and outwards to the temporomandibular joints.

The mandible, unlike that of the bones of the middle third, has a thick outer cortex and a central portion of cancellous bone and is a much more rigid structure.

The various muscle attachments to the mandible may cause displacement owing to spasm. Thus the temporalis and masseter muscles will tend to cause a forward and upward displacement of the vertical ramus when an angular fracture exists. The genial musculature will tend to rotate the mandible like a bucket handle with bilateral fractures of the body. The lateral pterygoids will tend to displace the fractured condyle forwards and medially. However, the mandible exists within a tight periosteal sheath, which will grant a certain stability except in a widely displaced compound fracture.

The inferior dental artery, veins and nerve pass through the length of the mandible from the lingula on the medial side of the vertical ramus to the mental foramen, supplying the mandibular and alveolar bone and the teeth. The mental branches form the entire sensory supply to the lower lip, with a less important vascular element. Damage to the nerve at the fracture leads to total or partial loss of sensation in the lower lip and corresponding teeth and alveolar mucosa.

Classification of fractures

The middle-third fractures involve, as described above, many different small bones; and, with the likelihood of comminution, a comprehensive classification is impossible. A French anatomist, René Le Fort, showed an interest in the patterns of facial bone fractures and in 1901 published a paper based on experimental trauma to cadavers followed by careful removal of the soft tissues.[1] He suggested a broad classification which is still in wide use today (Fig. 5.2). In using this it should be remembered that these fractures often occur together and may be unilateral or bilateral. A knowledge of the outline of these fractures is, however, most useful in understanding the midface structure, and subsequently in treatment planning.

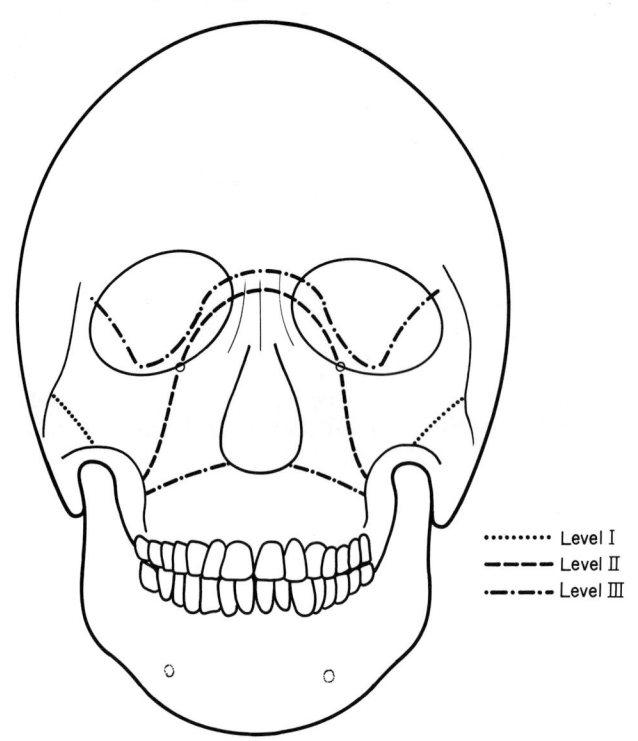

·········· Level I
 Level II
··· Level III

Fig. 5.2 The Le Fort lines of fracture.

The *Le Fort I* or low-level fracture of the middle third is where the entire tooth-bearing part of the true maxilla is separated horizontally from its attachments above the nasal floor. The fracture lines pass laterally across the anterior walls of the maxillary antra, continuing beneath the zygomatic buttress and posteriorly through the pterygoid plates. The fracture lines also pass through the lateral nasal walls and lower part of the nasal septum.

The *Le Fort II*, or pyramidal fracture, separates the central middle third, shaped from in front like a pyramid, from the base of the skull and the lateral middle third of the facial skeleton. The fracture lines pass high through the nasal septum, often involving the anterior cranial fossa centrally. Laterally they pass through the orbit across the medial walls towards the infraorbital margins, in the region of the infraorbital foraminae. They then pass down across the anterior walls of the maxillary antra towards the maxillary tuberosities, fracturing the pterygoid plates.

The *Le Fort III*, or high transverse fracture, separates the whole middle-third of the facial skeleton from the cranial base. The fracture lines run from the frontonasal fissure, involving the cribriform plate and ethmoids, posteriorly and inferiorly towards the optic foramen, reaching the posterior part of the inferior orbital fissure. The lines divide into the higher, which passes laterally across the orbital wall to the zygomatico-frontal suture, and the lower, passing downwards and posteriorly across the pterygomaxillary fissure, separating the pterygoid plates high at their attachments to the base of the skull.

To complete the classification of middle-third fractures, those involving the *zygomatic complex*, the *nasal complex* and *dentoalveolar* fractures need to be added (Fig. 5.3).

Mandibular fractures are easier to understand with a less complex osteology (Fig. 5.4). Lines of weakness exist in the mandible and largely determine the sites of indirect fracture. A blow insufficient to cause a fracture at the site of

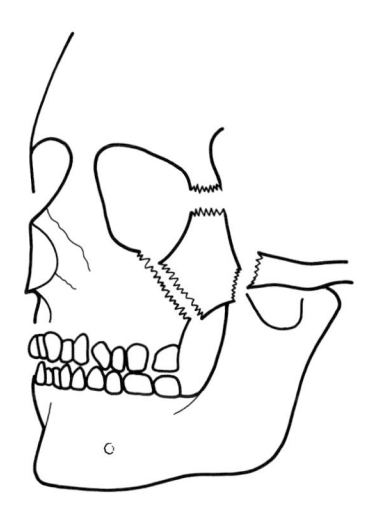

Fig. 5.3 The classical lines of fracture of the zygomatic complex.

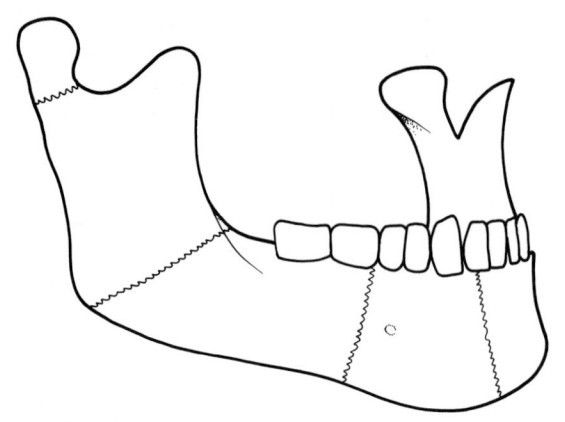

Fig. 5.4 Common sites of fracture of the mandible: the condylar neck, angle, body and parasymphyseal sites are marked.

trauma may lead to a 'contre-coup' fracture. Thus, the simple fracture of the condylar neck opposite the site of trauma is the commonest unilateral fracture. Bilateral condylar neck fractures are also seen with the point of trauma on the chin. Equally, a fracture of the angle or the horizontal body of the mandible, that part between the angle and the region of the canine tooth, may be accompanied by a fracture of the opposite condylar neck or angle. Fractures of the parasymphysis, which is the area between the canine teeth, may accompany fractures of the body, angle or condylar neck. Rarely the coronoid process is fractured.

Early management of facial fractures

The most important procedure in the management of a patient with a facial fracture is to ensure an *adequate airway*, particularly as many patients may have an associated head injury. This may involve anything from clearing debris from the mouth to the performance of a tracheostomy.

Initially a careful examination of the oral cavity and pharynx should be made, with removal of foreign bodies such as glass and fractured dentures, broken or grossly displaced teeth. This is best carried out with the help of a wide-bore blunt suction end and a good light held by an assistant. At this stage, particularly with unconscious patients, an *oral airway* may be useful if tolerated; but when the airway is at risk the passing of an *endotracheal tube* is more satisfactory. This, even in the most competent hands, can be extremely difficult in the acute situation with active bleeding and unstable jaws, in which case a *tracheostomy* is preferred.

In the majority of cases, even in unconscious patients, oral and pharyngeal toilet will be adequate, together with careful positioning of the head and neck, to maintain a good airway. The conscious patient sitting up with the face held forwards and bolstered will breathe comfortably. The semi- or unconscious patient may be better managed lying on the side with the neck extended.

In all cases supervision of the airway is essential in the early stages, and frequent aspiration is likely to be necessary.

Severe *haemorrhage*, as stated earlier, is not a common occurrence in facial fractures, particularly when there are no associated facial lacerations. The rare but alarming haemorrhage is that from the maxillary artery into the nasopharynx. It is seldom possible to visualize the site, and a post-nasal pack may be necessary to control the bleeding.

With most middle-third fractures the delicate soft tissue lining of the nose and paranasal sinuses is lacerated and a continuing *epistaxis* will be apparent, perpetuated by movement of the fractures. The airspace is gradually filled with clotted blood and a serous trickle only may follow. This should be distinguished from *cerebrospinal fluid rhinorrhoea*. It is wise, therefore, at an early stage, to know the haemoglobin concentration and to ascertain the patient's blood group. With the more severe injuries an intravenous line should always be established. Mandibular fractures rarely cause significant haemorrhage.

Thus, shock with peripheral vasoconstriction and hypovolaemia is unusual with the facially injured patient, and if it occurs it may indicate the presence of other injuries. The emotional concentration given quite naturally to severe facial injuries can be responsible for late diagnosis of other injuries.

Once a *stable airway* and *control of haemorrhage* are established, a full general examination is possible. Many patients with a severe maxillofacial injury will have sustained a head injury, with impairment of consciousness. An assessment of neurological function can be made on a simple scale such as that described by Teasdale and Jennett.[2] Additionally a brief ophthalmic examination should be made, noting pupillary size, equivalence and reaction to light neurologically, and any global injury.

The general examination should pay special attention to the cervical spine, abdomen and thorax for closed injuries. Violent deceleration injuries to the face, such as in a road traffic accident, may lead to cervical vertebral fracture or dislocation. These, in turn, may have already caused spinal cord compression, or may allow this to happen with injudicious cervical movements by the examiner.

The limbs may be traumatized and should be carefully examined for signs of fracture and consequent closed haemorrhage and neurological damage.

From this general examination a list of *priorities for treatment* can be drawn up. *It is common for the definitive reduction and fixation of facial fractures to be low on this list*, as they are not life-threatening once the airway is established. There is everything to gain in allowing the maxillofacially injured patient a period of stabilization following the trauma. In particular, the severity of any associated head injury can be established and its progression or regression monitored without the dangerous alterations of signs when a general anaesthetic is administered.

The closure of facial lacerations can often be carried out with local analgesia. This is a priority as the oedema that will develop over the subsequent 12 hours will make accurate closure more difficult.

If, for any reason, a general anaesthetic is administered, the opportunity for careful digital examination of the fractured facial bones and teeth cannot be missed. Impressions of the dentition can also be taken more easily under anaesthesia, for the construction of maxillofacial splints.

The diagnosis of facial fractures

A thorough examination of the facial bones and a detailed assessment of the presenting fractures is made. This must always include both *extra- and intra-oral examination*, and for those unfamiliar with the mouth some guidelines are laid down. The examiner should have available a strong light and a dental mirror or a series of wooden spatulae.

The observer will benefit by standing behind the head of the patient during the examination of the middle third, using thumbs and forefingers of both hands to palpate the bony outlines, while observing asymmetry. The bony outlines followed should commence with the zygomatic arches, from the zygomatic processes of the temporal bones, passing forwards to the lateral orbital and supraorbital margins. Deformity, asymmetry and in particular step defects can be noted. The palpation will then involve the lateral and infraorbital margins.

The commonest middle-third fracture is that of the *zygomatic complex*, which is characterized by a depression and loss of prominence of the 'cheekbone'. The zygomatic complex is classically fractured at or near the zygomatico-temporal, -frontal and -maxillary suture lines. Depending on the severity of displacement, one or all of these sites will exhibit a step. The degree of oedema and circumorbital ecchymosis may vary and will develop over the first 24 hours. An early reliable sign, not to be missed, is the development of a subconjunctival ecchymosis to the lateral of the affected eye, which appears to have no posterior limit. This is due to bleeding from the fracture of the lateral orbital wall tracking beneath the conjunctiva, and is unlike that of the localized conjunctival haemorrhage observed in the ordinary 'black eye'. This fracture is normally accompanied by ipsilateral infraorbital paraesthesia. There will usually be antral haemorrhage, presenting as an epistaxis on the affected side as the fracture involves the roof and lateral wall of the maxillary antrum. Intraorally there will be a submucosal ecchymosis apparent in the upper buccal sulcus above the teeth.

The isolated *zygomatic arch fracture* has none of the above features, presenting with a depression over the arch and a degree of trismus owing to the fractured arch impinging on the coronoid process of the mandible.

When step defects are encountered bilaterally in the infraorbital and/or the lateral orbital margins, it is likely that a *Le Fort II or III fracture* may exist. Classically, the Le Fort III fracture will have step defects at both zygomatico-temporal and zygomatico-frontal sutures, the Le Fort II at both zygomatico-maxillary sutures. They will develop bilateral circumorbital and subconjunctival ecchymosis and later an oedematous balloon face. It should be remembered that these fractures may not occur in their classical form and combinations will be seen.

The *nasal bones* are palpated for mobility, asymmetry and flattening. A fractured nose always results in epistaxis. In severe trauma the ethmoids and floor of the anterior cranial fossa may also be involved, with resulting *cerebrospinal fluid rhinorrhoea*. Similarly, Le Fort II and III fractures will lead to a cerebrospinal fluid leak. The identification of cerebrospinal fluid is complicated when bleeding, lacrimal secretions and nasal mucus are combined, dribbling from the nostrils. The simple test for the presence of glucose is not applicable as, although nasal mucus is free from glucose, lacrimal secretions are not, and in the first few days after injury it may be impossible to identify a positive cerebrospinal fluid leak, apart from the clinical observation of a persistent thin nasal discharge.

Intraorally the examiner should look for submucosal ecchymosis in the upper buccal sulci and for loose and broken teeth. Mobility of a group of teeth, commonly the incisors, reveals a dentoalveolar fracture. Rarely a midline split may be noted in the hard palate and mobility detected across the split.

The *occlusion* in the dentate patient may be disrupted by displacement of any of the Le Fort fractures. This displacement usually has a posterior component and, as mentioned above, leads to the maxillary molars gagging the occlusion open. Minor occlusal discrepancies are assessed by the specialist practitioner.

If there is uncertainty about the presence of a Le Fort fracture, the maxilla may be grasped with thumb and forefinger of the right hand, intraorally, around the stable teeth or alveolus and gently moved in an anteroposterior direction whilst spreading the palm of the left hand over the forehead, with the thumb and forefinger over the nasal bones to stabilize the upper-third. Mobility can be detected by this method unless there is severe impaction of the maxilla, but it is uncomfortable and usually avoidable.

With the higher-level and lateral middle-third fractures there is damage to the bony orbit, which may lead to global involvement or disruption to the origins of the ocular musculature. An early ophthalmological assessment is recommended if global damage is suspected, and, although eye movements are difficult to examine in the early stages, a record should be made of visual acuity, diplopia, pupillary action and level and degrees of enophthalmos and exophthalmos. The possibility of retrobulbar haemorrhage is strong, and, if any doubt exists, the eyes should be examined regularly in the post-traumatic and post-reduction period, as this complication can lead to compression of the posterior ciliary arteries with consequent blindness.[3]

The level of the globe of the eye is maintained by Lockwood's suspensory ligament passing from the lacrimal bone to Whitnall's tubercle on the orbital face of the zygomatic bone beneath the zygomatico-frontal suture. This tubercle may be lowered by the fracture and hence the pupillary level drops. When there is disruption of the orbital floor, as in an isolated *orbital floor fracture*, or a comminuted zygomatic fracture, the bony origin of the inferior oblique muscle may be displaced and the bulk of the inferior rectus muscle may, together with orbital fat, fall into the maxillary antrum, giving enophthalmos and diplopia.

Continuing the extraoral palpation, the angles and lower borders of the mandible should be felt for step defects. Local contusion and swelling, with accompanying pain, may lead to the clinical diagnosis of fracture. Mandibular opening and lateral movements may be restricted.

Intraorally the buccal and lingual sulci can be examined for ecchymosis present near a fracture site. The occlusal planes may show a step and the occlusion should be checked for abnormality. An assessment of displacing muscle pull on the fracture can be made clinically at this stage.

Fractures of the horizontal ramus, behind the mental foramen, may cause paraesthesia of the ipsilateral lower lip since the inferior alveolar nerve passes through the body of the mandible; and so manipulating a body fracture results in considerable pain.

60 *Facial fractures*

Radiographic examination

Radiographic examination should follow the clinical assessment of the facial injuries. In the early stages after injury it may not be in the patient's interests to have a prolonged session in the radiology department, where often large numbers of inappropriate films may be taken.

When facial fractures are suspected it is important that views at different angles are taken, so that the degree and direction of displacement of the skeletal components can be estimated. It is suggested that the following are taken as standard views:

1. 10° and 30° *occipitomental views*. These will show the degree of downward and backward displacement of the central and lateral middle-third. Fig. 5.5 shows a typical 15° view.

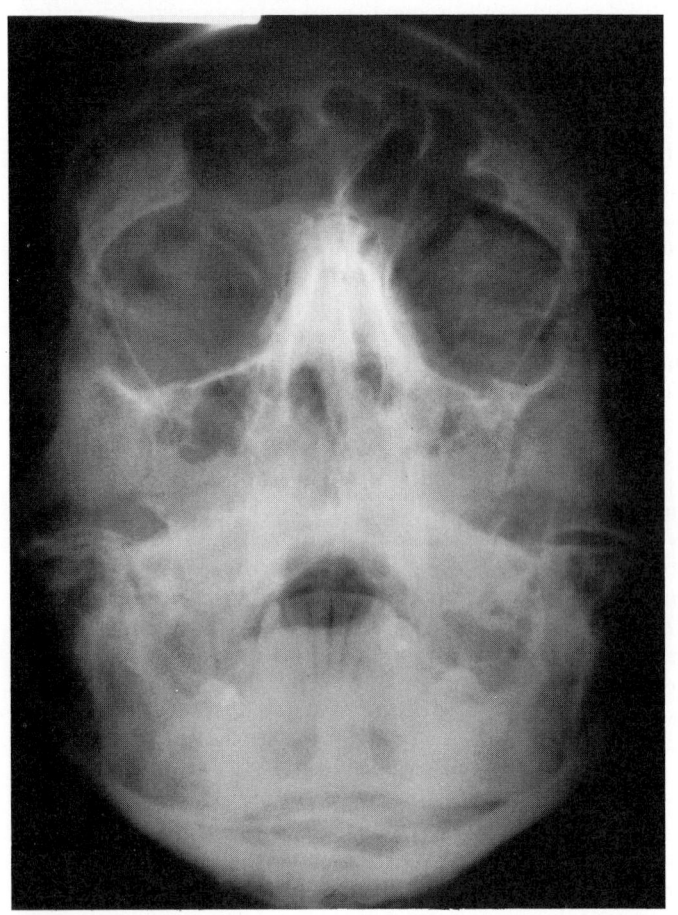

Fig. 5.5 A 15° occipitomental radiograph showing a Le Fort II fracture with a left Le Fort III fracture. Note that both maxillary antra are radio-opaque, filled with blood. The fracture lines cross both infraorbital margins with a large step on the left side. On the left a fracture line crossing the lateral orbital wall to the widened fronto-zygomatic suture can be seen.

2. *True lateral skull*, including the cervical spine. This will show the downward and backward displacement of the midface in central middle-third fractures. It will also be useful for diagnosing cervical spine and skull vault fractures and show vertical displacement of mandibular body fractures.
3. *Oblique lateral views of the mandibular rami*. These will reveal fractures in the vertical rami, the subcondylar regions and part of the horizontal rami.
4. *Posteroanterior of the mandible*. This shows fractures of the parasymphyseal region and the lateral displacement of fractures of the vertical and horizontal rami.
5. *Intraoral views*. In particular the upper standard occlusal of the maxilla if a split palate is suspected.

Other views may be necessary, as indicated, for mandibular condylar fractures and orbital floor fractures. These can be delayed until the general condition of the patient allows.

The roles of computerized tomography and nuclear magnetic resonance scanning in facial fractures are still being evaluated, but the results, particularly with the latter, are most encouraging.

Treatment guidelines

The early treatment as outlined above is directed towards *control of the airway and cessation of haemorrhage*.

Severe *pain* is not a feature of maxillofacial injuries, fortunately, as the administration of opiates would compound the respiratory difficulties suffered by the severely injured patient and mask any developing signs of head injury. Usually only *minor analgesics* and sedatives are necessary. *Local oral toilet*, removing crusting clots with suction where swallowing is painful, and *support of very mobile fractures* with circumdental wires will help maintain comfort.

The majority of fractures involving the facial bones are *compound*, involving an epithelial surface. This may be in the nasal passages, paranasal sinuses or the mucosa of the mouth. The facial skin may be involved where a laceration exists over a fracture. *Early administration of antibiotics*, preferably initially by intramuscular or intravenous routes, is necessary. Benzyl penicillin is administered initially for fractures of the mandible alone. If there is skin involvement or with middle-third fractures, a broader-spectrum antibiotic such as amoxycillin is chosen. Later, when the patient is able to take a soft diet, antibiotics can be given orally. Administration should continue for five days after the fractures have been stabilized.

The special cases where disruption of the dura is suspected should receive *prophylaxis against meningeal infection*. The regimen of sulphonamides has been largely superseded by combinations of ampicillin and flucloxacillin intravenously; this regimen should continue for one week after the definitive immobilization of the fracture or the cessation of overt cerebrospinal fluid rhinorrhoea.

The definitive treatment of fractures of the facial skeleton has two aims: *the restoration of normal bony facial contours*, as well as *the restoration of function*, allowing the jaws to move fully in articulation and mastication, and the eyes to move normally within the orbits. Reduction of the displaced zygoma may have no functional necessity, purely a cosmetic one, but the patient who has lost his cheekbone prominence is most unhappy and could rightly seek compensation if the diagnosis is missed.

Reduction, immobilization and rehabilitation form the baselines for treatment of a fractured bone, and this is precisely the same with facial fractures. In most cases the occlusion of the teeth is a useful guide to the successful reduction, and *intermaxillary fixation* is almost exclusively used, combined with other forms of immobilization. This fixation further threatens the airway and complicates oral feeding. Thus it is essential with the more severe facial fractures to leave a *nasopharyngeal airway* in position for the first postoperative 24 hours and to institute nasogastric or intravenous feeding.

The *principles of reduction* of the middle-third fracture are complicated as the complexity of the fractures means that the separated fragment is unlikely to exist as a single block. Re-establishing the occlusion in a Le Fort II and III fracture will correct the mandibulomaxillary relationship, and only eventual estimation will satisfactorily reduce the higher components of the middle-third fracture.

General endotracheal anaesthesia is necessary in most cases. Nasal intubation or tracheostomy allows the occlusion to be established, and the nasotracheal tube can be left as a nasopharyngeal tube at the end of the procedure.

The isolated *zygomatic complex fracture* or zygomatic arch fracture may be elevated indirectly by the elegant *Gillies' temporal approach*, which relies on the potential space beneath the temporal fascia which attaches to the zygomatic arch and the temporalis muscle, which passes to the coronoid process of the mandible.[4] An elevator is passed through a temporal incision which includes the temporal fascia, downwards, under the zygoma. Taking care not to compress the temporal bone, the zygoma can be lifted laterally.

A *bone hook* can be passed through a stab incision in the cheek and directed under the body of the zygoma to elevate it. This method gives a direct and more positive reduction.[5]

The re-establishment of normal contour and elimination of step defects are a guide to a correct reduction. If comminution has occurred or treatment is delayed, the reduced fracture may be unstable and direct or indirect fixation is necessary.

Transosseous wiring through incisions at the fronto-zygomatic fracture site and/or the infraorbital rim may be necessary. Alternatively, and occasionally in addition, *packing the maxillary sinus* with one-inch ribbon gauze impregnated with Whitehead's varnish, via a Caldwell Luc approach, may give better stabilization. Transosseous wires are commonly left in place. An antral pack should be removed after six weeks unless mobility is still apparent, as late contracture can occur with loss of prominence in the unstable zygomatic fracture.

Isolated *orbital floor fractures* can be treated using an antral pack often placed after lifting the orbital contents via an infraorbital incision. Alternatively, a silastic sheet can be inserted to cover the defect and support the orbital contents.

The *central middle third*, including the tooth-bearing part of the maxilla, can be reduced using disimpaction forceps, which grasp the maxillae with a blade in the nasal floor and the opposing blade in the mouth on the hard palate. These forceps (right and left) are used together to pull the maxilla into a reduced position. With a Le Fort I fracture this is the only reduction necessary, but as indicated the higher fractures will need additional reduction, using nasal septal forceps and digital pressure from behind the soft palate to pull the central block forwards.

The *Le Fort III fracture* involves fractures of the lateral middle-third as well, and the principles of reduction are to commence laterally, working centrally, finally reducing any nasoethmoidal component.

As discussed above, the more severe middle-third fracture is likely to be a combination of fractures involving partial disruption at all three Le Fort levels and the lateral middle-thirds. When planning the reduction and fixation, allowance must be made for this, and it is therefore not possible to give textbook rules for each fracture, only guidelines for treatment.

Similar constraints apply to fixation and only broad principles will be discussed. The importance of sandwiching fractured components of the central middle-third between the stable parts of the facial skeleton forms the basis of fixation and, using this principle, it is often not necessary to use direct methods of fixation.

Extraoral fixation can be carried out using osseous pins screwed into the supraorbital ridges, fixed by a system of rods and universal joints to a projection bar from an upper silver cap splint, constructed from an impression of the teeth by a maxillofacial technician. This holds the maxilla firmly to the cranium. To increase rigidity and to maintain correct occlusion, it is necessary to add mandibular pins and construct a box frame of rods (Fig. 5.6). The halo frame is an alternative method of fixation. This is secured directly to the skull by screwpins, which perforate the scalp and contact the outer cortical plate. A similar series of rods and joints can be used to form a framework of rigid support.

Internal suspension wires can be used for the fixation of more minor fractures of the middle-third. Circumzygomatic wires around the zygomatic arches are attached to the maxillary teeth or a cap splint. Frontomaxillary wires are passed through a hole drilled in the supraorbital ridges via an eyebrow incision if the zygomas are unstable. These wires pass beneath the zygoma to the maxillary cap splints.

The principles of mandibular fracture, reduction and fixation, follow similar lines. Again, the importance of the occlusion as a guide to correct reduction is stressed. Individual muscle pull will tend to displace mandibular fractures and direct *transosseous wiring or plating* may be necessary, to counteract this. Intermaxillary fixation, using eyelet wiring, arch bars, *cap splints or Gunning's splints* for the edentulous will achieve rigidity. Single fractures of the condylar neck may only need symptomatic treatment, and it is seldom necessary to carry out direct fixation of such a fracture.

With all facial fractures postoperative care of the airway is essential, and *wires or pins that form the intermaxillary fixation need to be clearly marked for easy release in an airways emergency.*

A *liquid* or *semi-solid diet* can be taken using a wide-bore straw or feeding cup, but this is laborious and frequent feeds are thus necessary. Supplements of vitamin C and iron may be added.

Oral hygiene can be difficult with fixation in place, and if possible all patients

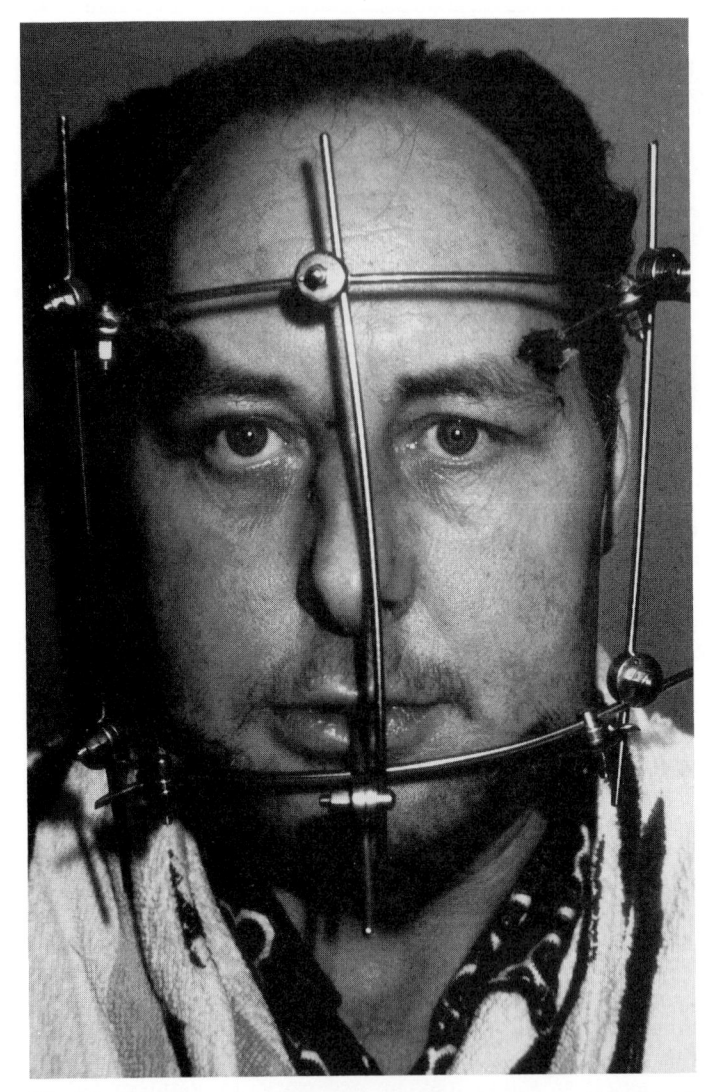

Fig. 5.6 A box frame in place 10 days following a high-level middle-third fracture. Note the supraorbital and mandibular osseous pins and the anterior projection bar attached intraorally to a maxillary dental cap splint.

should have specialist advice and assistance with this problem.

Rigid intermaxillary fixation needs to be maintained for three weeks in all cases to achieve bony union. This period will be increased by severe comminution and delay in initial treatment, but it is seldom necessary to maintain fixation for more than five weeks. Indeed, it may be counter-productive, as earlier introduction of moderate function will often lead to a more satisfactory union.

Late complications

Correct surgical management of the acute injury should lead to satisfactory restoration of appearance and function. Late complications are rare, but they include residual ophthalmic problems with neurological damage affecting movement, or mechanical disturbance due to deformity of the orbit. Other neurological complications, due to crush injuries, may lead to permanent facial anaesthesia or paraesthesia. Residual bony deformity is still seen, especially with the more severe middle-third fractures, and can be treated only with great difficulty by osteotomy and autogenous bone grafting, or using alloplastic onlay materials.

Conclusions

Facial fractures are complicated and challenging injuries from the initial care and diagnosis to the subsequent treatment and follow-up. They provide many problems for the initial care team, which continue with the specialist maxillofacial surgeon, and a knowledge of the principles of management is essential for any prospective surgeon.

References

1. (Le Fort R.), Tessier P. The classic reprint: experimental study of fractures of the upper jaw: 3. *Plast. Reconstr. Surg.* 1972; **50:** 600–7.
2. Teasdale G., Jennett B. Assessment of coma and impaired consciousness: a practical scale. *Lancet.* 1974; **2:** 81–4.
3. Ord R.A. Postoperative retrobulbar haemorrhage and blindness complicating trauma surgery. *Brit. J. Oral Surg.* 1981; **19:** 202–7.
4. Gillies H.D., Kilner T.P., Stone D. Fractures of the malar–zygomatic compound; with a description of a new x-ray position. *Brit. J. Surg.* 1927; **14:** 651–6.
5. Poswillo D. Reduction of the fractured malar by a traction hook. *Brit. J. Oral Surg.* 1976; **14:** 76–9.

Further reading

Rowe N.L., Williams J. *Maxillo-facial Injuries.* 2 vols. Edinburgh: Churchill Livingstone, 1985.
Banks P. *Killey's Fractures of the Middle Third of the Facial Skeleton.* 4th edn. London: John Wright, 1987.
Banks P. *Killey's Fractures of the Mandible.* 3rd edn. London: John Wright, 1983.

6

Cancer of the oral cavity: cheek, tongue and alveolar margins

Ashok R. Mehta, MS, FICS, and Samir A. Mehta, MS

The term 'oral cavity' refers to the lips, the mucosal lining of the cheeks, the floor of the mouth, the anterior two-thirds of the tongue, the upper and lower gingivae (gums) and the hard palate.

Cancers of the tongue, cheek and upper and lower alveolar margins present a unique set of problems because these sites are in continuity with the oropharynx. They constitute the beginning of the upper aerodigestive tract, and so important functions like mastication, swallowing, speech and respiration can be severely impaired by the development of a cancer or its treatment. Of all oral cancers at the Tata Memorial Hospital, cancers of the buccal mucosa account for 38 per cent, of the anterior tongue for 16 per cent, and of the lower alveolus for 15.7 per cent.[1]

The aim of treatment is, of course, to cure the maximum number of patients possible and to preserve or to restore their functions to near normal. Curative treatment of early cancers produces minimal cosmetic or functional deficits. There have been significant advances in recent years in reconstruction and rehabilitation following major resections for advanced cancers. Thirty per cent of our patients treated with an intent to cure are lost to follow-up, and nearly 80 per cent of all advanced cancers are likewise missing from the records. The latter group have in all probability succumbed to their disease.

Geographic pathology and mechanism

In India, head and neck cancers account for 30–40 per cent of cancers at all sites, compared with 5 per cent or less in the USA. Age-standardized incidence rates of oral cancer are given in Table 6.1.

A distinct predilection for cancer to arise in the buccal mucosa, tongue and alveolus, in tobacco chewers, reflects the widespread habit in our population whereby the tobacco is usually retained in the oral cavity for some time. Oral cancer accounts for about 10 per cent of all head and neck cancers (Table 6.2). In the West, alcohol and tobacco are together the main aetiological factors for oral cancers.

Nicotine and nor-nicotine are precursors of carcinogenic nitrosamines (NA). Tobacco also contains nitrates which are converted to nitrites by the enzyme nitrate reductase, present in the normal bacterial flora of the mouth. Thus when

Table 6.1 A selection of international age-standardized incidence rates (Extracted from *Cancer Incidence in Five Continents*, Vol. IV. Lyon: IARC, 1982)[2]

	Tongue Male	Female	Mouth Male	Female
India (Bombay)	10.2	4.1	5.8	5.8
UK (Birmingham)	0.8	0.5	1.4	0.6
USA (Connecticut)	3.3	1.0	4.9	1.6
GDR	0.7	0.2	0.9	0.3
South Australia	1.6	0.8	1.6	0.4

Table 6.2 Experience of head and neck cancers at Tata Memorial Hospital during 1985, showing the large number of oral cancers treated

Site	Number	Site	Number
Oral cavity	1128 (9.4%)	Nasopharynx	71 (0.6%)
Anterior tongue	264 (2.2%)	Larynx	441 (3.7%)
Lower alveolus	177 (1.5%)	Hypopharynx	743 (6.2%)
Upper alveolus	26 (0.2%)	Paranasal sinus	141 (1.2%)
Buccal mucosa	514 (4.3%)	Salivary glands	32 (0.3%)
Oropharynx	881 (7.3%)	Thyroid	125 (1.0%)

Percentage figures relate to *all* cancers (about 12 000 cases).

tobacco is chewed or held in the mouth, nitrites are formed, which then react with nicotine or nor-nicotine yielding NA.

The risk of developing cancer in the buccal mucosa is increased 7.7-fold for betel leaf chewers using tobacco, and three-fold when tobacco is not used.[3]

Premalignant conditions and clinical presentations

Leukoplakia

This term has been used for any white lesion in the oral cavity which cannot be rubbed off. Clinically it ranges from totally innocuous, homogeneous leukoplakia to dangerous speckled leukoplakia presenting as a thick, irregular, infiltrating lesion which may ulcerate. Histologically these lesions display various degrees of hyperkeratosis with or without dysplasia. These changes may progress to a carcinoma-in-situ or even an invasive cancer.[4] Toluidine Blue staining (see below) helps to identify the suspicious area for biopsy.

Homogeneous leukoplakia can be observed at regular follow-up. It is important to identify and eliminate any likely cause of irritation, such as tobacco chewing, smoking or sharp teeth. Speckled leukoplakia is best treated by local excision, by cryotherapy or by laser.

The prevalence of malignancy is 0.2–4 per cent in patients having leukoplakia.

Erythroplakia

Areas of deep reddening and atrophy of the mucosa, often associated with thick leukoplakia, is even more threatening and aggressive than leukoplakia. This condition must be considered premalignant.

Submucous fibrosis

Submucous fibrosis (SMF), an insidious chronic condition affecting the oral cavity, is endemic in Indians. Early symptoms include burning in the mouth, vesicular eruptions, ulceration of the mucosa, and recurrent attacks of stomatitis. Hot food and chillies are not tolerated. Late symptoms include severe fibrosis of the oral mucosa, the uvula, the soft palate, the tongue and the pharynx, resulting in severe trismus. The mucosa appears blanched and atrophic. Fibrotic bands can be felt in the buccal mucosa, coursing in vertical directions. Thirty per cent of oral cancers have associated SMF. Disturbances of speech and mastication occur later. Various forms of treatment such as intralesional corticosteroids, mechanical jaw stretching, excision and skin grafting have been of questionable benefit.[5]

Clinical presentations

A white patch, a non-healing ulcer and/or cervical lymph node enlargement are the usual presenting features of these cancers. The symptoms are negligible in the early stages, except for desquamation or a small ulcer causing mild irritation. Pain develops as the cancer progresses and may radiate to the ear.

Dysphagia, sialorrhoea, foul odour, bleeding, and ankyloglossia develop in later stages. Buccal mucosal cancer may lead to trismus and fungate on the skin of the cheek. Extensive nodal and, infrequently, distant metastases are seen in terminal cases.

Diagnostic procedures

Clinical

Examination of the entire oral cavity and the oropharynx, including mirror examination of the nasopharynx and laryngopharynx, should always be carried out in view of the multicentricity of these lesions. The extent of tumours is often under-estimated. It is far more reliable to palpate the underlying induration in the cheek and tongue than to measure the visible portion of the lesion.

Both sides of the neck are palpated for lymph node enlargement. The false-positive and false-negative rates vary between 15 and 30 per cent. Systemic examination is carried out to exclude metastases, though they occur infrequently and only in the late stages.

Radiology

The presence of mandibular invasion is an important factor affecting selection of treatment in intraoral carcinoma and ranges between 3 and 21 per cent.[6,7]

Clinical examination, conventional x-rays of the mandible and dental occlusal x-rays may demonstrate early involvement. Orthopantomographs are more reliable, although there are high percentages of false-positive and false-negative results. An orthopantomogram provides a panoramic view of the entire mandible and the upper alveolus with blurring out of the overlying soft tissues; it is taken on a single film measuring 4 x 10 inches.

A CT scan is more specific in detecting bone invasion.[8] The scan can also demonstrate occult, normal and abnormal lymph nodes in the neck.

Three-dimensional imaging is a new digital technology which renders a life-like anatomic display of the diagnostic information by interpolating two-dimensional CT scans. Three-dimensional reconstruction of the mandible can be used in planning ablative and reconstructive procedures. A plastic model of the mandible can be generated preoperatively, thereby improving the accuracy of a prosthesis of the resected bone. Also on the horizon is processing of the magnetic resonance imaging (MRI) data on these multidimensional images; this, too, should greatly facilitate three-dimensional reconstruction of the soft tissues.

Biopsy

Histological diagnosis is mandatory prior to undertaking any treatment. The tissue should be handled gently and should not be crushed. It should be placed quickly in the fixative solution (either formal saline or Bouin's fluid).

Toluidine Blue vital staining is used in extensive erythroplakia or leukoplakia to define the margins of the lesion for excision or for targeting the appropriate area for wedge biopsy. A solution (1–2%) is applied to the suspected lesion after the mucosa is gently dried with 1 per cent acetic acid (mucolytic agent). The dye stains the tumour nucleic acid.[9]

In an obvious growth or ulcer, a punch biopsy is obtained in the clinic. This does not require even a local anaesthetic. The preferred site is an edge of the lesion which includes normal mucosa, permitting the histopathologist to visualize the transition zone.

Excisional biopsy removes the entire lesion and is done for small accessible lesions.

Cytology

Cytological screening to facilitate diagnosis of early oral epithelial cancers produces high false-negative results. Its value is therefore restricted. It cannot reliably be used for mass screening, as in cancer of the uterine cervix.

Fine-needle aspiration cytology

Fine-needle aspiration cytology (FNAC) is being extensively used to establish a tissue diagnosis in suspected cervical lymph nodes. We do not advocate surgical biopsy of a lymph node in the neck.

The predictive value of a negative FNAC is low. A negative FNAC, therefore, does not indicate absence of malignant disease and should not lull a surgeon into complacency, which could have disastrous consequences. False-positive diagnoses in competent hands should be almost nil. The sensitivity in our hands is 90 per cent.

Histopathology

A carcinoma-in-situ (CIS) shows overt cytological criteria of malignancy without evidence of invasion across the basement membrane.

This is widely accepted as the preinvasive phase of cancer (stage 0), but whether it is an irreversible or progressive process is still debatable. Whenever CIS is diagnosed, the entire oral cavity must be carefully examined and additional biopsy specimens obtained to detect coexisting early invasive carcinoma or additional foci of CIS requiring prompt treatment.

Of these, 97 per cent are squamous cell carcinomas (SCC) (Table 6.3). They may be exophytic, verrucous (wart-like), infiltrative or ulcerative. The invasive pattern is associated with higher recurrence rates resulting from failure to obtain tumour-free margins at surgery.

SCC are further classified as *well-, moderately and poorly differentiated* (grades 1–4). Well-differentiated carcinomas are less prone to metastasize early and are curable by local excision, if they are treated before they grow to a large size. High-grade SCCs have a higher potential for early lymphatic dissemination.

Verrucous cancers lie somewhere between non-verrucous SCCs and the hyperplasias like leukoplakia. The term 'verrucous hyperplasia' can be very confusing to a clinician. These cancers present diagnostic problems owing to repeated negative biopsies. The entire lesion must be removed and examined microscopically before the presence of a carcinoma can be ruled out. Only 2 per cent of verrucous cancers develop lymph node metastases. Surgical excision is the treatment of choice. They respond poorly to radiation therapy and may result in anaplastic change.[10]

Table 6.3 Malignant tumours of the oral cavity and oropharynx at Tata Memorial Hospital, 1974–78

Subtypes	Numbers
Squamous cell carcinoma	4487 (96.82%)
Undifferentiated carcinoma	58 (1.25%)
Malignant melanoma	7 (0.15%)
Adenocarcinoma (salivary) (cylindroma)	57 (1.22%)
Malignant lymphoma	15 (0.32%)
Sarcoma	11 (0.24%)
	4635 (100.00%)

TNM staging

The TNM system of classification of malignant tumours is based on the anatomical extent of disease as determined clinically. It has three components:

- T : extent of primary tumour
- N : presence or absence and extent of regional lymph node metastases
- M : presence or absence of distant metastases.

The recording of accurate information of the extent of the disease helps in treatment planning, predicting the prognosis, evaluation of the results of treatment and exchange of information. The current TNM staging is given in Tables 6.4 and 6.5.

Table 6.4 TNM staging (UICC, 1988)

T Primary tumour	N Regional lymph nodes	M Distant metastases
Tx Tumour cannot be assessed	Nx Nodes cannot be assessed	Mx Metastasis cannot be assessed
T0 No evidence of primary tumour	N0 No nodal metastasis	M0 No distant metastases
Tis Carcinoma-in-situ (= CIS)	N1 Ipsilateral, single <3 cm	M1 Distant metastases
T1 2 cm or less	N2a Ipsilateral, single 3–6 cm	
T2 2–4 cm	N2b Ipsilateral, multiple <6 cm	
T3 >4 cm	N2c Bilateral, contralateral <6 cm	
T4 >4 cm, with involvement of antrum, pterygoid muscle, base of tongue or skin of cheek	N3 >6 cm	

Notes:
Direct extension of the primary tumour into lymph nodes is classified as lymph node metastasis.
Metastasis in any lymph node other than regional is classified as a distant metastasis.

Table 6.5 Stage grouping for tumours of the oral cavity (UICC, 1988)

Stage I	T1; N0; M0
Stage II	T2; N0; M0
Stage III	T3; N0; M0
	T1, T2 or T3; N1; M0
Stage IV	T4; N0 or N1; M0
	Any T; N2 or N3; M0
	Any T; any N; M1

General principles of treatment

An evaluation of the patient's general cardiopulmonary, hepatic and nutritional functions should be made at the first visit.

The three treatment choices are *radiation therapy*, *surgery*, and a *combination* of surgery with radiation therapy. *Chemotherapy* is used in advanced cancers which are not amenable to the conventional methods, or where they have failed to control the disease. Chemotherapy may also be used to potentiate the radiotherapuetic effect.

The treatment plan depends on the local extent of the disease, the involvement of the regional lymph nodes, the general condition of the patient, the functional and cosmetic disfigurement likely to be caused by surgery, and the psychological make-up of the patient. Multidisciplinary treatment is best suited for stage III and IV cancers. After the initial routine work-up and staging, a team consisting of the surgeon, plastic surgeon, radiation therapist and chemotherapist should assess the patient's treatment plan.

An understanding of patient selection and treatment results for each specific subset of tumours is essential in the search for an optimum treatment strategy. In patients with advanced disease and in those with positive lymph nodes in the neck, surgery is the method of choice to achieve long-term control. Current understanding of the biology of squamous cell cancers has identified numerous variables, and in practice single-modality treatment is fast being replaced by a combination of surgery and radiation therapy. The question of the optimum application of the two modalities has not been satisfactorily answered: surgery and radiation theraphy are complementary to each other, each having specific advantages with early and late consquences.

Surgery

Maintaining adequate surgical margins is the key to curing oral cancers. This can be achieved only by three-dimensional 'monobloc' excision of the primary tumour. Histologically, tumour extends a centimetre or more along the soft tissue planes. It is preferable to achieve at least 1 cm of tumour-free margin in relaxed or unstretched soft tissue. However, in practice one depends on frozen section of cut margins.

A T1 cancer directly on the bone is best treated by surgical removal: with aggressive radiation, ulceration and bone damage may result.

Infiltrative tumours are ideally suited to primary surgery.

T3 and T4 cancers and those with metastatic lymph nodes are generally treated surgically. Surgery has a distinct advantage in achieving long-term survival.

Residual or recurrent cancers following radiation therapy require radical surgery, depending on the anatomical site and extent of the tumour. Radical surgery often results in loss of the mucosal lining, the soft tissues and the mandible and/or maxilla. Small defects are primarily closed. Larger operative defects must be closed primarily using appropriate reconstructive techniques.

Radical neck dissection or one of its modifications is used to control regional nodes.

General surgical considerations

Local transoral excision is preferred only when there is Tis (CIS) or a superficial T1 lesion in an elderly person. The patient must be available for reliable and impeccable follow-up. Small localized cancers must not be treated as a trivial problem.[11]

T1 cancers of the buccal mucosa and tongue can be removed by surgery through the open mouth. Closure can be achieved by direct closure or by a split skin graft.

T1 or early T2 lesions of the upper alveolus can be treated with limited local resection and a split skin graft.

Surgery through the lower cheek flap offers good access for radical surgery.

In the past, it was presumed that lymphatics from intraoral cancer drained through the mandibular periosteum, which resulted in routine sacrifice of the uninvolved mandible. It is now well accepted that periosteal lymphatics are not involved unless there is a direct invasion by the tumour.[7] It is rational to perform *marginal mandibulectomy* (MM) to achieve tumour-free margins, and it is technically made possible by the use of high-speed cutting drills. We do not perform mandibular resection just to facilitate exposure for surgery or closure following resection.

If a primary tumour approaches the lingual plate, the alveolar process or even superficially erodes the lingual cortex, a marginal resection of the mandible is feasible (Figs. 6.1–6.4). This preserves the arch of the mandible and thus retains symmetry of the facial contour. Results with MM for cancer of the buccal mucosa show an overall local control rate of 79 per cent.[12]

Large primary tumours of the tongue not involving or approaching the mandible can be easily resected in a monobloc fashion via a mandibulotomy approach without violating oncological principles. *Median mandibulotomy with mandibular swing* can be performed without elevation of lower cheek flap, thus preserving the sensations of the skin of the chin on both sides. This offers the advantages of maintaining the facial contour and functions of the lower alveolus.[13] We are

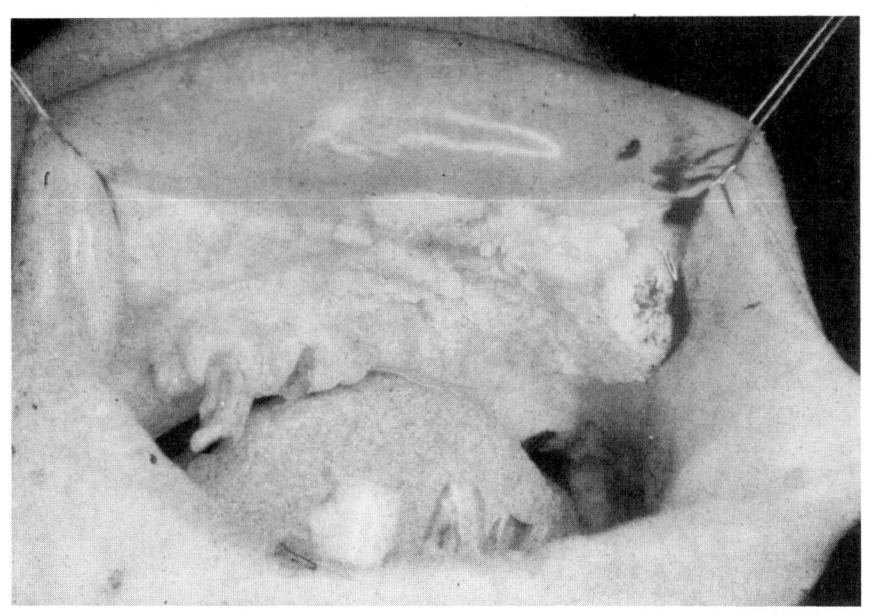

Fig. 6.1 Preoperative photograph showing the extent of verrucous cancer of the gingivolabial sulcus, involving alveolar mucosa of the anterior arch of the mandible.

74 *Cancer of the oral cavity*

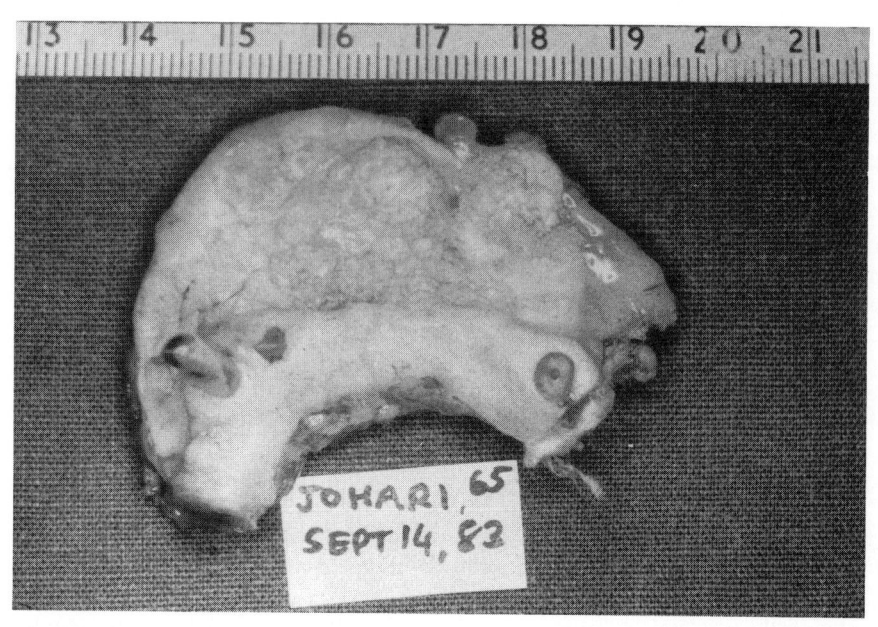

Fig. 6.2 A specimen of verrucous cancer of the gingivolabial sulcus extending to the lower alveolus, resected with marginal mandibulectomy.

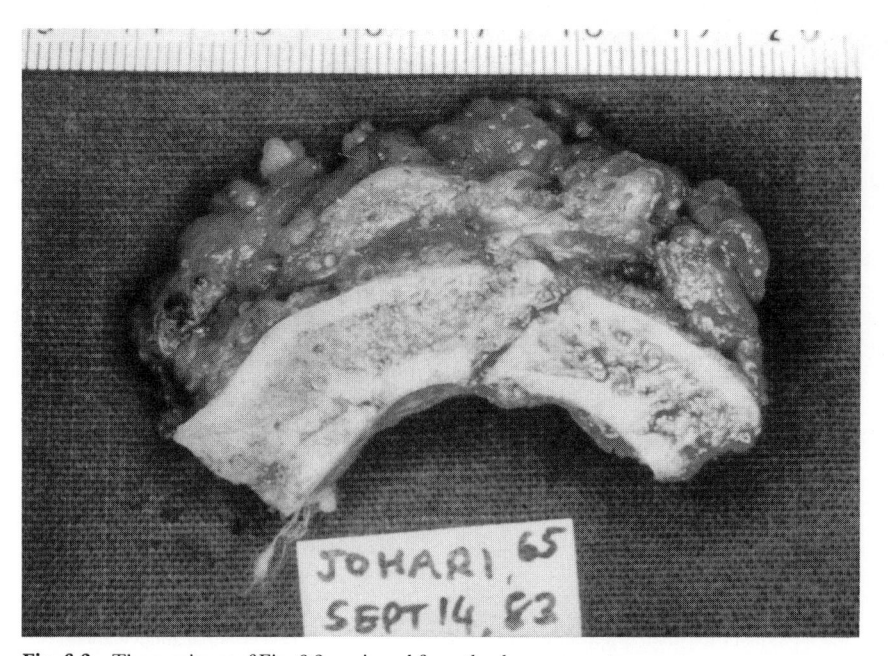

Fig. 6.3 The specimen of Fig. 6.2 as viewed from the deeper aspect.

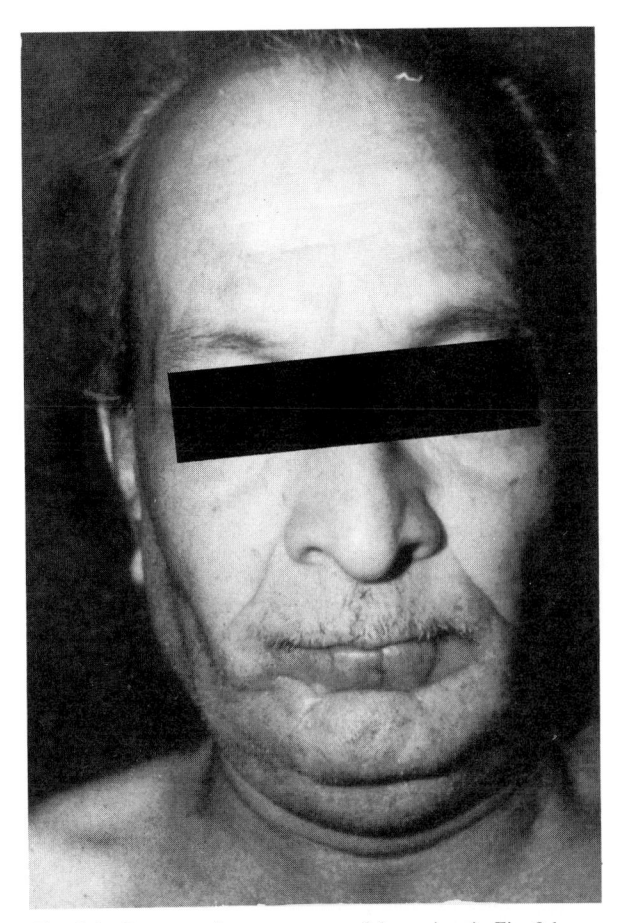

Fig. 6.4 Postoperative appearance of the patient in Fig. 6.1.

selectively using this approach for cancers of the lateral border of the tongue with involvement of the floor of the mouth, to get adequate margins of resection and to facilitate reconstruction to provide mobility of the tongue and improve the cosmetic result (Figs. 6.5–6.8).

The standard surgical approach to *advanced oral cancers* involving the cheek, lower alveolus and lymph nodes in the neck is to carry out an *en-bloc composite resection*, which includes a radical neck dissection, resection of half of the mandible, and full-thickness cheek resection or tongue resection depending on the site of the primary cancer in the oral cavity. Crile's incision or its modification is generally used for this approach. We prefer the McFee incision for its cosmetic superiority and safety, extending the upper incision in the midline to divide the lip.

76 *Cancer of the oral cavity*

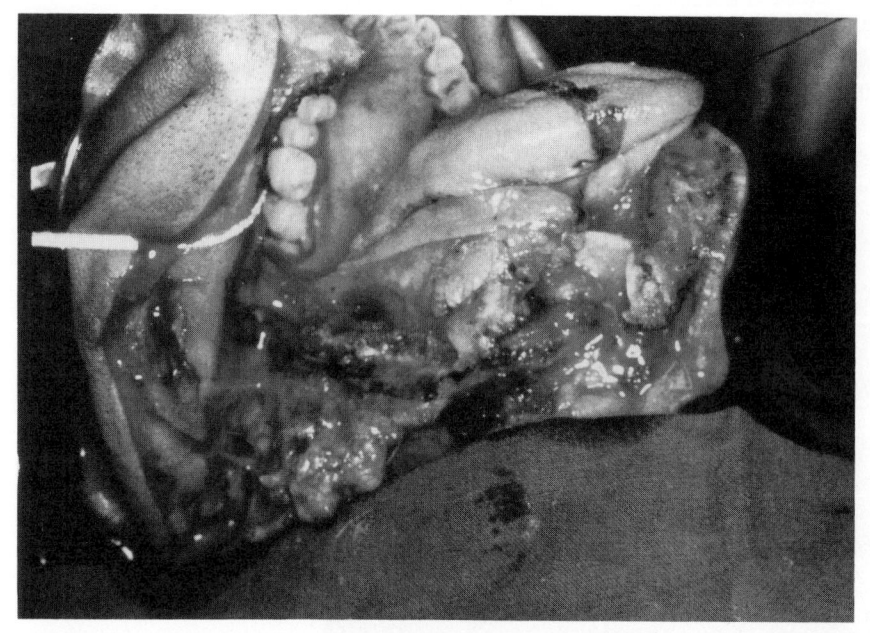

Fig. 6.5 Intraoperative view of cancer of the right lateral border and under-surface of the tongue, involving the floor of the mouth, as seen after mandibulotomy.

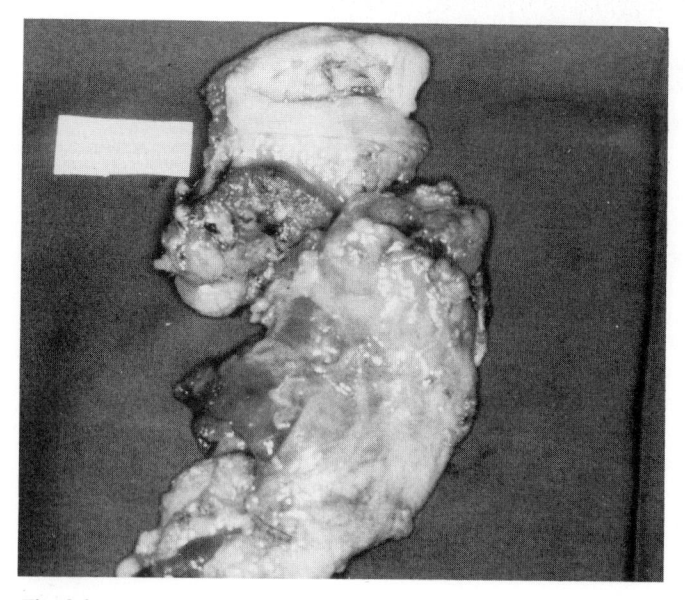

Fig. 6.6 A specimen delivered *en bloc*.

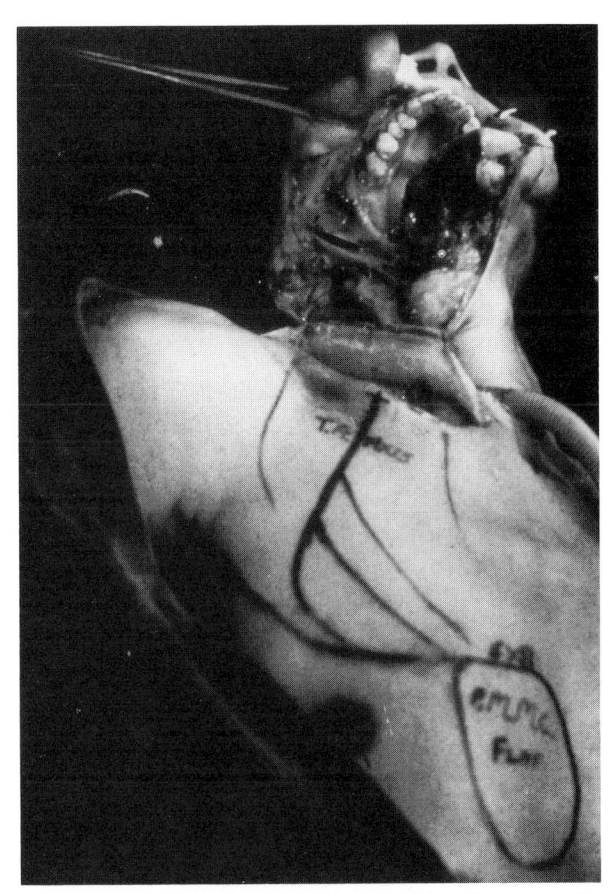

Fig. 6.7 The defect after the resection, and plan of reconstruction using a pectoralis major myocutaneous flap. Radical neck dissection was performed through a McFee incision.

Extent of neck dissection

Cervical lymph node involvement is reported in terms of five anatomic levels. Level I refers to nodes within the submandibular and submental triangles. Levels II, III and IV refer to the chain of nodes along the upper, middle and lower third of the jugular vein respectively. Level V describes nodes along the accessory nerve and within the posterior triangle.

The most important prognostic indicator in oral cancer is the presence or absence of cervical metastases. Identifying the presence of a node metastases and treating it appropriately in time is crucial for the management of oral cancers.

If the neck is positive for metastatic nodes, *radical neck dissection* (RND) is mandatory. In stages III and IV the neck must be accepted as potentially involved and must be treated. Most oral cancers initially metastasize to level I–III lymph nodes.

Modified neck dissection is finding more acceptance and preference over radical neck dissection in managing the N0 neck because of the severe morbidity of RND, such as shoulder dysfunction, poor cosmetic appearance, and facial oedema.[4]

The *supraomohyoid neck dissection*, which has minimal morbidity, provides most satisfactory sampling of the lymph nodes at levels I, II and III which are at the greatest risk. The extent of node clearance obtained allows accurate staging of the disease in the neck and easier selection of patients who need further treatment by radical neck dissection or adjuvant radiation therapy.[15] It gives comparable results with less surgical trauma.

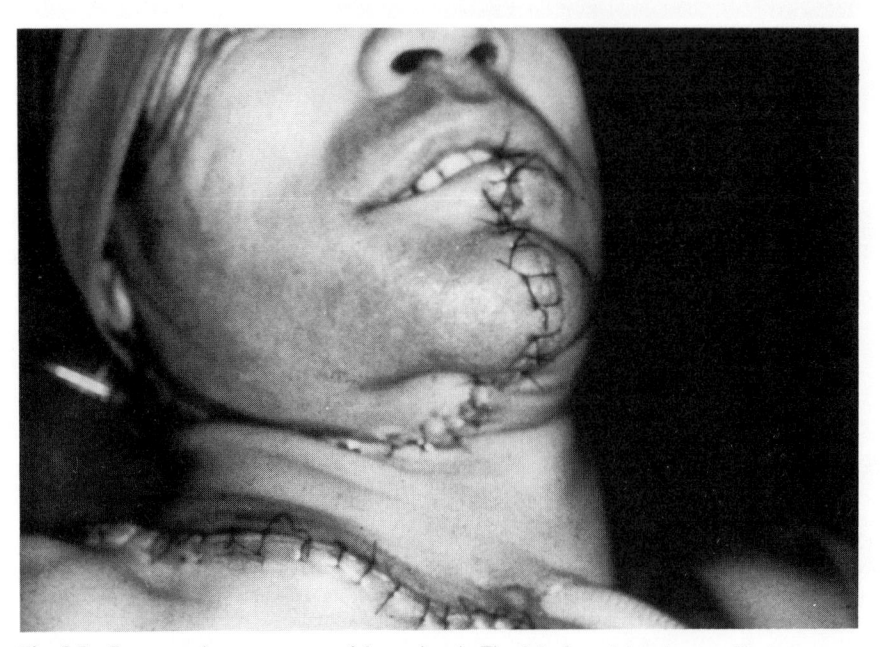

Fig. 6.8 Postoperative appearance of the patient in Fig. 6.5 after wiring the mandibulotomy.

Primary reconstruction

No therapy is acceptable unless it helps the patient to return to a near-normal social and functional existence. Reconstructive surgery, evolved over the last three decades, offers a reasonable chance of rehabilitating a patient after these formidable resections. Local flaps (e.g. the nasolabial flap), distant flaps (e.g. the forehead flap or deltopectoral flap), myocutaneous flaps (e.g. the pectoralis major myocutaneous flap—PMMC) are commonly used. Free flaps are occasionally used in our hospital. Currently the most commonly used are PMMC and DP flaps.[16]

Primary reconstruction is technically easier and needs less hospitalization than secondary reconstructive procedures, which have been largely abandoned. Replacement of the oral lining by selection of an appropriate flap adds to the mobility of the tongue and the mouth, facilitating speech and swallowing.

Reconstruction of anterior arch of mandible

When the anterior arch of the mandible is sacrificed it must be primarily reconstructed to prevent Andy Gump deformity and resulting incompetence of the oral closure, drooling of saliva and difficulty in speaking. The technique consists of transfer of composite osteomyocutaneous flaps with pectoralis major muscle with an attached segment of the fourth or fifth rib, providing two paddles of skin, one for an inner lining and one for the outer cover. The arch can also be reconstructed with transfer of composite tissue by microvascular techniques. An iliac crest based on the deep circumflex iliac vascular system or the radial forearm with a segment of radius are the two methods commonly used.[17,18]

Forehead flap

This flap, based on the anterior branch of the superficial temporal artery, was for many years the workhorse of head and neck surgeons. However, it is rarely used now owing to the unsightly cosmetic appearance of the grafted forehead and the need for a two-stage operation.

Deltopectoral flap

From the mid-1960s until the introduction of the PMMC (see below) in the late 1970s, this versatile flap based on the upper four perforating branches of the internal mammary artery was extensively used for reconstruction of oral defects. The disadvantages were the need for a second stage, and its significant rate of distal necrasis.

Pectoralis major myocutaneous flap

Introduction of the concept of vascular cutaneous territories of muscles carried on their vascular pedicles has led to the development of single-stage reconstruction to replace the multistage reconstructive procedures of the past.

The pectoralis major is most frequently used to carry a sizable area of skin from the chest wall, either as a single or bipedal flap, in one stage. This has revolutionized the reconstruction of oral defects. However, they are frequently bulky, and in obese patients the extreme bulk of the flap may make the operation technically difficult or impossible.

The skin island on a musculocutaneous flap is very loosely attached to the underlying muscle. Manipulation during flap elevation can avulse the tenuous areolar vascular attachments. The skin island should be sutured to the underlying muscle fascia prior to elevation of the muscle unit.

Osteomyocutaneous flap

This flap is used to close a composite defect in the soft tissues of the cheek and mandible. A pectoralis major osteomyocutaneous flap with underlying fourth or fifth rib is frequently used. All mandibular replacement requires effective fixation as well as adequate oral and external full-thickness soft-tissue coverage.

Free flaps

Advances in microsurgical techniques have led to the development of several procedures for the rehabilitation of the head and neck patient using free-tissue transfer. Groin flaps, dorsalis pedis flaps, and latissimus dorsi flaps can be used for soft-tissue reconstruction. Compound flaps (e.g. rib flaps, ilial crest flaps) for reconstruction of soft tissue and bone in a one-stage procedure have also been attempted. These are most complex reconstructive procedures. The principal complication is loss of patency of the vascular anastomosis and resulting flap necrosis.

Radiation therapy

RT has a clearly established role in the management of oral cancers. Exophytic rather than infiltrative tumours respond best to RT. The success of RT falls exponentially with increasing tumour bulk from T1 to T4, possibly owing to the large hypoxic cell population at the core. Bulky nodal metastases also exhibit a poor response rate.

The *principal advantages of radiotherapy* are:

1. preservation of tissue and function;
2. better cosmetic results;
3. more generous margins of treatment volume to cover potential areas of spread, including the regional lymphatics.

The *disadvantages of radiotherapy* are:

1. acute radiation side-effects such as painful mucositis, loss of taste, dry mouth, dysphagia and weight loss;
2. potential late complications of soft tissue and bone necrosis, carotid artery necrosis, carotid artery occlusive disease;
3. a protracted treatment course with external-beam irradiation.

A number of techniques are available. RT may be administered either alone or in conjunction with other modalities (surgery and chemotherapy).

External-beam radiotherapy utilizes megavoltage x-rays and electrons generated from x-ray machines, such as linear accelerators and betatrons, or gamma rays from cobalt ^{60}Co machines. Intraoral cones of different sizes and shapes may be used for electron-beam therapy of selective small superficial lesions in the oral cavity.

Brachytherapy utilizes interstitial implants and surface applicators of radioactive isotopes such as ^{102}Ir and ^{125}I. An after-loading technique is used in interstitial implants to minimize radiation exposure to medical personnel. The major advantage of brachytherapy is the physical dose distribution, which favours a higher total dose rate to the tumour than to the adjacent normal tissue, achieving a greater therapeutic ratio. Radiobiologically, the delivery of a therapeutic dose continuously over a short time interval may also be more efficacious than a course of conventional fractionated external-beam radiotherapy.

Dental prophylaxis

Dental sepsis increases discomfort and prejudices the ultimate success of radiation therapy, which should therefore be delayed until dental treatment (scaling, cleaning, extraction of septic teeth and healing of the sockets) is completed. Prophylactic extraction of teeth that come within the fields chosen for radiation therapy is strongly recommended. Late decay due to postradiation ischaemia may necessitate extraction. Sockets heal poorly and infection may result in radionecrosis of the mandible. This distressing complication may occasionally necessitate mandibular resection.

Treatment options with surgery and RT

Early cancers (T1 and T2) have comparable cure rates with radiation and surgery, RT having obvious cosmetic and functional advantages. For T3 and T4 lesions, RT is used preoperatively and postoperatively in combination with surgery.

Preoperative radiation therapy (35–50 Gy), followed within three weeks by radical surgery, has been tried and abandoned in most centres. It aimed at increasing the chances of cure and reducing the local recurrence rate. If this is done, excision must include the original tumour-bearing area, along with an adequate margin of normal tissue. Small conservative excisions following preoperative radiation therapy inevitably result in recurrent lesions.

For lesions involving the sites under consideration here, postoperative RT is preferred. The incidence of postoperative wound problems is significantly reduced, and improved local control rates are achieved. Furthermore, primary surgery provides detailed histopathological analysis of a specimen, enabling better prognostication and RT planning.

The optimum timing of postoperative RT is within six weeks of surgery; timing appears to influence cure rates significantly.

All primary T3/T4 lesions, and those which show neck node spread, are candidates for adjuvant RT.

Areas of known residual disease should receive 50–55 Gy in 5–6 weeks or 60–65 Gy in 6–7 weeks. A 'shrinking field' technique is used, wherein areas of residual disease receive higher doses.

Complications of radiation therapy

Acute side-effects of radiotherapy, such as mucositis, skin reaction, hair loss, alteration of taste, dry mouth, dysphagia and weight loss, are primarily due to the effects of radiation of the skin and mucosa, taste buds and salivary glands. These can be minimized by proper treatment planning: tailored blocks to spare normal tissues, an intraoral cone or an interstitial implant should be used whenever feasible. As a result of altered and decreased saliva following radiotherapy, patients are more prone to develop dental caries; this is minimized by good oral hygiene and topical fluoride applications. All patients should have dental evaluation and prophylaxis, as described earlier.

Chemotherapy

Single drugs

Methotrexate, cisplatin, bleomycin, and 5-fluorouracil are commonly used. Methotrexate is a widely used drug at a dose of 200 mg/m^2 as an I.V. infusion over six hours and repeated after 10 days, yielding response rates up to 80 per cent, with a complete response in 21 per cent of patients with advanced head and neck cancer.[19] The role of other drugs, including cyclophosphamide, hydroxyurea, vincristine, vinblastine, and mitomycin C, remains more uncertain. Response rates to a single drug vary between 30 and 50 per cent. The median duration of response is short.

Multiple drugs

Combination chemotherapy is most effective when used as the preoperative or preradiation treatment of locally advanced cases (anterior or induction chemotherapy); it is of less use for recurrent or metastatic disease. This is attributed to better vascularity and a favourable immune status in the untreated patients. Responses are, however, temporary.

Using cisplatinum (20 mg/m^2 daily for five days), methotrexate (20 mg/m^2 on days 1 and 8) and bleomycin (10 mg/m^2 on days 1 and 8), we have attained an overall response rate of 90 per cent at our hospital. A randomized trial using three cycles of induction cisplatinum and 5-fluorouracil infusion was reported to have an 85 per cent response rate, but without an overall survival benefit.[20]

The role of multimodal treatment

Chemotherapy is included as part of a multimodality treatment programme along with surgery and radiation therapy directed at cure of local or regional disease (Table 6.6).

These approaches are still considered experimental and are being tried in randomized trials. Multimodal treatment holds considerable promise for the future. Unfortunately, it does not yet have a proven role for the treatment of oral cancer in the clinical setting.

Table 6.6 Strategies for the use of chemotherapy in a multimodal treatment regimen

Palliative

1. For recurrent primary and neck nodes disease
2. For metastatic disease

Curative or long-term control as primary treatment

1. Chemotherapy prior to surgery or radiation therapy to reduce tumour burden (anterior chemotherapy)
2. Chemotherapy simultaneous with radiotherapy as a radiosensitizer
3. Postoperative adjuvant chemotherapy for minimal residual disease

Prognostic factors

There is no significant difference in the five-year survival rates for different sites, but the survival rate drops for larger cancers as they extend posteriorly into the oropharynx. Patients with early node-negative cancers (stages I and II) have better five-year survivals than those with advanced cancers.

The presence of metastatic lymph nodes in the neck is of grave prognostic significance. A linear relationship exists between the T-stage and N-stage; 50–60 per cent of patients with T3–T4 tumours have metastases in neck nodes. The survival rate drops from 60–80 per cent for N0 to 10–40 per cent for N+.

The survival rates for more advanced cancers which are bulky and invasive and have lymph nodes metastases remain distressingly low and have not changed appreciably.

A retrospective study of 162 cases of T4 cancer of the buccal mucosa, treated surgically, showed that tumour differentiation formed the most important preoperative prognostic parameter. All patients with poorly differentiated tumours developed loco-regional recurrences, even when surgery was followed by postoperative radiotherapy.[15]

The disease-free survival (DFS) rate for surgically treated T2 tumours is 57 per cent and for T3 it is 43 per cent. The DFS goes up to 60 per cent by combining surgery and postoperative radiation therapy, and for T4 tumours the cure rate is 35 per cent, compared with 21 per cent for surgery alone and 13 per cent for radiation therapy alone. The rate of surgical salvage in radiotherapy failures is only 6 per cent. The 'inoperable' T4 cancers constitute more than half of the entire group of T4 buccal mucosa cancers seen at our institution.

References

1. Rao D.N., Ganesh B. Epidemiological aspects of H&N cancer. In: Desai P.B., Rao R.S. (eds.): *Current Trends in the Management of H&N Cancer*. Bombay: Tata Memorial Hospital, 1988: 6–10.
2. Paymaster J.C. Oral and pharyngeal cancer in India. In: Conley J. (ed.): *Cancer of Head and Neck*. Washington: Butterworths, 1967: 308–16.
3. Jussawalla D.J., Deshpande V.A. Evaluation of cancer risk in tobacco chewers and smokers: an epidemiologic assessment. *Cancer*. 1972; **28:** 244–52.
4. Khafif R.A., Rafla S., Kopel S. Tumours of the head and neck. Therapeutic guidelines: site-specific. In: *Current Guidelines for the Management of Cancer*. Orlando: Academic Press, 1986: 29–30.
5. Mehta F.S., Daftary D.K., Sahiar B.E. A correlative histocytological study of epithelial atypia in leukoplakia and submucous fibrosis lesions amongst Indian villagers in a mass screening programme. *Ind. J. Cancer*. 1970; **7:** 18–23.
6. Whitehouse G.H. Radiological bone changes produced by intraoral squamous cancer involving the lower alveolus. *Clin. Otolaryngol*. 1976; **1:** 45–52.
7. Marchetta F.C., Sako K., Murphy J.B. The periosteum of the mandible and intraoral carcinoma. *Amer. J. Surg*. 1971; **122:** 11–13.
8. Close L.G., Merkel M., Burns D.K., Schaefer S.D. Computer tomography in the assessment of mandibular invasion by intraoral carcinoma. *Ann. Otol. Laryngol*. 1986; **95:** 383–8.
9. Myers E.N. The toluidine blue test in lesions of the oral cavity. *CA*. 1970; **20:** 134–9.
10. McDonald J.S., Crissman J.D., Gluckman J.L. Verrucous carcinoma of the oral cavity. *Head Neck Surg*. 1982; **5:** 22–8.
11. Marchetta F.C., Sako K., Razack M.S. Management of 'localised' oral cancer. *Amer. J. Surg*. 1977; **134:** 448–9.

12. Pradhan S.A., Rajpal R.M. Marginal mandibulectomy in the management of squamous cancer of the oral cavity. *Ind. J. Cancer.* 1987; **24:** 167–71.
13. Spiro R.H., Gerold F.P., Strong E.W. Mandibular swing approach for oral and oropharyngeal tumors. *Head Neck Surg.* 1981; **3:** 371–8.
14. Byers R.M., Wolf P.F., Shallenberger R. The modified neck dissection: a study of 967 cases from 1970 to 1980. Presented at the Fifth Joint Meeting of the American Society for H&N Surgery and the Society of H&N Surgeons, 5–8 May 1985, Dorado, Puerto Rico (Meeting abstract, p.126).
15. Pradhan S.A. Surgery for cancer of the buccal mucosa. In: Desai P.B., Rao R.S. (eds.): *Current Trends in the Management of H&N Cancer.* Bombay: Tata Memorial Hospital, 1988: 53–61.
16. Ariyan S. Pectoralis major, sternomastoid, and other musculocutaneous flaps for head and neck reconstruction. *Clin. Plas. Surg.* 1980; **7:** 89–98.
17. Taylor G.I., Townsend P., Corlett R. Superiority of the deep circumflex iliac vessels as a supply for groin flaps. II: Clinical work. *Plas. Reconst. Surg.* 1979; **64:** 745–9.
18. Soutar D.S., Scheker L.R., Tanner N.S.B., *et al.* The radial forearm flap: a versatile method of oral reconstruction. *Brit. J. Plas. Surg.* 1983; **36:** 1–8.
19. Advani S.H., Mehta A.R., Rao R.S., *et al.* Moderate dose methotrexate in H&N cancer. *Oncology.* 1981; **38:** 329.
20. Toohil R.J., Anderson T., Byhardt R.W., *et al.* Cisplatin and fluorouracil as neoadjuvant therapy in head and neck cancer. *Arch. Otolaryngol. Head Neck Surg.* 1987; **113:** 758–61.

7

Cancer of the thyroid

Tom S. Reeve, CBE, MBBS, FRACS, FACS, DDU, FRACR(Hon), and Leigh Delbridge, MD, BSc(Med), FRACS

Thyroid cancer is among the least common forms of malignancy, being responsible for less than 0.5 per cent of all cancer deaths in Western countries. Nonetheless the disease has always attracted considerable interest and controversy for a number of reasons. Firstly, the disease tends to occur primarily in a younger age group in whom it generally has an excellent prognosis when appropriately treated. Secondly, whilst thyroid cancer is rare, nodular thyroid disease, either single nodules or multinodular goitre, is very common in the community, and so the question of accurate diagnosis and the role of surgery for presumed thyroid cancer is a clinical reality frequently encountered by surgeons.

Most discussion centres around two questions. Firstly, what is the most accurate preoperative diagnostic modality in the patient in whom the diagnosis of thyroid cancer is suspected clinically; in particular, what is the role of imaging techniques such as nuclear and ultrasound scans, when compared with fine-needle aspiration biopsy and cytology? Secondly, in the young patient with differentiated thyroid cancer, what is the most appropriate form of surgical therapy when the advantages of total thyroidectomy in terms of improved disease control are compared with the potential risk of increased morbidity from the operation?

Pathology of thyroid cancer

Epidemiology and pathogenesis

Thyroid cancer is a common autopsy finding. Small deposits of clinically single papillary cancer have been reported in up to 20 per cent of some autopsy findings,[1] the true incidence probably reflecting the diligence with which a microscopic search is made of the gland. Thyroid cancer presenting as a clinical problem, however, is uncommon, with the reported incidence ranging from 2 to 10 cases per 100 000 per year in Western societies. Death from thyroid cancer is even rarer, with reported rates ranging from only 0.30 to 0.60 per 100 000 in the UK and USA.[2]

Thyroid malignancy is primarily a disease of the young to middle-aged female patient. There are a number of specific risk factors associated with the onset of thyroid cancer. Previous irradiation is one of the most important factors, the best documented examples being previous irradiation to the head and neck region, usually in the form of treatment for acne or for thymic enlargement in children,[3] and occasionally as the result of radioactive fallout.[4] Endemic goitre is also thought to be a factor in the pathogenesis of thyroid cancer. Death rates due to thyroid cancer are high in endemic goitre areas, one of the proposed mechanisms being the relationship with elevated TSH levels. The reliability of such statistics has, however, been called into question by Riccabona,[2] who points out that it may simply be that, in endemic goitre areas, patients tend to present later, with more advanced and less-favourable tumours, occurring within longstanding multinodular goitres.

Other epidemiological factors include genetic influences, with documented examples of 'thyroid cancer' families quite distinct from the MEN syndrome,[2] thyrotoxicosis due to Graves' disease, and probably Hashimoto's thyroiditis.[5]

Classification

The generally accepted histological classification of thyroid tumours is that established by the WHO as shown in Table 7.1. In clinical practice, the commonly encountered thyroid tumours are differentiated thyroid carcinoma

Table 7.1 WHO histological classification of thyroid tumours

I	*Epithelial tumours*	
	(A) Benign	
		1. Follicular adenoma
		2. Others
	(B) Malignant	
		1. Follicular carcinoma
		2. Papillary carcinoma
		3. Squamous cell carcinoma
		4. Undifferentiated (anaplastic) carcinoma
		(a) spindle cell type
		(b) giant cell type
		(c) small cell type
		5. Medullary carcinoma
II	*Non-epithelial tumours*	
	(A) Benign	
	(B) Malignant	
		1. Fibrosarcoma
		2. Others
III	*Miscellaneous tumours*	
		1. Carcinosarcoma
		2. Malignant haemangioendothelioma
		3. Malignant lymphoma
		4. Teratoma
IV	*Secondary tumours*	
V	*Unclassified tumours*	
VI	*Tumour-like lesions*	

(papillary, mixed, follicular), anaplastic carcinoma, medullary carcinoma and lymphoma. With the exception of lymphoma and medullary carcinoma, recent evidence has shown that the remaining tumours are all of follicular cell origin and that we are, in fact, looking at a spectrum of one disease, rather than a series of separate disease processes. Thus, whilst it is convenient for classification purposes to divide differentiated thyroid cancer into its varying histological patterns for discussion purposes, and indeed whilst most patients will demonstrate one type of tumour predominantly, there are numerous clinical examples of all types being demonstrated at different sites, or at different times in the one patient.[6]

Differentiated thyroid cancer

Papillary carcinoma is characterized by papillary structures consisting of a fibrovascular stalk covered with a single layer of epithelial cells. The tumour cells possess pale nuclei which are frequently overlapping. Psammoma bodies (laminated calcified bodies) are characteristic of papillary carcinoma. Follicular carcinomas are cytologically indistinguishable from follicular adenomas, showing a uniform structure of thyroid follicles with variable degrees of proliferation. The diagnosis of malignancy rests entirely on the finding of vascular or capsular invasion, or the presence of lymph node or distant metastases. Mixed carcinomas contain features of both papillary and follicular patterns. All three types can, and do, metastasize via the bloodstream to distant sites such as lung and bone, or via lymphatics to regional nodes. In addition, all three types will take up radio-iodine once all normal thyroid tissue has been removed surgically. The major biological difference in these tumours relates to the fact that follicular tumours tend to present more commonly in the older population, whilst papillary and mixed tumours are a disease of the young. Thus the apparent 'worse' prognosis of follicular cancer can be explained very largely on the basis of the patient's age (Fig. 7.1). In our own series, age at presentation was the single most important prognostic factor in differentiated thyroid cancer.[7]

Anaplastic cancer

Anaplastic cancer is now generally regarded as being dedifferentiated papillary or follicular thyroid cancer,[8] and commonly presents in one of three forms: spindle cell tumours, giant cell undifferentiated tumours, and small cell undifferentiated tumours. It is one of the most aggressive of all malignancies and infiltrates the surrounding tissues.

Medullary thyroid cancer

These tumours arise from the parafollicular C cells of the thyroid and are characterized, both clinically and on immunocytochemistry, by the secretion of calcitonin. The tumour cells are arranged in sheets or cords. It may occur as a sporadic finding, or as part of the MEN II syndrome.

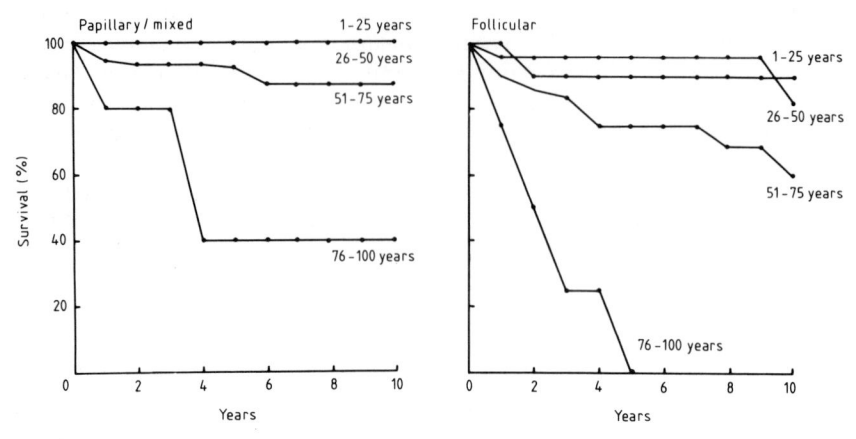

Fig. 7.1 Ten-year cumulative survival for patients with papillary/mixed forms of differentiated thyroid cancer compared with those with follicular forms, showing a similar worsening prognosis with increasing age in both groups. (Reproduced from reference 7 with the kind permission of Blackwell Scientific, Australia)

Thyroid lymphoma

Thyroid lymphoma is thought to arise in lymphoid infiltrates associated with pre-existing Hashimoto's thyroiditis. It presents the same histological and clinical spectrum as lymphoma arising in other sites.

Presentation

Malignancy in the thyroid is distinctly uncommon and may well be overlooked unless the examining physician is alert to the nuances of presentation. Thyroid carcinoma does not necessarily present with clear-cut signs or symptoms that indicate the diagnosis. Given its comparative rarity when compared with the multinodular goitre, it is necessary for clinicians to hone their clinical and diagnostic skills if the tell-tale subtleties that may prove of more value in diagnosis than many of the available diagnostic aids, are not to be missed.

The only clearly apparent sign of thyroid malignancy is rapid and progressive growth of a single thyroid nodule or a dominant nodule within a multinodular goitre. Whilst it is conventional wisdom that thyroid carcinoma arises in single nodules, and the presence of a multinodular goitre militates against this diagnosis, in our own unit at the University of Sydney just under half of all thyroid malignancies arose in other than true single nodules. The important clinical feature is therefore not the presence or otherwise of a multinodular goitre, but whether there is a dominant single area of nodularity, the so-called 'solitoma'. In addition, relying on clinical decisions may be misleading as about 50 per cent of patients with clinically single nodules are found at surgery to have a multinodular goitre with a single dominant nodule.

Accurate physical examination is crucial since, as will be discussed, the most important diagnostic test currently available is a fine-needle aspiration biopsy. The value of this test depends entirely on the accuracy of sampling by the physician, which is, in turn, dependent on his placing the needle within the substance of the nodule in question. The normal thyroid (with the exception of the isthmus in thin people) is not visible to the clinician, although the manoeuvre of having the patient swallow may reveal nodules not otherwise seen.

It is important to emphasize several points in the physical examination. While most texts promote examination from behind the patient, we believe that examination of the thyroid is more precise from the front, with the combination of the patient and examiner facing each other, fixing one side of the thyroid with the thumb posterior to the sternomastoid while palpation of the other lobe is carried out by the opposite thumb. This not only allows a combination of simultaneous inspection and palpation, but greatly enhances the accuracy of subsequent positioning of the fine-needle, which must of course be done from the front of the patient.

Thyroid nodules containing cancer are commonly firm to hard and, given time, will become fixed through invasion to underlying structures. Fixation to skin is rare. In the young, lymph node involvement may precede the appearance of a nodule. Such nodes may lie in either the posterior or anterior triangle and can frequently be felt deep to the clavicle. Unlike some other malignancies, there is no orderly pattern of lymph node involvement. The random pattern of nodal affection is one of the characteristic features of the disease.

Diffuse thyroid involvement is usually seen in the elderly and signifies the presence of undifferentiated or anaplastic malignancy. Primary lymphoma of the thyroid may also present with identical clinical signs. Such lesions are usually fixed to underlying structures and are frequently associated with symptoms of tracheal compression or recurrent laryngeal nerve involvement. In contrast, in the young patient with a single nodule, recurrent laryngeal nerve palsy is more commonly associated with compression from a benign nodule rather than signifying malignant invasion. If the patient presents with a lesion that the physician considers may be anaplastic, but has been present for a longer period of time than would normally be considered usual, the diagnosis of medullary carcinoma must be considered.

All single or dominant thyroid nodules should be investigated, as will be outlined. Nonetheless, clinical acumen should remain paramount and, if there is concern regarding the presence of malignancy despite negative investigations, surgical therapy should still be offered. If a nodule is palpable, then it should not be regarded as being 'occult' if it is subsequently found to contain cancer. On the other hand, it is recognized that impalpable occult cancers can occur, not infrequently, in the presence of a benign thyroid nodule.

Investigations

Clinical and laboratory assessment

Selection for surgery depends initially upon a careful history taking, the identification of recognized risk factors and a complete physical examination.[9]

Patients with nodular thyroid disease who have significant risk factors, such as previous neck irradiation, should be submitted to surgery regardless of the results of further investigations. Likewise, the presence of symptoms, such as dysphagia or respiratory obstruction, are an absolute indication for surgery. Similarly, the removal of a very large nodule may well be indicated for cosmetic reasons, even in the absence of symptoms. This will now leave a significant group of patients, with nodular thyroid disease, who are asymptomatic, in which the only real concern is whether or not they contain malignancy.

Laboratory tests of thyroid function are essential preoperatively in order to rule out the presence of unsuspected thyrotoxicosis, but otherwise are of no use in the diagnosis of malignancy. The only laboratory investigation which may be of value is the measurement of serum calcitonin to detect medullary cancer. Since this is a relatively uncommon condition, however, routine measurement is probably not cost-effective and should be reserved for a specific indication such as a positive family history, or suspicious physical findings.

Imaging techniques

One of the major changes that has occurred in the past decade has been in the role of imaging procedures in the diagnosis of thyroid cancer. Prior to this time, the principal modalities upon which patients have been selected for surgery have been by isotope scans and ultrasound. This has been based on the belief that malignancy is more likely if the scan shows a 'cold' lesion or there is a 'solid' component to the lesion on ultrasound.

The reported accuracy of isotope scanning varies greatly. In a review by Ashcraft and Van Herle,[10] malignant disease was found in 16 per cent of cold nodules and 9 per cent of warm nodules. In a review of five years of unselected thyroid scans for clinically single nodules at Royal North Shore Hospital,[11] Wiseman found a 10.5 per cent incidence of malignancy in 'cold' nodules and a 10.2 per cent incidence in 'functioning' nodules. Thus reliance on a 'cold' scan to predict malignancy will lead to a significant incidence of thyroidectomies where cancer is not found, whilst a 'warm' scan in no way reliably excludes malignancy. Most authors would now agree that isotope scans are quite unnecessary in the assessment of the euthyroid patient with a solitary or dominant thyroid nodule,[9] except in the proven thyrotoxic patient.

Similar conclusions can be reached about the use of ultrasound in single thyroid nodules. In a concurrent review by Ashcraft and Van Herle,[12] 21 per cent of solid lesions, 12 per cent of cystic/solid lesions and 7 per cent of cystic lesions were malignant at operation. At Royal North Shore Hospital in a review of 520 ultrasounds for single nodules, the presence of a solid component was associated with malignancy in only 6.4 per cent of cases.[11] In addition, needle aspiration, as will be discussed, is a reliable technique for the detection of cystic change within a thyroid nodule and has the added advantage of providing cytological information. It has been stated that one of the values of ultrasound scanning is in the differentiation of single nodules from multinodular goitre. Whilst this may be true, such a distinction is not clinically relevant. If the patient has a dominant nodule, then the presence or otherwise of underlying multinodular change within the thyroid gland has no bearing on the risk of malignancy in that nodule.

Whilst the reported data vary from institution to institution based on the experience of those performing the investigations, it is clear that both isotope scans and ultrasounds have significant limitations in identifying malignant lesions in patients being selected for surgery. For this reason, in our unit, neither is now used routinely in the investigation of nodular thyroid disease.

Fine-needle aspiration biopsy

Fine-needle aspiration biopsy of thyroid nodules is a simple, safe and effective technique for assessing the likelihood of malignancy in thyroid nodules. It is painless, complication-free and can be performed in the office setting as part of the initial consultation. Indeed there are many who believe that fine-needle aspiration biopsy should be considered simply as an extension of the routine physical examination. That is not to say that there are not limitations to the technique: it requires careful technique to avoid sampling errors, an experienced cytologist to provide expert interpretation of the smears, and an appreciation of the significance and limitation of the reports provided.

The technique was popularized by the Swedes in the 1950s[13,14] but has only recently achieved acceptance worldwide. A 23- or 21-gauge needle attached to a 10 ml syringe held in a special hand-grip is inserted into the centre of the nodule and several passes made whilst suction is maintained. The aspirate is smeared on to slides, air-dried and stained. In our unit, reports are classified into one of four groups depending on their cytological characteristics, namely: inadequate; benign; atypical; or malignant. The important features are summarized in Table 7.2.

It is important to appreciate some of the limitations of the technique. For

Table 7.2 Commonly seen features of each classification of fine-needle aspirates of thyroid nodules

Aspirate	Typical features
Inadequate	Few or no follicular cells present

Benign
  Colloid nodule
  Thyroiditis
  Cystic degeneration
	Colloid with scant to moderate cellularity; other features (e.g. lymphocytes) in thyroiditis

Atypical
  Follicular adenoma
  Follicular carcinoma
	Scant colloid and cellular specimen with numerous microfollicular structures; oncocytes predominate in Hurthle cell neoplasm

Malignant
  Papillary carcinoma
 	
  Medullary carcinoma
  Anaplastic carcinoma
  Lymphoma
  Metastases
	Papillary: papillary and follicular cell clusters; intranuclear inclusions; psammoma bodies
	Medullary: solid cell clusters with spindle-shaped cells
	Anaplastic: necrosis with pleomorphic or multinucleated cells
	Lymphoma: resemble Non-Hodgkins cells
	Metastatic: resemble primary

example, it is impossible to differentiate on cytological grounds between a benign follicular adenoma and a follicular carcinoma—both will show an atypical follicular pattern (Fig. 7.2). This distinction is made histologically on the grounds of capsular or vascular invasion, and even then, may be exceedingly difficult. This is not a major consideration, however, as all follicular neoplasms should be regarded as potentially malignant and selected for surgical excision.[9] The major benefit is differentiating the benign colloid nodule, which shows a benign pattern, from cellular tumours.

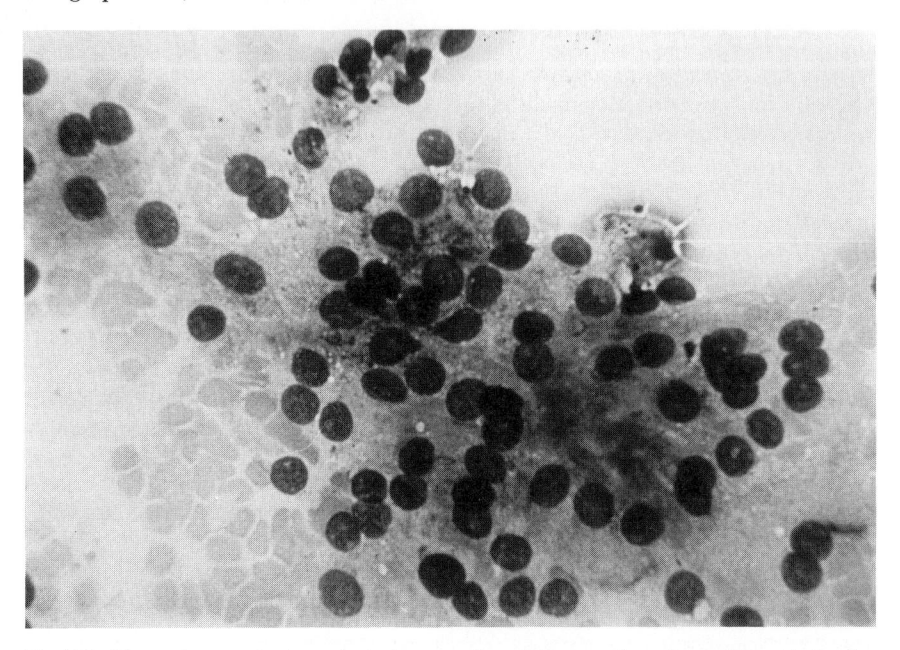

Fig. 7.2 Photomicrograph of a cytological preparation of a fine-needle aspirate of thyroid, showing an atypical follicular pattern.

The accuracy of fine-needle aspiration is relatively constant. In our own unit, the percentage incidence of malignancy in each category has been: malignant, 83; atypical, 26; inadequate, 7; benign, 2. As in most other series, the false-negative rate is low and so patients with a benign pattern can avoid a thyroidectomy if there are no other indications for surgery. In our own unit, and in other centres, the introduction of fine-needle aspiration biopsy as the decision point for single nodules has resulted in a significant reduction in the number of patients undergoing thyroidectomy as a biopsy for benign disease.[15]

It has been argued that in smaller centres, where cytological expertise is lacking, fine-needle aspiration biopsy can not be relied on. It has been shown however that, even in small county hospitals, good quality reports can be obtained with a degree of commitment and a relatively short period of training by a cytologist. In addition, the use of air-dried specimens means that the aspiration can be performed anywhere and the slides sent to major centres for reporting.

Management

Surgical management

Discussion of the management of differentiated thyroid cancer tends to produce more flame than heat. Essential to an understanding of the problem is the fact that thyroid cancer may take many decades before recurrence becomes clinically apparent. In addition, thyroid cancer has no real defined cytological or histological markers to identify patients whose disease will turn out to be more aggressive. The only clear factors are age at presentation and sex, with elderly males being the most prone to aggressive disease. The longest duration between presentation and death observed in our unit was 50 years in a patient who had had a near-total thyroidectomy followed by thyroid suppression at 15 years of age for a papillary cancer, and who subsequently died with metastatic papillary cancer of the lung at age 65. Whilst some authors claim that papillary cancer is benign, those dying from the disease would probably disagree.

The management of differentiated thyroid cancer is relatively clear-cut, and simple surgical principles should prevail. The first step is resection of the involved organ as a total thyroidectomy together with any involved lymph nodes.

The minimal initial operation must be a lobectomy as a biopsy. There is no place for subtotal lobectomy or enucleation of a nodule, as the risk to the recurrent laryngeal nerve should a completion thyroidectomy be required is unacceptable. The isthmus should be taken in order to clear the trachea. If fine-needle aspiration cytology was positive for malignancy preoperatively, a total thyroidectomy should be performed regardless. If not, the specimen is submitted to frozen section and, if this is positive for malignancy, the surgeon should proceed to a completion total thyroidectomy.

Few would argue with the role of total thyroidectomy in the management of the follicular form of differentiated thyroid cancer as there is documented improvement in the survival rate.[16] We believe that, since there are no real differences in the biological behaviour of the different types of thyroid cancer, there is no logic in proposing different forms of management. In this situation, total thyroidectomy fulfils a number of functions:[7]

1. It removes all intraglandular malignancy.
2. It reduces the risk of local recurrence.
3. It reduces the risk of transition to anaplastic forms.
4. It allows the evaluation and subsequent treatment of functional metastases.

There are, in fact, a number of compelling arguments for removing all thyroid tissue even for papillary tumours. Between 30 and 82 per cent of such tumours are multicentric. Whilst not all such microscopic foci of tumour develop into clinical tumours, local recurrence rates of between 5 and 24 per cent have been reported, and when this occurs, subsequent mortality may be as high as 40 per cent.[17] In addition, there is evidence that thyroid cancers may progress to higher grade tumours with time and that anaplastic cancer may well derive from untreated differentiated cancers.[18]

There are numerous cases of localized cancers which, on subsequent radio-iodine scanning after total thyroidectomy, show diffuse interstitial replacement of the lung parenchyma with functioning metastases that were not apparent either clinically or on x-ray imaging.[19] The presence of small remnants of normal thyroid tissue effectively prevents the evaluation of metastases by radio-iodine, as all the tracer is taken up by the remaining normal tissue. Attempts to ablate large remnants of normal thyroid tissue carry a significant risk of inducing malignancies such as leukaemia, owing to the production of radioactive thyroxine from the remnant thyroid during the initial ablative dose.

The only real argument against total thyroidectomy relates to the risk of surgical complications. While criticism is raised that many surgeons are not comfortable with total thyroidectomy, that cannot be accepted as a reasonable stance. With experience the operation of total thyroidectomy can be performed as safely as lesser operations. The risk of bilateral nerve palsy or permanent hypoparathyroidism when total thyroidectomy is undertaken for small tumours in one lobe is exceedingly small when carried out by experienced surgeons.[20] The most important factor is surgical technique. Damage to both the recurrent laryngeal nerves and to the blood supply of the parathyroid glands can be minimized by employing the 'capsular' technique,[21] with careful dissection on the capsule and ligation and division of the small tertiary vessels as shown in Fig. 7.3.

For these reasons we recommend, along with many other authors,[7,20,22,23] that total thyroidectomy is the appropriate procedure for the initial management of all forms of differentiated thyroid cancer.

Lymph node involvement

Lymph node involvement should be assessed preoperatively and, if localized, removal by 'berry picking' is permissible. Paratracheal nodes can be locally excised with preservation of the recurrent laryngeal nerve. Lateral cervical nodes may require a modified neck dissection with preservation of sternomastoid muscles, accessory nerve and internal jugular vein. There is no evidence that aggressive neck dissection for involved lymph nodes offers any survival advantage or reduces the risk of local recurrence when compared with simple excision.[24]

Anaplastic cancer

Whilst all patients with this form of thyroid cancer have usually died from their disease within one or two years, aggressive surgery should still be performed if possible. Removal of the local tumour mass may be the only means of avoiding the alternative of strangulation, and a reasonable remission may be obtained with a combination of chemotherapy and external-beam irradiation. Tracheostomy, however, should be avoided as it may well become the track for a fungating tumour.

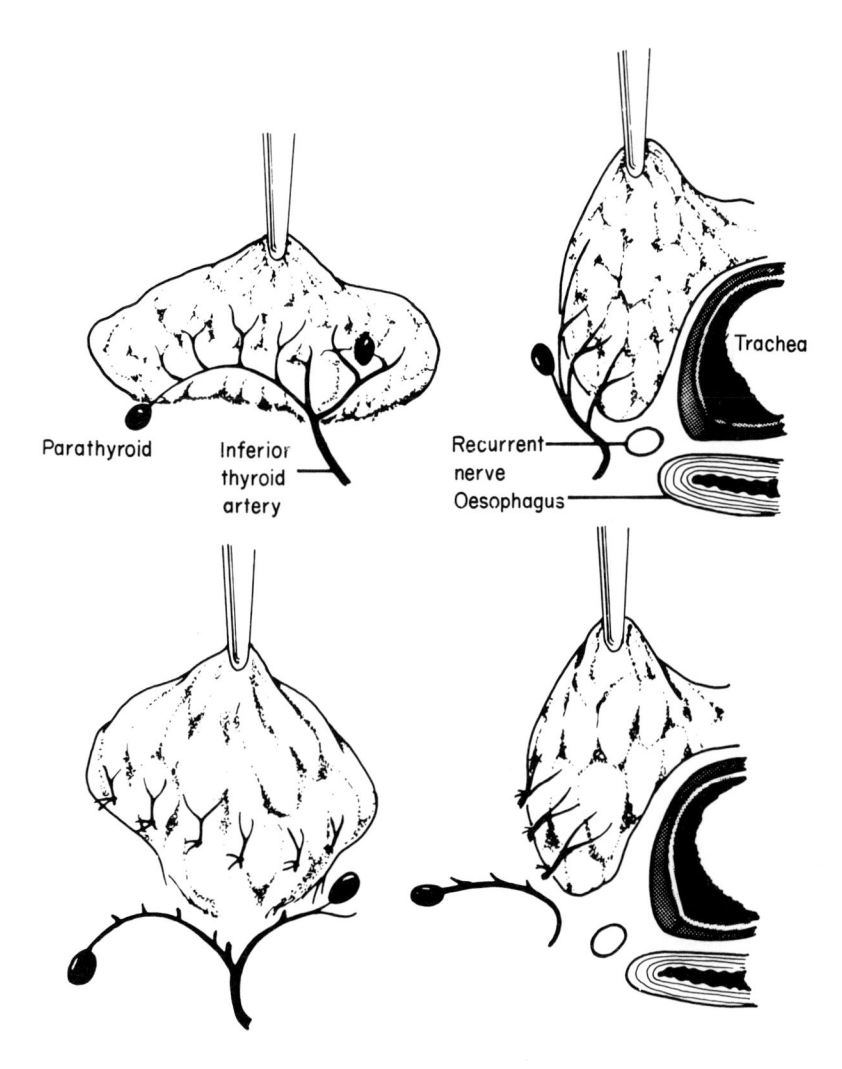

Fig. 7.3 Dissection used during the capsular technique for thyroidectomy, with ligation and division of the small tertiary vessels on the gland, preserving the blood supply to the parathyroid glands and protecting the recurrent laryngeal nerve. (Reproduced from reference 21 with the kind permission of J. B. Lippincott Co., Philadelphia)

Medullary cancer

The diagnosis of this disease can usually be confirmed preoperatively on fine-needle aspiration, and confirmed by demonstrating elevated serum calcitonin levels. Total thyroidectomy is indicated, together with a central node dissection. Adequate clearance of tumour at the first procedure is usually the only chance these patients have to achieve long-term survival.

Lymphoma

Surgery is necessary only to establish the diagnosis, if this cannot be achieved by fine-needle aspiration biopsy, or to relieve a compromised airway. Chemotherapy and radiotherapy provide the best form of definitive treatment.

Radio-iodine therapy

Following total thyroidectomy, complete ablation of all residual normal thyroid tissue should be achieved by an ablative dose of 6 GBq (150 mCi) of ^{131}I. In our hands, although every effort is made to perform a total thyroidectomy, complete removal of all tissue such that no uptake is seen on the initial postoperative 200 MBq (5 mCi) scan, is achieved in only 3 per cent of cases. If lower scan doses are used, significant residual tissue in the neck may be missed. Only after all normal thyroid tissue has been ablated can microscopic metastatic disease be detected. In our experience, 26 per cent of patients have required more than one ablative dose to remove all residual tissue following total thyroidectomy. Our current protocol employs scanning of patients off thyroxine therapy at regular intervals, initially every six months then gradually increasing to every two years. Thyroglobulin is measured both on and off thyroxine in order to assist with the detection of recurrent metastatic disease. The duration of hypothyroidism can be minimized by changing patients over to triiodothyronine therapy six weeks prior to the scan date, then withdrawing this medication 10 days beforehand.

It has been argued that follow-up scans are not required and that simple follow-up with repeated serum thyroglobulin estimations is all that is required.[25] In our experience, however, a significant number of patients (10 out of 363 treated so far) will have a negative thyroglobulin level, even off thyroxine, in the presence of a positive scan. The discriminatory value of thyroglobulin alone is even poorer when suppressive doses of thyroxine are being taken.

The morbidity arising from routine radio-iodine ablation is very low, and justifies its continuing use as the benefits outweigh the risks. Whilst the induction of haematological malignancies remains a possibility, Emrich and Creutzig[26] have demonstrated that this really only occurs in patients with widespread bony metastases and following multiple cumulative doses, and that therapy below 60 GBq (1.5 Ci) is without long-term hazard to the patient. In our experience with 363 patients treated with ablative radio-iodine, there have been only two cases of lymphoma and one case of leukaemia, all associated with multiple doses. On the other hand, in our series the relative survival (compared with an age- and sex-matched Australian population) of young patients with differentiated thyroid cancer so treated is 99 per cent (Fig. 7.4).

Future directions

The introduction of measurement of DNA content in assessing the prognosis in patients with thyroid cancer of follicular cell origin is one of the promising future directions in the management of thyroid cancer. Histologic appearances and pathological classification appear to have little bearing on subsequent survival,

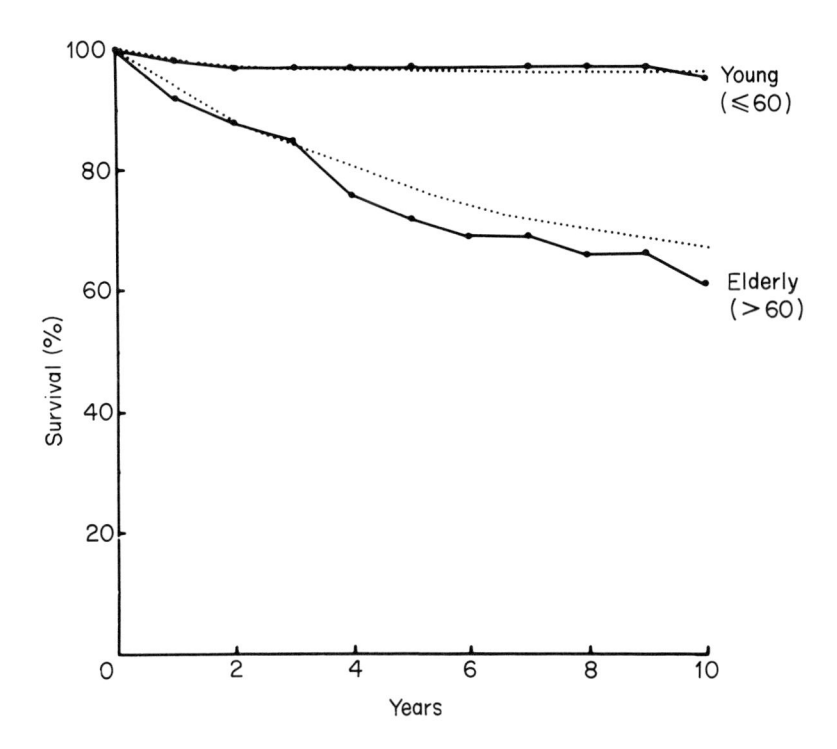

Fig. 7.4 Cumulative survival of young and older patients with differentiated thyroid cancer, compared with an age- and sex-matched Australian population. (Reproduced from reference 7 with the kind permission of Blackwell Scientific, Australia)

whereas there is increasing evidence that measurement of DNA content may well be an accurate predictor of biologic behaviour. Cohn et al.[27] were able to show that, for papillary thyroid cancer, DNA content predicted survival absolutely, with no deaths in patients with a diploid pattern on cytometry, all the deaths occurring when an aneuploid DNA pattern was demonstrated. Similar results have been obtained for follicular cancers.[28] The ability to determine DNA content on fine-needle aspirates may well determine future surgical approaches, with diploid tumours being treated by simple lobectomy with more radical surgery being reserved for aneuploid thyroid cancer.

Conclusions

Whereas nodular thyroid disease is common in most communities, thyroid cancer remains a rare disorder. The first problem facing the surgeon is to be able to differentiate those thyroid nodules requiring surgical excision from those which are benign and do not require treatment. While standard teaching has emphasized appearances on nuclear scans and ultrasound, these modalities have now largely been replaced by the use of fine-needle aspiration biopsy, enabling direct cytological examination of the tumour. Once diagnosed, appropriate therapy is best achieved by maintaining sound surgical principles, removing the affected organ by total thyroidectomy, followed by radio-iodine therapy to ablate all functioning thyroid cells. Surgeons should equip themselves to become comfortable with thyroid anatomy and pathology so that they can perform total thyroidectomy safely with a low morbidity. To do less than this, and attempt to ablate any excess of remnant thyroid tissue, leads to an unacceptable body burden of ^{131}I for the young patient.

References

1. Williams E.D. Pathology and natural history. In: Duncan E. (ed.): *Thyroid Cancer*. Berlin: Springer, 1980.
2. Riccabona G. *Thyroid Cancer: Its Epidemiology, Clinical Features and Treatment*. Berlin: Springer-Verlag, 1987.
3. Koroff J.M., DeGroot L.J. The management of radiation-induced tumours of the thyroid. *Clinics Endocrin. Metab.* 1981; **10:** 299–315.
4. Conrad, R.A., Dobyns B.M., Jutow W.W. Thyroid neoplasia as a late effect of exposure to radioactive iodine in the fallout. *JAMA*. 1970; **214:** 316–24.
5. McLeod M.K., East M.E., Burney R.E., Harnes J.K., Thompson N.W. Hashimoto's thyroiditis revisited: the association with thyroid cancer remains obscure. *World J. Surg.* 1988; **12:** 509–16.
6. Schlumberger M., Tubiana M., deVathaire F., *et al*. Long term results of treatment of 283 patients with lung metastases from differentiated thyroid cancer. *J. Clin. Endocrin. Metab.* 1986; **63:** 960–7.
7. Reeve T.S., Delbridge L., Crummer P. Total thyroidectomy in the management of differentiated thyroid cancer: a review of 258 cases. *Aust. NZ J. Surg.* 1986; **56:** 829–33.
8. Lennquist S. Surgical strategy in thyroid cancer: a review. *Acta Chir. Scand.* 1986; **152:** 321–38.
9. Wheeler M.H. Indications and strategy for surgery of thyroid nodules. *Prog. Surg.* 1988; **19:** 1–20.
10. Ashcraft M.W., van Herle A.J. Management of thyroid nodules. II: Scanning techniques, thyroid suppressive therapy and fine needle aspiration. *Head Neck Surg.* 1981; **3:** 297–322.
11. Wiseman J.C. Nuclear and ultrasound imaging of the thyroid. In: Shizume K., Imura H., Shimizu M. (eds.): *Endocrinology* (Proceedings of the 7th Asia and Oceania Congress of Endocrinology). Amsterdam: Excerpta Medica, 1983: 474–8.
12. Ashcraft M.W., van Herle A.J. Management of thyroid nodules. I: History and physical examination, blood tests, x-ray tests and ultrasonography. *Head Neck Surg.* 1981; **3:** 216–30.
13. Soderstrom N. Aspiration biopsy puncture of goitres for aspiration biopsy. *Acta Med. Scand.* 1952; **144:** 237–44.
14. Lowhagen T., Willems J.S., Lundell G., Sunblad R., Granberg P.O. Aspiration biopsy cytology in diagnosis of thyroid cancer. *World J. Surg.* 1981; **5:** 61–73.
15. Reeve T.S., Delbridge L., Sloan D., Crummer P. The impact of fine needle aspiration biopsy on surgery for single thyroid nodules. *Med. J. Aust.* 1986; **145:** 308–10.
16. Bierwaltes W.H., Nishiyama R.H., Thompson N.W., Copp J.E., Kubo A. Survival time and cure in papillary and follicular thyroid cancer with distant metastases: statistics following University of Michigan therapy. *J. Nucl. Med.* 1982; **23:** 561–8.
17. Tollefson H.R., Shah J.P., Huvos A.G. Papillary carcinoma of the thyroid: clinical recurrence in the thyroid gland after initial surgical treatment. *Amer. J. Surg.* 1972; **124:** 468–72.
18. Nishiyama R.H., Dunn E.L., Thompson N.W. Anaplastic spindle-cell and giant cell tumors of the thyroid gland. *Cancer*. 1972; **30:** 113–27.
19. Grant S., Luttrell B., Reeve T.S., *et al*. Thyroglobulin may be undetectable in serum of patients with metastatic disease secondary to differentiated thyroid carcinoma. *Cancer*. 1984; **54:** 1625–8.
20. Perzik S.L. The place of total thyroidectomy in the management of 909 patients with thyroid disease. *Amer. J. Surg.* 1976; **132:** 480–3.

21. Reeve T.S., Delbridge L., Cohen A., Crummer P. Total thyroidectomy: the preferred option for multinodular goiter. *Ann. Surg.* 1988; **206:** 782–6.
22. Clark O.H. Total thyroidectomy—the treatment of choice for patients with differentiated thyroid cancer. *Ann. Surg.* 1982; **196:** 361–70.
23. Reeve T.S., Delbridge L. Thyroid cancers of follicular cell origin: the place of radical or limited surgery. *Prog. Surg.* 1988; **19:** 78–88.
24. Mazzaferi L.E., Young R.L. Papillary carcinoma—a 10-year follow-up report of the impact of therapy in 576 patients. *Amer. J. Med.* 1981; **70:** 511–18.
25. Schlumberger M., Fragu P., Parmentier C., Tubiana M. Thyroglobulin assay in the follow-up of patients with differentiated thyroid carcinoma: comparison of its value in patients with or without normal residual thyroid tissue. *Acta Endocrinol.* 1981; **98:** 215–21.
26. Emrich D., Creutzig H. Benefits and risk of radio-iodine therapy in differentiated thyroid carcinoma. *Prog. Surg.* 1988; **19:** 133–46.
27. Cohn K., Backdahl M., Forsslund G., *et al.* Prognostic value of nuclear DNA content in papillary thyroid carcinoma. *World J. Surg.* 1984; **8:** 474–80.
28. Backdahl M., Auer G., Forsslund G., *et al.* Prognostic value of nuclear DNA content in follicular thyroid tumours. *Acta Chir. Scand.* 1986; **152:** 1–7.

8

Avoiding bowel ostomies

R.J. Nicholls, MChir, FRCS

Introduction

There are two general indications for constructing a stoma. Firstly, a stoma is inevitable after operations which remove the anal sphincter mechanism. Secondly, a stoma may be indicated to divert the faecal stream owing to the presence of distal pathology. In the former circumstance, the stoma is permanent and usually constructed from the terminal or end part of the intestine. In the latter, the aim and hope is that it will be temporary and is often (although by no means always) formed from a loop of intestine.

Stoma avoidance has been a major theme in gastrointestinal surgery for many years, and notable achievements in reducing the incidence of colostomy and ileostomy have been made. It has become a topic of such interest that plastic procedures to replace anal sphincter function after total rectal excision have even been described. It may well be in future that these will prove to be satisfactory, but at the present time this is doubtful. A well-fashioned stoma with good aftercare support is a very satisfactory solution for most patients. Any attempt to avoid a stoma must offer an improved quality of life.

The type of pathology is the fundamental constraint when choosing between a stoma or no stoma in a particular circumstance. In cancer, for example, it is the surgeon's first duty to select the procedure with the greatest chance of eradicating the disease; avoiding a stoma takes second place. An operation which avoids a stoma at the expense of adequate cancer treatment is unacceptable because the consequence of local treatment failure is usually death. In colitis the same principle is generally true, but since disease-related failure is less serious for the patient, it may be reasonable in certain cases to try a stoma-avoiding procedure in the hope that function will be satisfactory.

The results of surgery depend more upon tactics than the skill of execution. Mistakes in choosing the type of procedure and its timing will profoundly influence subsequent events, however beautifully the operation was done. This is especially true when deciding between total rectal excision and a sphincter-preserving procedure for rectal cancer. It is therefore essential to define criteria to allow the choice to be made as safely as possible.

Much attention has been directed to avoiding a permanent stoma. Temporary stomas, however, cause morbidity and mortality, they are unpleasant for the patient and increase the cost of treatment. Developments in anastomotic technique have led to a fall in the number of cases defunctioned after major restorative resections. In malignant large bowel obstruction, extended resections and more recently lasers are available as a means of reducing the need for a stoma.

Avoidance of a permanent colostomy

A permanent end colostomy is required after total rectal excision with removal of the anal sphincter mechanism. There are three diseases in which this operation may be necessary: these include rectal cancer, anal cancer and Crohn's disease.

Rectal cancer

The decision between total rectal excision and a sphincter-preserving operation is based on criteria which are now reasonably well established. The evidence suggests that stage for stage survival and local recurrence rates after each type of procedure are similar if the criteria are observed.[1-4] The three most important factors are all pathological and include (a) the level of the tumour, (b) the degree of local spread, and (c) the presence of distant metastases. The level of the tumour and extent of local spread will determine whether adequate local clearance without removal of the anal sphincter can be achieved.

Level of tumour

The clearance obtained by both total rectal excision and anterior resection is the same, proximally along the bowel, within the lymphovascular pedicle and at the lateral margins of the growth. It is in the length of rectum distal to the growth that there is a difference. Pathological studies have shown that malignant spread below the lower border of the macroscopic extent of tumour is limited,[5-7] being less than 2 cm in over 95 per cent of cases. Clinical studies have shown little relationship between the length of distal margin of rectal wall below the tumour and survival or local recurrence.[8-10] The conclusion from these studies is that a distal margin of 2 cm is likely to be satisfactory. In the case of carcinomas within 8 cm of the anal verge, this means that growths down to 7 cm, or occasionally 6 cm, may well be suitable for an anterior resection since the anal canal will still be fully preserved.

Extent of local spread

Local recurrence in the presence of an anastomosis is most undesirable. A palliative colostomy is often needed, and discharge of blood and mucus per anum can be very troublesome. Thus it is unwise to carry out an anterior resection in a case where local recurrence seems likely. There is a direct relationship between the degree of local spread and the incidence of local recurrence. This was first reported by Dukes and Bussey[11] on pathological examination of resected specimens. Local recurrence is also related to the level of tumour, being more likely the more distal the growth.[12] Local recurrence is a most important source of morbidity and with few exceptions patients with local recurrence will die of their disease. This may be because most have disseminated disease as well. In the study of Berge *et al.*, only 8 per cent of local recurrences observed at post mortem were found to exist without distant metastases.[13]

In a recent study it was possible to predict the occurrence of local recurrence after surgery with a high level of confidence from the histopathological examination of the lateral margin of the tumour.[14] Of 51 patients followed for two years, 13 had had lateral margin involvement, of whom 11 subsequently developed local recurrence. This compared with only one case in the remaining 38 without lateral margin involvement.

Distant metastases

Low anterior resection, especially when it involves a coloanal anastomosis, has a fairly high risk of anastomotic complications (10–40 per cent). The risk is three times greater in patients with disseminated disease.[15] When life expectancy is limited perhaps to months, complications with or without a defunctioning stoma offer poor palliation, and bowel function is often poor for several months where the anastomosis is low. A Hartmann's operation in this circumstance offers the patient as short a hospitalization as possible and may well be the preferred option.

Other factors

The degree of histological differentiation is related to pathological stage, which influences survival. Anaplastic tumours have a high incidence of local recurrence.[16] However, no difference in survival was observed in patients with poorly differentiated middle-third carcinomas after either anterior resection or total rectal excision.[17] Histological differentiation is probably a less important factor than was previously thought, although a preoperative grade of anaplasia in a biopsy is likely to signal a Dukes C lesion. The wishes of the patient as, too, the desire of the surgeon should be subordinate to what is possible in terms of the pathology. The build of the patient only very rarely precludes a restorative operation. Techniques allowing an anastomosis between colon and lower rectum or anal canal have been available for many years.

Preoperative selection

Digital examination and sigmoidoscopy will enable the level of the tumour to be determined. In general a tumour lying above or at the upper border of the prostate can be treated by anterior resection. Digital examination can also gauge local extent.[18] Preoperative clinical staging is accurate in 70–80 per cent of cases in placing tumours into two groups, which include: locally not extensive (stage 1) and locally extensive (stage 2).[19] These correlate well with subsequent local recurrence rates. Imaging by computed tomography is useful in showing extensive spread with invasion of neighbouring organs, but intraluminal ultrasound is clearly the most sensitive and specific means of assessing local spread. This has been discussed fully in Chapter 12. Correlation between ultrasound stage based on the TNM classification and the histopathological extent is approximately 95 per cent.[20,21] Histological examination of a preoperative biopsy will enable the degree of differentiation to be determined.

Anterior resection

In recent years the incidence of anterior resection has risen at the expense of total rectal excision owing to the development in anastomotic techniques and to the appreciation that survival and local failure rates are similar after each operation when applied to upper and middle rectal carcinomas.

Modern anastomotic techniques include colorectal and coloanal anastomosis by hand suture or staples. There is evidence that leakage after hand suture is surgeon-related,[22] ranging from 5 to over 30 per cent. Leakage of stapled anastomosis is probably not significantly different[23,24] and occurred in 9.8 per cent in a large survey of American surgeons.[25] The double-stapled technique since the introduction of the EEA-Premium instrument (American Autosutures) is very satisfactory and undoubtedly speeds the procedure, although with the disadvantage of high cost.

There is a remarkable difference in local recurrence rates reported in different series (Table 8.1). Phillips *et al.* reported the results in 4228 patients operated

Table 8.1 Pelvic local recurrence rates after major resection of middle and lower third rectal carcinoma

Reference		Operation	Number of patients	Local recurrence (%)
26	Gilbertsen (1960)	AP	89	36
12	Morson *et al.* (1963)	AP	1115	12
27	Pilipsen *et al.* (1984)	AP + RA	330	30
4	Williams and Johnston (1984)	AP	83	8
		AR	71	11
16	Phillips *et al.* (1984)	AP	478	12
		AR	370	18
10	Williams (1985)	AR	74	14
		AP (matched)		19
28	Hurst *et al.* (1982)	AR	34	32
29	Heald and Ryall (1986)	AR	115	2.6

on by nearly 100 surgeons partaking in the St Mary's Hospital Large Bowel Cancer Project and produced evidence suggesting that local recurrence was surgeon-related.[15] High local recurrence rates may be related to attempting anterior resection in growths in the lower third,[28] and they may be lower when the entire mesorectum is removed with the rectum.[29] This latter manoeuvre may minimize local recurrence rates, but local recurrence occurs after total rectal excision in which the mesorectum is also removed. Clearly pathological factors are more important than technicalities.

Functional results

The more distal the anastomosis, the more likely it is that there will be frequency of defaecation with some urgency. Loss of the rectal reservoir with an already impaired anal sphincter may result in incontinence. Pull-through or endoanal procedures may themselves damage the sphincter. Functional disturbances tend to improve with the passage of time[30] but do not resolve in all cases. More attention has been given to continence than to the frequency of defaecation, and it is only in recent years, with the development of ileoanal procedures, that this latter aspect of function has been given due recognition. Lazorthes et al.[31] and Parc et al.[32] describe the use of a colonic reservoir with coloanal anastomosis for reconstruction after anterior resection. When compared with patients having a straight coloanal operation, stool frequency at one year was significantly less in the reservoir (2.4 and 3.6 respectively).[33] An inverse relationship between capacitance and frequency of defaecation was also demonstrated. The patients also had normal continence. These data suggest that the use of a reservoir can improve function.

Frequency values were not given by Parks and Percy in their paper on coloanal anastomosis.[34] A clinical and physiological comparison of 13 reservoir and 15 straight coloanal patients has suggested that the reservoir eliminates the few cases of marked frequency that occur in the latter group.[34]

Continence has been better studied, and after low anterior resection about 20 per cent of patients have some soiling postoperatively, with a further 10 per cent having difficulty in holding flatus.[35] In the 76 patients reported by Parks and Percy,[34] continence was normal in 50 per cent and satisfactory in a further 46 per cent. Only one patient required a colostomy for incontinence.

Local excision

About 5 per cent of tumours in the lower rectum are suitable for local treatment which is an alternative to total rectal excision and not to anterior resection. The criteria for selection are based on factors which indicate whether or not loco-regional spread has occurred. By digital examination and intraluminal ultrasound it is possible to identify tumours confined to the rectal wall, less than 3 cm in diameter and accessible to treatment in 95 per cent of cases. The presence of regional nodal enlargement and of a poorly differentiated tumour on the preoperative biopsy are contraindications to local excision.

Surgical removal (taking the full thickness of the rectal wall) offers a specimen which is examined by the pathologist. Evidence of penetration of the bowel wall or of vascular or lymphatic invasion should lead to an immediate total rectal excision. With this policy, cancer-specific five-year survival rates of 95 per cent can be obtained.[36,37] Other techniques, including contact radiotherapy,[38] electrocoagulation[39] and laser destruction,[40] do not yield a specimen but refinements of imaging technology may make histological examination less important in the future.

Anal cancer

For many years most cancers of both the anal canal and the anal margin were treated by total rectal excision. Only those of an early local stage (T1, TNM[41]) were deemed suitable for local excision, with overall five-year survival rates in this group of 45–77 per cent being reported.[42–44]

For many years radical external radiotherapy has been offered in some centres as an alternative to total rectal excision. Overall five-year survival rates ranging from 42 per cent[45] to 59 per cent[46] have been reported, with others recording rates in between.[47] Papillon, using a split course technique of external and interstitial radiotherapy, obtained a five-year crude survival rate of 65 per cent.[38]

More recently, combined chemotherapy and radiotherapy have been used following the first report by Nigro[48] of remarkable tumour regression with a combination of external irradiation (30 Gy) and fluorouracil and mitomycin C. With this treatment the surgical component has diminished to an excision biopsy of the tumour site six weeks after the end of treatment. Rectal excision is then used only as a salvage procedure on failure of chemoradiotherapy. Of 104 patients treated, 20 have died and only 13 had recurrence.[49] Trials comparing chemoradiotherapy with radiotherapy alone are in progress (EORTC, UKCCCR).

Total rectal excision in anal cancer does not appear to produce improved survival over radiotherapy. Radiotherapy does not always result in avoidance of a stoma and sphincter damage by the tumour, and treatment is sufficient for a long-term colostomy to be necessary in about 20 per cent of cases.[38]

Avoidance of a permanent ileostomy

A permanent ileostomy is necessary after proctocolectomy or after proctetomy in a case previously submitted to colectomy. The operation is indicated in patients with inflammatory bowel disease, diffuse neoplastic disease of the large bowel, and occasionally in functional bowel disease (e.g. constipation).

Inflammatory bowel disease

It is now possible with few exceptions to avoid a permanent stoma in patients with *ulcerative colitis*. Two operations are available.

Colectomy with ileorectal anastomosis

For many years this was the only alternative to proctocolectomy with permanent ileostomy in ulcerative colitis. Aylett[50] carried out the procedure in over 90 per cent of cases, but others have been more selective, submitting 30–40 per cent of patients to the procedure.[51,52] Others with a rate of 10 per cent have been very cautious in its use.[53] Besides this evident surgeon-related bias, it is possible to identify criteria for selection based upon the state of the anorectum.

Indications for colectomy with ileorectal anastomosis include the presence of mild inflammation only in a pliant distensible rectum, an adequate anal sphincter, and the absence of severe dysplasia or malignant transformation anywhere in the large bowel.

There is no need to cover the procedure with a temporary stoma. Complications are infrequent. In a series of 125 patients treated at one hospital, there was one postoperative death and three other disease-related deaths.[51]

Complications. Thirty-three patients (28 per cent) had had the rectum excised for persisting inflammation,[18] bleeding,[1] technical failure[5] and neoplastic transformation.[6] Failure was usually late, occurring months to years postoperatively. Information on function is scanty, but 17 per cent of patients with an intact ileorectal anastomosis had a frequency of defaecation per 24 hours of seven or more. About half the patients required antidiarrhoeal medication, and about 20 per cent experienced occasional episodes of incontinence. Others have reported failure rates ranging from less than 10 per cent to 40 per cent.[50] As with the intact large bowel in ulcerative colitis, patients with an ileorectal anastomosis are at risk of developing cancer in the rectal stump. Baker *et al.* reported a 5 per cent rate at 20 years among Aylett's cases.[54] Regular postoperative surveillance is therefore essential in these patients.

Restorative proctocolectomy with ileal reservoir

Ravitch and Sabiston described an operation for familial adenomatosis in which the entire large bowel was removed and an ileoanal anastomosis constructed.[55] Function in terms of frequency and urgency were satisfactory in only about 50 per cent of cases,[56,57] owing to the absence of an adequate 'neorectal' reservoir.[58]

The addition by Parks of an *ileal reservoir* to create capacitance has greatly improved function,[59] and the operation is now well established in the treatment of ulcerative colitis and familial adenomatous polyposis.

Indications. Case selection is important. Patients should be motivated to avoid a permanent ileostomy and should understand the possible complications and other disadvantages that can occur. Medical indications include a diagnosis of ulcerative colitis or familial adenomatous polyposis, where a conventional proctocolectomy would otherwise be necessary, and an adequate anal sphincter.

Crohn's disease is a contraindication, and patients with severe acute colitis or those on high doses of steroids should be treated initially by colectomy with ileostomy and preservation of the rectal stump. The presence of cancer is not a contraindication provided a radical clearance is possible.

Technique. The patient is placed in the Trendelenburg position with legs raised. A routine colectomy is carried out in continuity with full mobilization of the rectum. A close rectal dissection avoids sexual nerve dysfunction.[60] The gut tube is divided at the level of the anorectal junction and the specimen removed. There is no need to leave a rectal stump. Mobility of the mesentery sufficient to bring the terminal ileum to the level of the dentate line is tested by a trial descent before making the reservoir.

Several types of reservoir have been described, including the three-loop,[59] two-loop[61] and four-loop[62] designs (Fig. 8.1). The aim should be to produce a reservoir of adequate capacity which can be joined directly to the anal stump without any interposed segment of small bowel. This latter requirement avoids the failure of spontaneous evacuation which occurred in over 50 per cent of three-loop designs in an early report.[63]

With construction of the reservoir, the residual mucosa is stripped from the

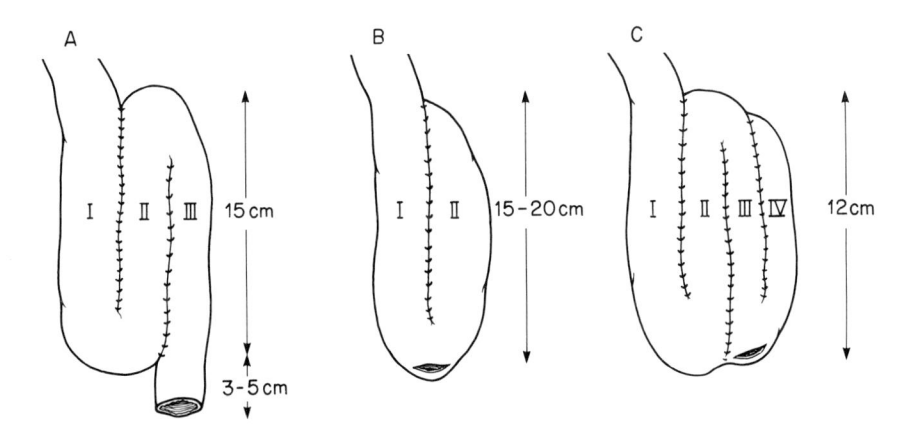

Fig. 8.1 Three-, two- and four-loop intestinal pouches. (Reproduced from reference 62 with the kind permission of Butterworth Scientific)

anal stump and an ileoanal anastomosis carried out. This can be done by hand or with the stapler. A temporary loop ileostomy is then made. This is closed about eight weeks later after healing of the anastomosis has occurred.

There is a controversy as to whether the mucosa in the upper anal canal (transitional zone) should be preserved or excised. It is argued that sensory receptors in this area are important for function.[64] However, preserving a significant amount of mucosa might increase the late risk of malignant transformation.

Results. The results from some published series are shown in Table 8.2. The operative mortality has been low (below 1 per cent). Failure, defined as the need to establish a permanent ileostomy, has ranged from 3 to over 20 per cent. In most large series it is around 5–10 per cent. The most important complications include intestinal obstruction due to adhesions, and some degree of breakdown of the ileoanal anastomosis; both occur in about 10 per cent of cases.

Frequency is inversely related to the capacitance of the reservoir.[66] There

Table 8.2 The results of restorative proctocolectomy with ileal reservoir. (Reproduced from reference 65 with the kind permission of Springer–Verlag, New York)

	Number of patients	Operative death	Laparotomy for obstruction	Pelvic sepsis	Frequency /24 hours mean	Antidiarrhoeal medication (%)
Dozois	188	0	16	9	7.2	40
Rothenberger and Goldberg	91	0	16	21	6	46
Utsunomiya	55	1	4	12	4.5	–
Cohen	125	0	4	10	6–8	70
Nicholls	119	1	14	22	4	23
Hulten	32	0	2	4	5	72
Total	611	2 (0.3%)	56 (9%)	78 (13%)		

is some variation in frequency between series, with a range of mean capacity from 4 to 7 or more times per 24 hours. Night evacuation is probably a more sensitive guide to frequency, which in the author's series occurs one or more times per week in about 20 per cent of patients. Urgency does not appear to be a problem postoperatively, and normal continence occurs in 70–90 per cent of cases. At night minor leakage requiring a pad occurs in 5–40 per cent of patients according to the series reported. In the early years, catheterization of the reservoir per anum was necessary for defaecation in a high proportion of patients having a three-loop reservoir construction.[63] This can be almost completely avoided using a reservoir without the distal ileal segment which was a feature of the original three-loop design. Function tends to improve up to 12 months from closure of the ileostomy.

Long-term follow-up has failed to reveal dysplasia, but about 10–15 per cent of patients develop an inflammation of the reservoir which is symptomatic. 'Pouchitis' can be defined by clinical, endoscopic and histopathological criteria.[77] About 5 per cent of all patients require vitamin B_{12} injections, and several more require iron supplements. About 90 per cent of patients consider the result to be good when questioned on a variety of daily activities and personal feelings.[68]

Diffuse neoplastic disease

Occasionally complete removal of the large bowel may be necessary in cases with several metachronous tumours, but familial adenomatous polyposis is responsible for the largest number of patients in this group. The choice between colectomy with ileorectal anastomosis and restorative proctocolectomy should depend on the assessment of the cancer risk in a given patient. In adolescents this is extremely low. There is therefore every reason to recommend colectomy with ileorectal anastomosis here. The operation is simple, complications are uncommon, function is reasonable and total treatment time is sufficiently short to allow recovery to occur during a school holiday. In the patient over 25 years the risk of cancer rises to a point where about 50 per cent of untreated 35-year-olds are likely already to have formed a cancer. A restorative proctocolectomy in the older patient should eliminate this risk. Only where there is a carcinoma in the lower rectum will a proctocolectomy with permanent ileostomy be necessary.

Constipation

When surgery is applied to idiopathic constipation, colectomy with ileorectal anastomosis leads to a significant improvement in about 60 per cent of patients.[69] In some cases of failure, the inability to defaecate becomes so intolerable that an ileostomy is contemplated. In this circumstance a restorative proctocolectomy is a viable alternative.

Crohn's disease

Avoidance of stomas in Crohn's disease is substantially due to the location of the disease. Where there is rectal inflammation uncontrollable by medical treatment associated with anal sepsis or ulceration, there is little hope of avoiding a permanent stoma. However, in selected cases with anal fistulation or rectovaginal fistula, Lee[70] recommended complete defunctioning using a split ileostomy in which overflow of faeces from proximal to distal limbs of the stoma was impossible. In a series of 29 patients with rectovaginal or severe anorectal fistula, the operation led to improvement or healing in 20 per cent of the cases. Subsequent reversal was possible in some patients, and six (20 per cent) did not have a stoma at the time of the review. Others, however, have had disappointing results with defunctioning.[71]

Temporary stoma avoidance in bowel obstruction

The traditional three-stage approach to acute left-sided large bowel obstruction, which involves performing a colostomy initially, has been challenged in recent years. Obstruction is a common presentation, with up to 30–40 per cent of patients presenting in this condition.[72] Approximately half of these patients will already have disseminated disease, and there is a low incidence of Dukes A cases in obstruction. The patients are often old and weak from water and electrolyte depletion, racked with advanced tumour and operated on at night by a junior surgeon, so it is not surprising that treatment mortality rates are high around 20 per cent.

Information obtained from the Large Bowel Cancer Project has shown no difference in the in-hospital mortality rates among patients treated by staged resection (22 per cent) and those by primary resection (19 per cent). There was, however, an increased mortality in patients operated on by trainee surgeons.[73] A primary resection policy offers considerable advantages in stoma avoidance and shortness of inpatient stay. The use of on-table lavage with primary anastomosis is associated with an acceptably low mortality and morbidity. In a series of 61 obstructed cases, mortality was 8 per cent and anastomotic leakage occurred in 7 per cent. The mean hospital stay was 13 days.[74]

There is no evidence to suggest that survival rates after staged or primary resection are different.[75] Thus there is every indication for aiming to perform a resection with primary anastomosis in these cases. An experienced surgeon and team using on-table lavage might be expected to reduce the death and complication rate.

Resection with primary anastomosis of non-right-sided growths can also be achieved by an extended right hemicolectomy. Tumours in the transverse colon or more distal can be removed with all proximal dilated colon, and an anastomosis between the terminal ileum and the collapsed intestine distal to the obstruction can be carried out.

A recent approach to acute obstruction has been to use intraluminal laser treatment to recanalize the bowel at the point of obstruction. This will lead to the patient's general recovery, allowing a subsequent formal one-stage resection. There is now experience of laser treatment in patients with obstructive symptoms due to inoperable tumour. At one month after treatment approximately 80 per cent of surviving patients have good palliation, but this rate steadily declines to around 40 per cent among those still alive at 12 months.[76,77]

Complications include death in about 1 per cent, mostly due to perforation, and an incidence of abscess, fistula or bleeding in a further 5 per cent.

References

1. Slanetz C.A., Herter F.P., Grinnell R.S. Anterior resection versus abdominoperineal resection for cancer of the rectum and rectosigmoid: an analysis of 524 cases. *Amer. J. Surg.* 1972; **123:** 110–17.
2. Lockhart-Mummery H.E., Ritchie J.K., Hawley P.R. The results of surgical treatment for carcinoma of the rectum at St Mark's Hospital from 1948–1972. *Brit. J. Surg.* 1976; **63:** 673–7.
3. Nicholls R.J., Ritchie J.K., Wadsworth J., Parks A.G. Total excision or restorative resection for carcinoma of the middle third of the rectum. *Brit. J. Surg.* 1979; **69:** 404–9.
4. Williams N.S., Johnston D. Survival and recurrence after sphincter saving resection and abdominoperineal resection for carcinoma of the middle third of the rectum. *Brit. J. Surg.* 1984; **71:** 278–82.
5. Westhues A. Uber die Entstehung und vermeidunt des locanen Rektum Karzinom. *Rezidevs Arch. Klin. Chir.* 1930; **161:** 582–97.
6. Quer E.A., Dahlin D.C., Mayo C.W. Retrograde intramural spread of carcinoma of the rectum and rectosigmoid: a microscopic study. *Surg. Gyn. Obst.* 1953; **46:** 24–30.
7. Penfold J.C.B. A comparison of restorative resection of carcinoma of the middle third of the rectum with abdominoperineal excision. *Aust. NZ J. Surg.* 1974; **44:** 354–6.
8. Wilson S.M., Beahrs O.H. The curative treatment of carcinoma of the sigmoid, rectosigmoid and rectum. *Ann. Surg.* 1975; **183:** 556–65.
9. Pollett W.G., Nicholls R.J. Relationship between the extent of distal clearance and survival and local recurrence rates after curative anterior resection for carcinoma of the rectum. *Ann. Surg.* 1983; **198:** 159–63.
10. Williams N.S., Durdey P., Johnston D. The outcome following sphincter-saving resection and abdominoperineal resection for low rectal cancer. *Brit. J. Surg.* 1985; **72:** 595–8.
11. Dukes C.E., Bussey H.J.R. The spread of rectal cancer and its effect on prognosis. *Brit. J. Can.* 1958; **12:** 209–20.
12. Morson B.C., Vaughan E.G., Bussey H.J.R. Pelvic recurrence after excision of the rectum for carcinoma. *Brit. Med. J.* 1963; **2:** 13–18.
13. Berge T., Ekelund G., Mellner C., *et al*. Carcinoma of the colon and rectum in a defined population: an epidemiological, clinical and postmortem investigation of colorectal carcinoma. *Acta Chir. Scand.* 1973; **438:** 1–86.
14. Quirke P., Durdey P., Dixon M.F., Williams N.S. Local recurrence of rectal adenocarcinoma due to inadequate surgical resection: histopathological study of lateral tumour spread and surgical excision. *Lancet.* 1986; **i:** 996–9.
15. Vandertoll D.J., Beahrs O.H. Carcinoma of the rectum and low sigmoid: evaluation of anterior resection of 1776 favorable lesions. *Arch. Surg.* 1965; **90:** 793–8.
16. Phillips R.K.S., Hittinger R., Blesovsky L., Fry J.S., Fielding L.P. Local recurrence following 'curative' surgery for large bowel cancer. 1: The overall picture. *Brit. J. Surg.* 1984; **71:** 12–16.
17. Elliot M.S., Todd I.P., Nicholls R.J. Radical restorative surgery for poorly differentiated carcinoma of the mid-rectum. *Brit. J. Surg.* 1982; **69:** 273–4.
18. Mason A.Y. Malignant tumours of the rectum: local excision. *Clin. Gastroenterol.* 1975; **4:** 582–93.
19. Nicholls R.J., Galloway D.J., Mason A.Y., Boyle P. Clinical local staging of rectal cancer. *Brit. J. Surg.* 1985; **72** (Suppl): 51–2.
20. Hildebrandt U., Feifel G., Schwartz H.P., Scherr O. Endorectal ultrasound: instrumentation and clinical aspects. *Int. J. Colorectal Dis.* 1986; **1:** 203–7.
21. Beynon J., Foy D.M.A., Roc A.M., Temple L.N., Mortensen N.J.McC. Endoluminal ultrasound in the assessment of local invasion in rectal cancer. *Brit. J. Surg.* 1986; **73:** 474–7.
22. Fielding L.P., Stewart-Brown S., Blesovsky L., *et al*. Anastomotic integrity after operations for large bowel cancer: a multicentre study. *Brit. Med. J.* 1980; **281:** 411–14.
23. Beart R.W., Kelly K.A. Randomised prospective evaluation of the EEA stapler for colorectal anastomosis. *Amer. J. Surg.* 1981; **141:** 143–7.
24. McGinn F.P., Gartell D.C., Clifford P.C., *et al*. Staples or sutures for low colorectal

anastomoses: a prospective randomised trial. *Brit. J. Surg.* 1985; **72:** 603–5.
25. Smith L.E. Anastomosis with EEA stapler after anterior colonic resection. *Dis. Colon Rect.* 1981; **24:** 236–42.
26. Gilbertsen V.A. Adenocarcinoma of the rectum: incidence and locations of recurrent tumor following operations for cure. *Ann. Surg.* 1960; **151:** 340–8.
27. Pilipsen S.J., Heilweil M., Quan S.H.Q., et al. Patterns of pelvic recurrence following definitive resection of rectal cancer. *Cancer.* 1984; **53:** 1354–62.
28. Hurst P.A., Prout W.G., Kelly J.M., et al. Local recurrence after low anterior resection using the staple gun. *Brit. J. Surg.* 1982; **69:** 275–6.
29. Heald R.J., Ryall R.D.H. Recurrence and survival after total mesorectal excision for rectal cancer. *Lancet.* 1986; **ii:** 1479–82.
30. Bennett R.S. The place of pull-through operations in the treatment of carcinoma of the rectum. *Dis. Colon Rect.* 1976; **19:** 420–4.
31. Lazorthes F., Fages P., Chiotasso P., et al. Resection of the rectum with construction of colonic reservoir and colon and anastomosis for carcinoma of the rectum. *Brit. J. Surg.* 1986; **73:** 136–8.
32. Parc R., Tiret E., Frileux P., et al. Resection and colo-anal anastomosis with colonic reservoir for rectal cancer. *Brit. J. Surg.* 1986; **73:** 139–41.
33. Nicholls R.J., Lubowski D.Z., Donaldson D.R. Comparison of straight and reservoir coloanal anastomosis following rectal excision for benign and malignant conditions. *Brit. J. Surg.* 1988; **75:** 318–20.
34. Parks A.G., Percy J.P. Resection and sutured coloanal anastomosis for rectal carcinoma. *Brit. J. Surg.* 1982; **69:** 301–4.
35. Goligher J.C., Duthie H.L., De Dombal F.T., et al. Abdomino-anal pullthrough for tumours of the mid-third of the rectum. *Brit. J. Surg.* 1965; **52:** 328–35.
36. Whiteway J., Nicholls R.J., Morson B.C. The role of surgical local excision in the treatment of rectal cancer. *Brit. J. Surg.* 1985; **72:** 694–7.
37. Hermanek P., Gall F.P. Early (microinvasive) colorectal carcinoma: pathology, diagnosis, surgical treatment. *Int. J. Colorectal Dis.* 1986; **1:** 79–84.
38. Papillon J. Radiation therapy in the conservative management of cancers of the low rectum and anal canal. *Int. J. Colorectal Dis.* 1986; **1:** 251–5.
39. Madden J.L., Kandalaft S. Clinical evaluation electrocoagulation in the treatment of cancer of the rectum. *Amer. J. Surg.* 1971; **122:** 347–51.
40. Brunetaud J.M., Mosquet L., Houcke M., et al. Villous adenoma of the rectum: results of endoscopic treatment with argon and Nd: YAG lasers. *Gastroenterology.* 1985; **89:** 832–7.
41. Papillon J. *Rectal and Anal Cancers.* Berlin: Springer-Verlag, 1982: 124–5.
42. Greenall M.J., Quan S.H.Q., Urmacher C., et al. Treatment of epidermoid carcinoma of the anal canal. *Surg. Gyn. Obs.* 1985; **161:** 502–17.
43. Borman B., Moertel C.G., O'Connell M.G., et al. Carcinoma of the anal canal: a clinical and pathological study of 188 cases. *Cancer.* 1984; **54:** 114–25.
44. Pinna Pintor M., Nicholls R.J., Northover J.M.A. The surgical treatment of anal carcinoma. *Brit. J. Surg.* 1989; **78:** 806–810.
45. Eschwege F., Breteau N., Chavy A., et al. Complication de la radiotherapie transcutanee des epitheliomas due canal anal. *Gastroenterol. Clin. Biol.* (Paris). 1979; **3:** 183–6.
46. Cummins B., Keane T., Thomas G., et al. Results and toxicity of the treatment of anal canal carcinoma by radiation therapy or irradation therapy and chemotherapy. *Cancer.* 1984; **56:** 2062–8.
47. Rousseau J., Mathieu G., Fenton J. Resultats et complications de la radiotherapie des epitheliomas du canal anal: étude de 128 cas traites de 1956 à 1970. *Gastroenterol. Clin. Biol.* (Paris). 1979; **3** 207–8.
48. Nigro N.D., Vaitkevicius V.R., Considine B. Combined therapy for cancer of the anal canal: a preliminary report. *Dis. Colon Rect.* 1974; **17:** 354–6.
49. Nigro N.D. An evaluation of combined therapy for squamous cell cancer of the anal canal. *Dis. Colon Rect.* 1984; **27:** 763–6.
50. Aylett S.O. Three hundred cases of diffuse ulcerative colitis treated by total colectomy and ileorectal anastomosis. *Brit. Med. J.* 1966; **1:** 1001–5.
51. Hawley P.R. Ileorectal anastomosis. *Brit. J. Surg.* 1985; **72** (Suppl): 75–82.
52. Jones P.F., Munro A., Ewan S.W.B. Colectomy and ileorectal anastomosis for colitis: report on a personal series with a critical review. *Brit. J. Surg.* 1977; **64:** 615–23.

53. Adson A.A., Cooperman A.M., Farrow G.M. Ileorectostomy for ulcerative diseases of the colon. *Arch. Surg.* 1972; **104**: 424–8.
54. Baker W., Glass R.E., Ritchie J.K., *et al.* Cancer of the rectum following colectomy and ileorectal anastomosis for ulcerative colitis. *Brit. J. Surg.* 1978; **65**: 862–8.
55. Ravitch M.M., Sabiston D.C. Anal ileostomy with preservation of the sphincter: a proposed operation in patients requiring total colectomy for benign lesions. *Surg. Gyn. Obst.* 1947; **84**: 1095–9.
56. Valiente M., Bacon H. Construction of a puch using 'pantaloon' technique for pull-through of ileum following total colectomy: a report of experimental work and results. *Amer. J. Surg.* 1955; **90**: 742–50.
57. Telander R.L., Perrault J. Total colectomy with rectal mucosectomy and ileoanal anastomosis in young patients: its use for ulcerative colitis and familial polyposis. *Arch. Surg.* 1981; **116**: 623–7.
58. Heppel J., Kelly K.A., Phillips S.F., *et al.* Physiologic aspects of continence after colectomy, mucosal proctectomy and endorectal ileoanal anastomosis. *Ann. Surg.* 1982; **195**: 435–9.
59. Parks A.G., Nicholls R.J. Proctocolectomy without ileostomy for ulcerative colitis. *Brit. Med. J.* 1978; **2**: 85–8.
60. Leicester R.J., Ritchie J.K., Wadsworth J., *et al.* Sexual function and perineal wound healing after intersphincteric excision of the rectum for inflammatory bowel disease. *Dis. Colon Rect.* 1984; **27**: 244–8.
61. Utsunomiya J., Iwama T., Imajo M., *et al.* Total colectomy, mucosal proctectomy, and ileoanal anastomosis. *Dis. Colon Rect.* 1980; **23**: 459–66.
62. Nicholls R.J., Pezim M.E. Restorative proctocolectomy with ileal reservoir for ulcerative colitis and familial adenomatous polyposis; a comparison of three reservoir designs. *Brit. J. Surg.* 1985; **72** 470–2.
63. Nicholls R.J., Pescatori M., Motson R.W. Restorative proctocolectomy with a three-loop ileal reservoir for ulcerative colitis and familial polyposis. *Ann. Surg.* 1984; **199**: 383–8.
64. Johnston D., Holdsworth P.J., Nasmyth D.G., *et al.* Preservation of the entire anal canal in conservative proctocolectomy for ulcerative colitis: a pilot study comparing end-to-end ileoanal anastomosis without mucosal resection with mucosal proctectomy and endoanal anastomosis. *Brit. J. Surg.* 1987; **74**: 940–4.
65. Dozois R.R., Goldberg S., Rothenberger D., *et al.* Symposium: Restorative proctocolectomy with ileal reservoir. *Int. J. Colorectal Dis.* 1986; **1**: 2–19.
66. Nicholls R.J., Moskowitz R.L., Shepherd N.A. Restorative proctocolectomy with ileal reservoir. *Brit. J. Surg.* 1985; **72** (Suppl): 76–7.
67. Moskowitz R.L., Shepherd N.A., Nicholls R.J. An assessment of inflammation in the reservoir after restorative proctocolectomy with ileoanal ileal reservoir. *Int. J. Colorectal Dis.* 1986; **1**: 167–74.
68. Pezim M.E., Nicholls R.J. Quality of life after restorative proctocolectomy. *Brit. J. Surg.* 1985; **72**: 31–3.
69. Kamm M.A. The surgical treatment of severe idiopathic constipation. *Int. J. Colorectal Dis.* 1987; **2**: 229–35.
70. Harper P.H., Kettlewell M.G.W., Leed E.C.G. The effect of split ileostomy on perianal Crohn's disease. *Brit. J. Surg.* 1982; **69**: 608–10.
71. Lockhart Mummery H.E. Anal lesions in Crohn's disease. *Brit. J. Surg.* 1985; **72**: (Suppl): 95–6.
72. Gill P.G., Morris P.J. The survival of patients with colorectal cancer treated in a regional hospital. *Brit. J. Surg.* 1978; **65**: 17.
73. Fielding L.P., Wells B.W. Survival after primary and staged resection for large bowel obstruction caused by cancer. *Brit. J. Surg.* 1974; **61**: 16.
74. Koruth N.M., Krukowski Z.H., Youngson G.G., *et al.* Intra-operative colonic irrigation in the management of left-sided large bowel emergencies. *Brit. J. Surg.* 1985; **72**: 708–11.
75. Phillips R.K.S., Hittinger R., Fry J.S., *et al.* Malignant large bowel obstruction. *Brit. J. Surg.* 1985; **72**: 296–302.
76. Mathus-Vliegen E.M.H., Tytgat G.N.T. Nd: YAG laser photocoagulation in gastroenterology—its role in palliation of colorectal cancer. *Lasers Med. Sci.* 1986; **1**: 75–80.
77. Bown S.G., Barr H., Matthewson K., *et al.* Endoscopic treatment of inoperable colorectal cancer with the Nd: YAG laser. *Brit. J. Surg.* 1986; **73**: 949–52.

9

New thoughts and methods in colorectal cancer

Neil Mortensen, MD, FRCS

Although some would argue that the outcome following surgery for colorectal cancer has changed little over the past 20 years,[1] there is an undeniable sense of optimism in the air. Earlier diagnosis, better staging, expert surgery and the use of adjuvant therapy in some cases have made the management of colorectal cancer an exciting area of surgical endeavour. Although technological advances are playing their part, there is still the challenge for the surgeon that what happens during the operation has a decisive influence on immediate and longer term outcome.

Staging and operability

Before embarking on what may be a demanding and difficult operation for the patient and surgeon, it is common sense to find out as much as possible about a colorectal cancer. Accurate clinical staging involves not only locating the tumour precisely, but also assessing the degree of local invasion, the presence or absence of any involved lymph nodes, and assessing metastatic spread, particularly to the liver. All these factors, together with the age and general health of the patient, must be weighed in the balance before a decision can be made concerning the choice of procedure.

The primary tumour

Above the peritoneal reflection the depth of local invasion of a colonic cancer is less important than below it in the rectum. A barium enema or colonoscopy will give information about the size of a tumour and the degree of obstruction it may be causing; but unless there is a large fixed mass, further imaging by CT scanning or external ultrasound will not yield information which is likely to change surgical decision-making. For the same reasons routine intravenous urograms have been abandoned.

In the rectum things are very different. Here there is less space for local invasion and there are many important local structures. Inappropriate or incomplete surgery has grave consequences and local recurrence is very difficult to manage. For those tumours within reach, digital rectal examination has been the traditional method for assessing local invasion by feeling for the size and extent of a cancer, and the degree to which it is tethered or fixed within the pelvis. Experienced surgeons can also palpate the mesorectum through the rectal wall for enlarged lymph nodes. This important examination may be easier with the patient sedated or anaesthetized. The information is used not only to decide what can be achieved oncologically, but also technically—whether the patient can be offered a restorative sphincter-saving resection or an abdominoperineal excision and a permanent colostomy, to identify patients suitable for local treatment, and define those at high risk of local recurrence where combined surgery and radiotherapy might be considered. Sigmoidoscopy determines the level of the tumour above the anal verge and its intraluminal appearance, but cannot assess the extent of local spread or the presence of lymph node involvement. York Mason[2] proposed a clinical staging system based on digital rectal examination; the examiner moves the tumour to assess the degree of local invasion (Fig. 9.1). Freely mobile tumours were those involving the mucosa and submucosa only. Tethered tumours, where there was a degree of resistance to movement, were those penetrating into the muscularis propria. Greater degrees of fixity indicated local invasion beyond the rectal wall; and when a tumour was completely fixed, involvement of adjacent organs, such as bladder, was likely.

This proposed system was tested prospectively in an important paper by Nicholls *et al*.[3] Clinical findings were compared with the results of pathological examination of the resected specimen. Gross degrees of spread were accurately predicted by digital examination in around 80 per cent of cases, but invasion within the rectal wall and early local spread less so. Not surprisingly the expert clinicians in the study were more accurate than the 'non-expert' registrars.

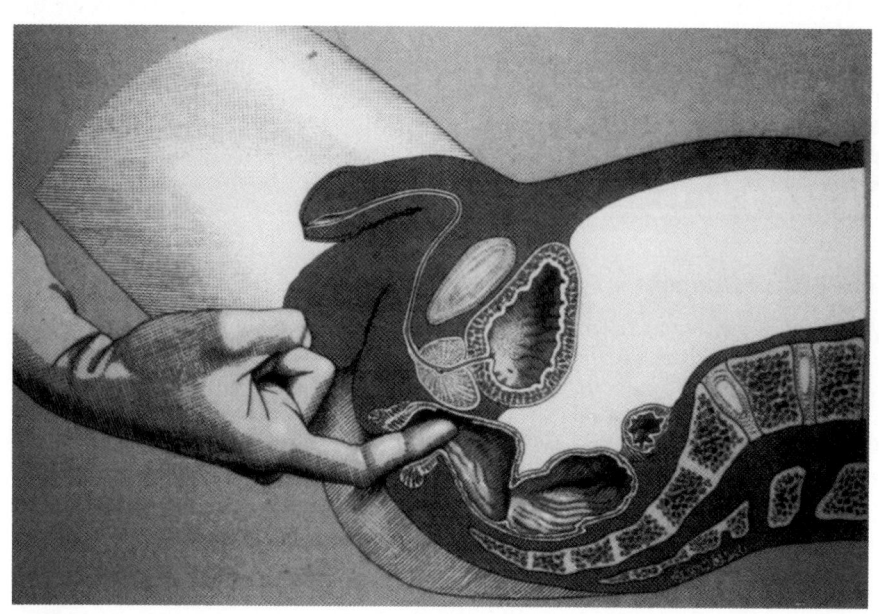

Fig. 9.1 Rectal examination. This is still the most widely used method for assessing a rectal cancer prior to surgery. The tip of the index finger is used to push the lower edge of the tumour and assess mobility. Deep palpation posteriorly may detect enlarged lymph nodes in the mesorectum.

Lymph node involvement was predicted in around 65 per cent of cases by the experts. In the same study, computed tomography (CT) scans identified extensive local invasion in 90 per cent of cases, but for earlier degrees of spread and nodal involvement they were no better than digital examination.

Radiological techniques in staging rectal cancer

Endosonography of the rectum

This technique was first introduced in the 1950s, but because of technical limitations was not used in routine clinical practice until 1983. The first application was transrectal scanning of the prostate for prostatic malignancy, but it soon became clear that rectal cancer could also be imaged.[4] A transducer with a high frequency (5.5 or 7 MHz) and short focal length is mounted on a rotating rod and covered with a water-filled latex balloon to give good acoustic contact with the tumour. In an unanaesthetized patient the probe is inserted into the rectum, the balloon inflated and the complete length of the tumour examined by varying the amount of water in the balloon and moving the probe longitudinally (Fig. 9.2). For tumours high in the rectum the probe can be placed at the exact point to be examined through an adapted rectoscope. The rotating transducer provides a radial image of the rectum and surrounding structures. Early interpretation of the images was controversial, but there is now general agreement that five ultrasonic layers can usually be identified both in

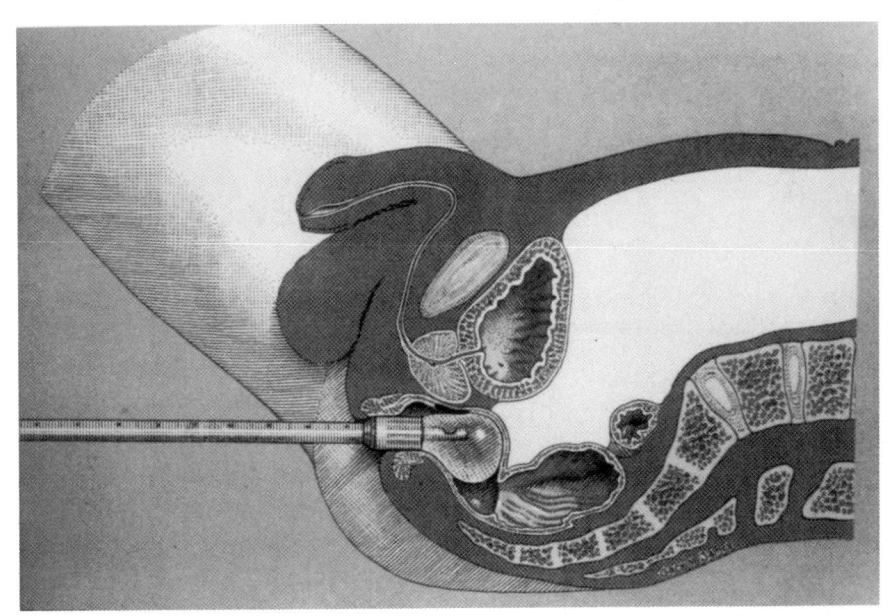

Fig. 9.2 Rectal endosonography. A water-filled balloon surrounds the rotating transducer which will give a transverse section through the rectum at right-angles to its axis. The probe is moved up and down, and the volume of water in the balloon varied to give the optimum ultrasound image of any lesion.

the rectum[5] and upper gastrointestinal tract (Fig. 9.3). *These five layers correspond more or less to the five histological layers of the rectum*:

Layer 1: hyperechoic—the interface between the balloon, its contained water, and the mucosal surface
Layer 2: hypoechoic—combined image produced by the mucosa and muscularis mucosae
Layer 3: hyperechoic—submucosa–muscularis propria interface
Layer 4: hypoechoic—muscularis propria
Layer 5: hyperechoic—interface between the muscularis propria and perirectal fat or serosa if present.

Using this interpretation of the image disruption of the individual layers implies disruption of the corresponding histological layer by invasive tumour (Fig. 9.4). Accuracies of around 90 per cent in predicting the degree of local invasion have been achieved using rectal endosonography, and when compared with computed tomography (CT) and digital examination[6] endosonography is the most accurate technique for staging rectal cancer.[3–5] It is relatively cheap, and

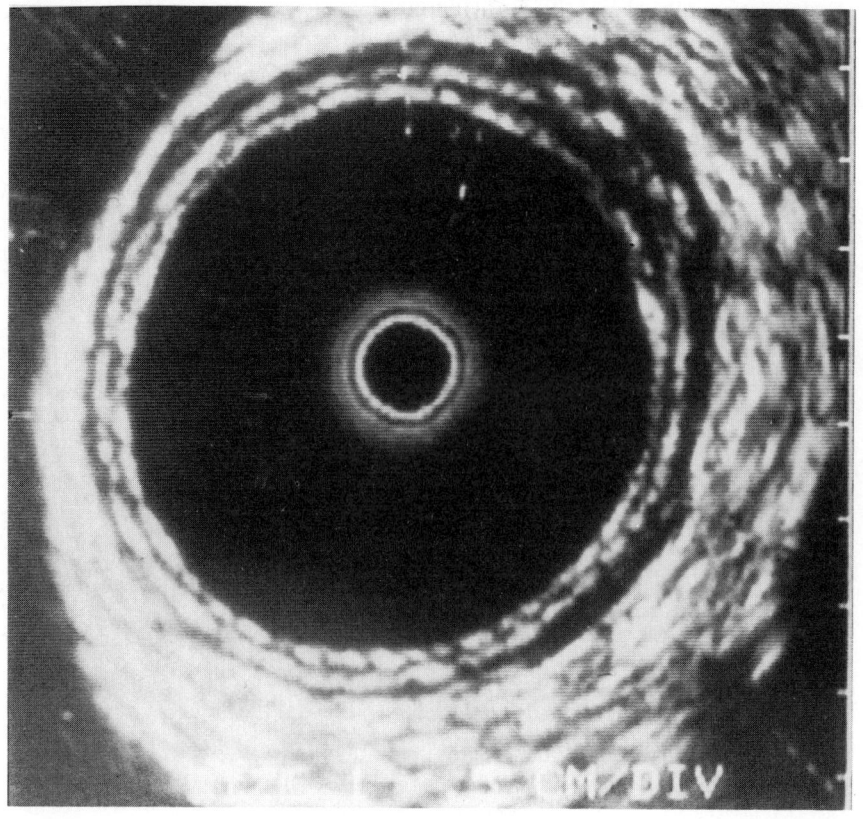

Fig. 9.3 A rectal endosonogram, showing the usual ultrasound appearance of gut wall. The five layers have been shown to correspond with the anatomical layers of normal gut wall.

easy to learn. The major problem is in stenotic tumours where the transducer cannot easily be passed through the tumour.

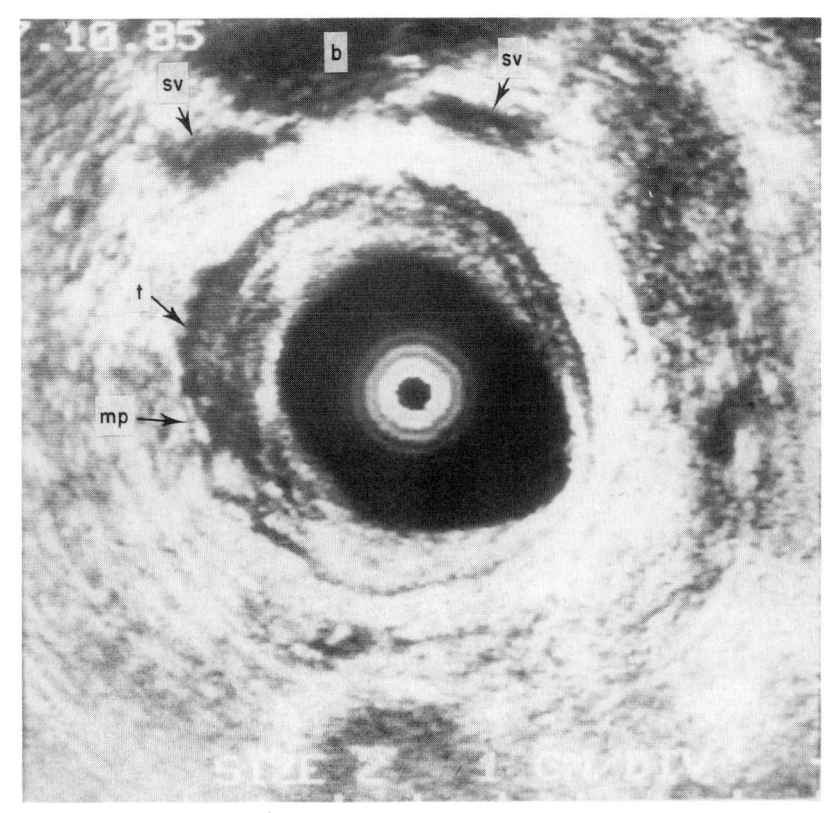

Fig. 9.4 A rectal endosonogram. Anteriorly are the seminal vesicles (sv) and the base of the bladder (b). There is a tumour involving the anterior quadrants of the rectal wall (t). The muscularis propria (mp) has been disrupted (arrow) and the tumour is invading into perirectal fat.

Other radiological techniques

CT scanning can identify extensive local invasion[3,7,8] but is less accurate and more expensive than digital examination and rectal endosonography. The cardinal sign on CT scans is of perirectal fat involvement. Nuclear magnetic resonance (NMR) shows promise,[9] but as yet is no more helpful than CT scanning in preoperative assessment. With experience and technical refinements accuracy may improve.

Lymph node involvement

Although involved and enlarged lymph nodes may be palpated, rectal endosonography would seem to be the most accurate of the methods currently available.[10] It can of course only record enlargement, but for nodes of 0.5 cm in diameter or greater an accuracy of 80 per cent has been reported. Nodes are seen as hypoechoic rounded lesions in the mesorectum (Fig. 9.5), and with practice can be readily recognized and distinguished from pelvic blood vessels.

Using CT scanning, lymph node enlargement of 1 cm or greater can be detected, but again this is not specific for nodal metastases.[11] There is not much information on NMR and lymph node assessment as yet,[9] and there do not appear to be any advantages over CT. Since all these methods can only demonstrate non-specific enlargement of lymph nodes, there has been a renewed interest in lymphoscintigraphy. Using a conventional technique and comparing scans with histopathology from resected specimens, reliable mesorectal node imaging is now possible.[11] Specific targetting of tumour bearing lymph nodes using monoclonal antibody immunoscintigraphy shows great potential but so far cannot be used in clinical management.

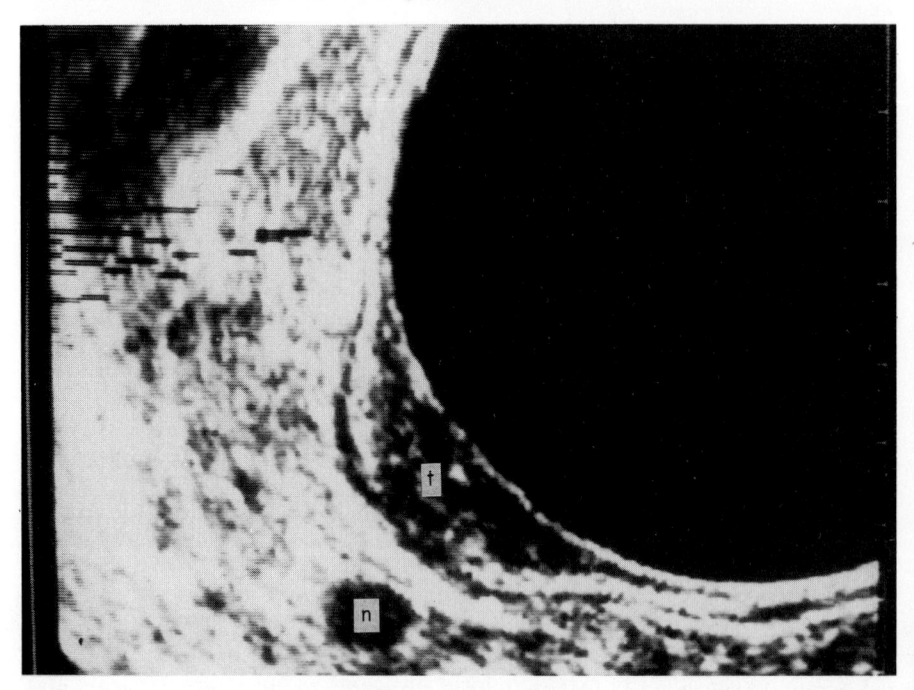

Fig. 9.5 A rectal endosonogram. An early tumour (t) with a lymph node (n) lying nearby in the mesorectum.

Distant metastases

The most common site for distant metastases from colorectal cancer is the liver. Conventional methods of assessment of the liver will include preoperative liver ultrasound and CT scanning, both with an accuracy in expert hands of around 75 per cent.

Finlay and McArdle[13] have demonstrated, by high-resolution close-cut CT scanning, occult hepatic metastases in 24 per cent of patients having a 'curative' resection for colorectal cancer. These would be patients where both preoperative imaging and palpation of the liver intraoperatively were negative. The presence or absence of these occult hepatic metastases at the time of surgery predicted the majority of deaths from disseminated disease (Fig. 9.6). Their method, however, involving numerous liver sections, was time-consuming and cannot be applied routinely in preoperative staging.

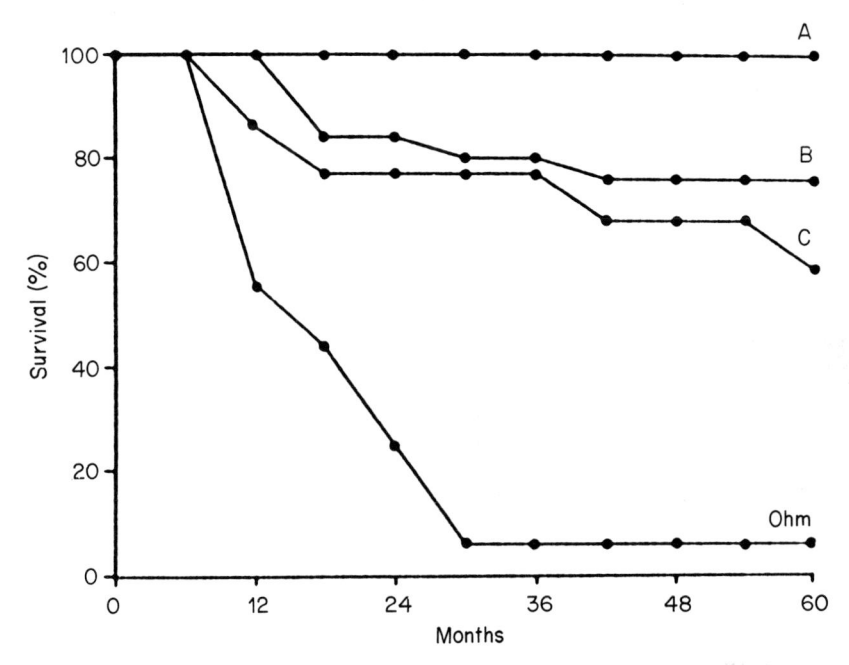

Fig. 9.6 Survival curves for colorectal cancer patients with and without occult hepatic metastases (OHM). (Reproduced from reference 13 with the kind permission of Butterworth Scientific)

Another technique for detecting early spread has been reported—the hepatic perfusion index[14]—but large-scale studies are not yet available.

Intraoperative liver ultrasound scanning using a high-frequency short-focal-length transducer directly in contact with the liver is now believed to be the most accurate method for the detection of liver metastases. A hand-held probe is systematically passed over the liver, segment by segment. Metastases are echopoor and can be readily distinguished from the brighter echogenic normal liver tissue and the tubular structures of intrahepatic veins and bile ducts (Fig. 9.7). Moreover, their relationship to hepatic veins allows an immediate assessment of operability. Machi et al.[17] have reported using intraoperative scanning during 33 operations for colorectal cancer, and in 15 per cent hepatic metastases were discovered which had not been detected by conventional preoperative techniques or palpation. Most of these tumours were 1 cm in size and non-palpable. This promising work is being vigorously pursued in a number of centres, and if small metastases can be detected much earlier, then staging will become more accurate, allowing selection of patients for hepatic resection or chemotherapy with a greater hope of success.[16]

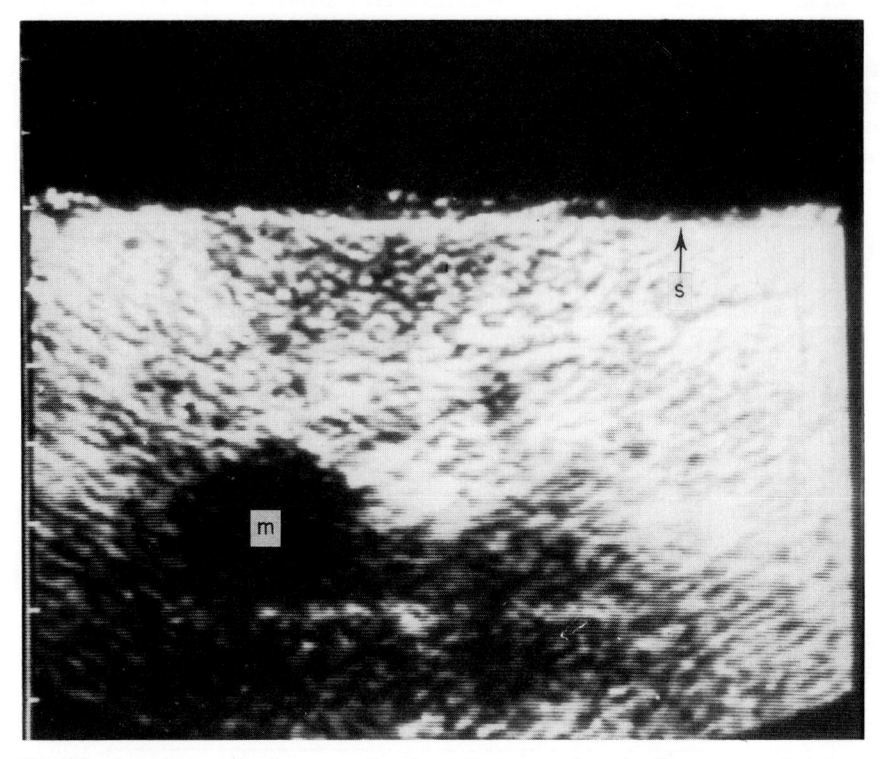

120 *New thoughts and methods in colorectal cancer*

Fig. 9.7 An intraoperative liver scan of a colorectal cancer patient. A solitary metastasis (m) can be seen beneath the liver surface (S).

The detection of liver metastases during colonic surgery is not generally an indication for immediate resection unless isolated secondaries are found on the liver surface. Here an enucleation is sufficient. For larger lesions within the liver substance, however, a biopsy is taken to confirm the diagnosis and the colonic resection specimen then subsequently assessed for adequacy of excision of the primary tumour. A CT scan of the liver and hepatic arteriograpy will give further useful information about the hepatic anatomy prior to resection, and some surgeons advocate waiting several months before offering liver surgery to be sure that more widespread metastases have not developed.[17] The operative management of these lesions is outside the scope of this chapter.

The biology of the primary tumour

Local and distant metastatic spread is only one indicator of the aggressiveness of a tumour and its likely response to treatment and outcome. It has been traditional to grade a rectal biopsy in rectal cancer patients, and those with biopsies showing poorly differentiated tumours in the middle or lower third of the rectum are not offered a restorative sphincter-saving procedure on the grounds that distal intramural spread and local recurrence are more likely. Recent studies on the accuracy of preoperative biopsies have demonstrated a poor correlation between biopsy grade and resection specimen grade. This is partly a sampling problem since accuracy can be improved by taking multiple biopsies, and partly observer error since there is a wide range of interpretation when the same biopsy is shown to a group of experienced histopathologists.[8]

In order to overcome these problems other cellular characteristics have been examined for their possible prognostic value. Tumour cell DNA content has been studied using DNA flow cytometry.[8,18] Aneuploid tumours carry a poorer prognosis and are associated with an increased risk of local recurrence.

Sulphomucin staining of colonic epithelial goblet cells is common adjacent to large bowel cancers and is associated with increased colonic mucosal cell kinetics. The presence of sulphomucin staining at the site of an anastomosis is also associated with an increased risk of local recurrence after apparently curative resection.[19]

These and other aspects of colorectal cancer biology may play an increasing role in assessing operability.

The operation

Since colorectal cancers are so common, their surgical excision can easily become something of a mechanical routine. There are, however, a number of crucial events during surgery which may determine the outcome. These are: the general effects of any operation, the detail of the local surgical excision, and the effects of manipulation of the tumour on the development of distant metastases.

As well as surgical trauma, there is the effect of anaesthesia, the use of antibiotics and analgesics, and in some cases blood transfusion. All these factors can diminish immune responsiveness at least experimentally.[20] There has been a great deal of interest recently in the role of allogeneic blood transfusion in colorectal cancer patients, with perhaps predictably conflicting conclusions. Some reports have shown that cancer recurrence is greater in transfused patients and that there is a survival advantage of the order of 30 per cent in non-transfused patients.[21] If this effect is confined to intraoperative transfusion and not perioperative blood transfusion, it might suggest that transfusion is simply a marker for biologically aggressive tumours—the bulky tumour in the pelvis, more difficult to remove and more likely to result in greater amounts of blood loss. Most of the studies refer to blood transfusion, which may implicate stored whole blood, packed cells, or fresh blood, and the particular factors responsible for immunosuppression have not been identified. The issue has generated a great deal of research and clinical interest, and the results of new studies may have a major impact on clinical practice. Traditionally, preoperative anaemia has been corrected, and modest operative blood loss replaced, but these may turn out to be quite the wrong things to do. Operative technique may have to be changed to minimize blood loss, and even autotransfusion could be introduced.

Excision of the primary tumour

An ideal curative operation for colorectal cancer would have carefully defined limits of excision of colon and mesenteric lymphatics. No such definition exists, although there is a consensus about tumours above the sigmoid colon. Since functional impairment is less of a problem here, wide excision together with a lymphadenectomy to the apex of the colic artery supplying that segment is the usual technique. The situation is more complicated where there is either a very small or a large locally invasive tumour. Bulky cancers invading abdominal wall, bladder or pancreas should wherever possible be resected *en-bloc*. Local invasion does not imply incurability, and a five-year survival of 30–50 per cent can be expected after extended *en-bloc* resection. Small tumours such as flat villous lesions with early malignant change may be treated by more local 'sleeve' resections, but this should include the local lymph nodes.

The polyp cancer problem

Large polyps can be removed by colonoscopic polypectomy, and the larger the polyp, the greater the incidence of malignant change. The histological report of invasion of the stalk in a malignant polyp raises another controversial issue. Is polypectomy sufficient if excision is complete, and is there any appreciable incidence of lymph node metastases from these small cancers? In the UK excision is judged complete if there is no tumour at the diathermy burn mark, if there is no lymphatic invasion, and if the polyp cancer is well or moderately well differentiated. In these circumstances the chance of lymph node involvement is less than 1 per cent.[22] If these criteria are not met the patient should be offered a conventional resection to include local lymph nodes. Some would still argue, however, that the incidence of the involved nodes has been underestimated and that, with the exception of very early submucosal invasion, a resection should always be offered as the safest policy.

Tumours in the sigmoid and rectum

For cancers of the sigmoid colon a more-or-less wide excision is carried out up to the level of the left colic artery. Some authors claim that the additional 4–5 cm of mesenteric node area included when resection is at the origin of the inferior mesenteric artery confers an added survival advantage, but this is not certain. A more extensive para-aortic lymph node dissection has also been proposed, but no clear advantage has been demonstrated.[20]

The 'no-touch' technique

Handling a cancer may spread the tumour by increasing the numbers of cancer cells in lymphatic and venous pathways. Turnbull in 1967 described the 'no-touch' technique in which the vascular pedicle leading away from the tumour is ligated prior to mobilizing it.[23] A significantly higher five-year survival rate was found in patients with Dukes C cancers compared with historical controls. The study provoked a great deal of interest and controversy since it was not randomized, and the extent of resection was not the same for the controls. A more recent randomized study from the Netherlands[24] has looked at the effect of 'no touch' on the development of subsequent metastases. Of course a crucial problem for any study like this is accurate staging. Patients with Dukes D lesions were excluded as far as possible. Liver metastases developed in 20 per cent of patients after a conventional resection compared with 7 per cent after 'no-touch', but with a mean follow-up of 58 months this difference has so far failed to reach statistical significance. Nevertheless, it would seem that using such a relatively simple change in technique may well prevent or delay metastasis.

The pelvic dissection: oncological considerations

A cancer of the rectum poses very special problems. Here in the narrow pelvis the technical demands made on the surgeon are much greater. There are opposing claims of adequate margins of excision and preservation of function. What is the gain in saving the patient a colostomy only to put him at higher risk of local recurrence? Whilst the technical details of restorative surgery are dealt with in another chapter, the oncological details will be discussed here.

Since it is now possible to carry out restorative procedures in patients with cancers of the middle and lower thirds of the rectum, what are the specific details which must be followed to avoid recurrence?

Lymph normally drains proximally, allowing a smaller distal resection margin, although lateral and retrograde drainage occurs occasionally in the lower rectum because of lymphatic blockage. Traditionally a 5 cm rule determined the safe margin of colon or rectum distal to a tumour, but recent studies have demonstrated that distal longtitudinal intramural tumour invasion rarely exceeds 1–2 cm, and that a distal margin of 2 cm is sufficient.[25] A minority of tumours with greater degrees of distal spread are usually inoperable and histologically poorly differentiated.

It is not just a matter of how much bowel is left distal to the tumour, however, but also how much mesorectum is removed. In a narrow pelvis with a bulky tumour there is a tendency for the surgeon to come in on the bowel beyond the cancer. Heald et al.[26] have drawn our attention to the importance of complete mesorectal excision, and failure to excise it all as a cause of local recurrence (Fig. 9.8). The lateral resection margins, too, not routinely reported by most pathologists are a sensitive indicator of recurrence. There are often tiny lateral margins amounting to only a few millimetres or less. In one series a careful study by repeated sectioning showed that 27 per cent of rectal resections had gone through the edge or satellites of tumour.[27] All but one of these developed local recurrence, whilst there was only one recurrence in those with a clear margin. Some authors have advocated either on-table frozen sections of the pelvic side walls, or even instant cytological imprints, to assess adequacy of clearance.

If the tumour is necessarily so close to the margins of excision, what are the important steps in a pelvic dissection? The patient must be in the modified lithotomy Trendelenburg position. An experienced surgeon and an experienced assistant together with good lighting from both overhead and fibrelight retractors are essential. The optimal dissection is in the mesorectal plane between the mesorectal and presacral fascia. This seems to act as a 'natural barrier' to any but the most advanced tumours. Staying in this plane also minimizes the risk of damage to pelvic nerves and the resulting problems with bladder and sexual function. It should be developed by sharp dissection

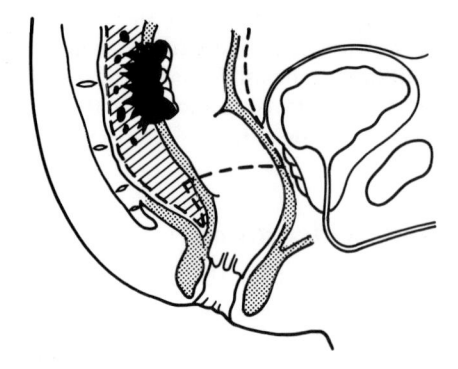

Fig. 9.8 Total mesorectal excision for rectal cancer. Note that this includes the wodge of fatty mesorectum in the cul-de-sac at the pelvic floor. (Reproduced from reference 26 with the kind permission of Butterworth Scientific)

under direct vision, diathermizing any small vessels to keep the pelvis perfectly dry. Gentle traction on the rectum helps the development of the plane, but it should not be by tearing and not blindly with a hand. All the mesorectum is removed in tumours of the middle or lower third of the rectum, even if this means making a lower anastomosis than might otherwise have been necessary.

It is likely that some of the worryingly high local recurrence figures presented in early papers on stapling techniques may have arisen because these principles were not upheld in the attempt to make ever lower anastomoses. Careful comparison of figures looking at abdominoperineal excision and anterior restorative resection has not shown higher recurrence rates, and some stapling series have exceptionally low rates.[28]

Exfoliated colorectal cancer cells

Having accomplished a successful mobilization of the rectum deep in the pelvis, it is important to avoid the potential complication of implantation metastasis. Clearly, inadvertent rupture of the specimen during mobilization, or spillage of luminal contents into the pelvis during rectal transection, may be implicated. There is now good evidence that viable exfoliated cancer cells can be found some distance away from the tumour both proximally and distally.[29] These can implant at the anastomosis site, or within the pelvis, as a potential cause of both intra- and extra-luminal recurrence.

Many clinical studies support the efficacy of irrigating or swabbing out the lumen of both bowel ends before constructing an anastomosis. Mercuric perchloride 0.2 per cent was at one time the preferred irrigation solution, but toxicity and even the occasional mortality have limited its use now. Cytotoxicity testing *in vitro* has shown that colorectal cancer cells can be rapidly killed with 5 per cent concentrations of both chlorhexidine-cetrimide and povidone-iodine.[29] I recommend thorough cleansing of the bowel ends with one of these reagents. Also, during anterior resection of the rectum a clamp should be placed across the bowel below the tumour, and the distal rectal stump irrigated through a large Foley catheter passed per anum at the beginning of the operation. It is also worth placing 60 ml of irrigant in the rectum prior to tying a perianal pursestring in patients having an abdominoperineal excision of the rectum, to minimize spillage implantation from inadvertent rupture of the rectum.

Adjuvant therapy

Even if the surgeon is aware of all the factors liable to predispose to recurrence, and is as radical as possible, it is unlikely that complete local clearance of microscopic disease will always be feasible. Radiotherapy seems the most likely choice of adjuvant therapy, though the trials have yielded conflicting and often disappointing results.[30] Patients with fixed or partially fixed tumours in the pelvis seem to have benefited most from radiotherapy, and since they have macroscopic local spread, those with residual microscopic disease might be expected to do even better if only they could be specially selected. This would require an enormous increase in the workload of pathology departments, but prospective trials in this area might be very fruitful.

Palliative surgery

In some 20 per cent of patients only palliative surgery of the primary tumour is possible at presentation. The mortality of resection for locally advanced lesions in elderly patients is high. The alternative of a proximal diverting colostomy can only relieve obstructive symptoms, and any surgical procedure involves a prolonged recovery period encroaching on a limited prognosis, and the major handicap of a colostomy in an elderly patient. Local palliative procedures as an alternative to major resections will be employed increasingly as the hospital population becomes more elderly. Local radiotherapy, cryotherapy and electrocoagulation have all been used, but none very widely. Two recent techniques are particularly worth considering.

Lasers are being tested in the endoscopic recanalization of advanced obstructing tumours of the oesophagus and major airways. In similar fashion Nd YAG lasers have been used for endoscopic palliation of advanced tumours of the rectum and distal sigmoid: Bown *et al.*[31] have reported results of laser treatment in 17 patients. They were prepared as for a conventional colonoscopy and given intravenous sedation or analgesia as necessary. None required a general anaesthetic. The laser was used to vapourize the most protuberant or identifiable areas and coagulate the underlying area. Tissue necrosed by the laser sloughs to a depth of 2–3 mm a few days after treatment, and therefore care must be taken at the junction with normal colorectum to avoid perforation. Because of inaccessibility, poor visualization or sheer bulk of tumour, treatment may have to be repeated two or three times at two-weekly intervals as a day case. The mortality from surgery for obstructed colorectal cancers is at least twice that of non-obstructed cases, and lasers offer the possibility of preliminary recanlization followed by safer elective resection. At the present time, however, lasers are expensive and not widely available.

A cheaper, 'low tech' method of achieving palliative endoscopic resection has been described by Berry et al.[32] A urological resectoscope can be used to chip away at a rectal cancer, irrigating the lumen with fluid in a similar manner to a prostatic resection. Good palliative results can be achieved, but the patient requires a short general anaesthetic.

Concluding comment

The surgeon in training will be understandably put out when denied the opportunity to 'have a go' at a colonic or anterior resection. Such is the complexity of issues surrounding the successful surgical management of these tumours, particularly in the pelvis, that they will be increasingly concentrated in the hands of specialist surgical teams. A standardized method of assessment taking into account clinical and pathological characteristics of colorectal cancers has been proposed,[33] and standardization of the individual operative details of resection to minimize surgeon to surgeon variability will also be important in improving results. Although earlier detection of colorectal cancers by faecal occult blood screening[34] may improve the outlook, and practice in the future, surgeons will be dealing with established disease for many years to come, and it is salutary to remember that the detail of the surgical technique still plays a crucial role in determining outcome.

References

1. Phillips R.K.S., Hittinger R., Blesovsky L., Fry J.S., Fielding L.P. Local recurrence following curative surgery for large bowel cancer. 1: The overall picture. *Brit. J. Surg.* 1984; **71:** 12–16.
2. York Mason A. Rectal cancer: the spectrum of selective surgery. *Proc. R. Soc. Med.* 1976; **69:** 237–44.
3. Nicholls R.J., York Mason A., Morson B.C., Dixon A.K., Kelsey Fry I. The clinical staging of rectal cancer. *Brit. J. Surg.* 1982; **69:** 404–9.
4. Beynon J., Foy D.M.A., Roe A.M., Temple L.N., Mortensen N.J.McC. Endoluminal ultrasound in the assessment of local invasion in rectal cancer. *Brit. J. Surg.* 1986; **73:** 474–7.
5. Beynon J., Foy D.M.A., Temple L.N., Channer J.L., Virjee J., Mortensen N.J.McC. The endoscopic appearances of normal colon and rectum. *Dis. Colon Rect.* 1986; **29:** 810–13.
6. Beynon J., Mortensen N.J.McC., Foy D.M.A., Channer J.L., Virjee J., Goddard P. Preoperative assessment of local invasion in rectal cancer: digital examination, endoluminal sonography or computed tomography? *Brit. J. Surg.* 1986; **73:** 1015–17.
7. Zheng G., Eddleston B., Schofield P.F., Johnson R.J., James R.D. Computed tomographic scanning in rectal carcinoma. *J. R. Soc. Med.* 1984; **77:** 915–20.
8. Williams N.S., Durdey P., Quirke P., et al. Preoperative staging of rectal neoplasm and its impact on clinical management. *Brit. J. Surg.* 1985; **72:** 868–74.
9. Hodgman C.G., Maccarty R.L., Wolff B.G., et al. Preoperative staging of rectal carcinoma by computed tomography and 0.15T magnetic resonance imaging. *Dis. Colon Rect.* 1986; **29:** 446–50.
10. Hildebrandt U., Feifel G. Preoperative staging of rectal cancer by intrarectal ultrasound. *Dis. Colon Rect.* 1985; **29:** 42–6.
11. Dixon A.K., Kelsey Fry I., Morson B.C., et al. Preoperative computed tomography in carcinoma of the rectum. *Brit. J. Radiol.* 1982; **54:** 655–9.
12. Reasbeck P.G., Manktelow A., McArthur A.M., Packer S.G.K., Berkeley B.B. An evaluation of pelvic lymphoscintigraphy in the staging of colorectal cancer. *Brit. J. Surg.* 1984; **71:** 936–40.
13. Finlay I.G., McArdle C.S. Occult hepatic metastases in colorectal carcinoma. *Brit. J. Surg.* 1985; **72:** 128–30.

14. Leveson S.H., Wiggins P.A., Giles G.R., Parkin A., Robinson P.J. Deranged liver blood flow patterns in the detection of liver metastases. *Brit. J. Surg.* 1985; **72:** 128–30.
15. Machi J., Isomoto H., Kurohiji T., *et al.* Detection of unrecognized liver metastases from colorectal cancers by routine use of operative ultrasonography. *Dis. Colon Rect.* 1986; **29:** 405–9.
16. Taylor I. Colorectal liver metastases—to treat or not to treat? *Brit. J. Surg.* 1985; **72:** 511–16.
17. Ekberg H., Tranberg K.G., Andersson R., *et al.* Determinants of survival in liver resection for colorectal secondaries. *Brit. J. Surg.* 1986; **73:** 727–31.
18. Armitage N.C., Robins R.A., Evans D.F., Turner D.R., Baldwin R.W., Hardcastle J.D. The influence of tumour cell DNA abnormalities on survival in colorectal cancer. *Brit. J. Surg.* 1985; **72:** 828–30.
19. Wood C.B., Dawson P.M., Habib N.A. The sialomucin content of colonic resection margins. *Dis. Colon Rect.* 1985; **28:** 260–1.
20. Jeekel J. Curative resection of primary colorectal cancer. *Brit. J. Surg.* 1986; **73:** 687–8.
21. Taylor R.M.R., Parrott N.R. Red alert. *Brit. J. Surg.* 1988; **75:** 1049–50.
22. Day D.W., Morson B.C. The polyp problem. In: Hunt R.H., Waye J.D. (eds.): *Colonoscopy.* London: Chapman & Hall, 1981; 301–26.
23. Turnbull R.B., Kyle K., Watson F.R., Spratt J. Cancer of the colon: the influence of the no-touch technique on survival rates. *Ann. Surg.* 1967; **166:** 420–7.
24. Wiggers T., Jeekel J., Arends J.W., *et al.* No touch isolation technique in colon cancer: a controlled prospective trial. *Brit. J. Surg.* 1988; **75:** 409–15.
25. Williams N.S., Dixon M.F., Johnston D. Re-appraisal of the 5 centimetre rule of distal excision for carcinoma of the rectum. *Brit. J. Surg.* 1983; **70:** 150–4.
26. Heald R.J., Husband E.M., Ryall R.D.H. The mesorectum in rectal cancer surgery—the clue to pelvic recurrence? *Brit. J. Surg.* 1982; **69:** 613–16.
27. Quirke P., Durdey P., Dixon M.F., Williams N.S. Local recurrence of rectal adenocarcinoma due to inadequate surgical resection. *Lancet.* 1986; **2:** 996–9.
28. Williams N.S. The rationale for preservation of the anal sphincter in patients with low rectal cancer. *Brit. J. Surg.* 1984; **71:** 575–81.
29. Umpleby H.C., Williamson R.C.N. Anastomotic recurrence in large bowel cancer. *Brit. J. Surg.* 1987; **74:** 873–8.
30. Cummings B.J. A critical review of adjuvant pre-operative radiation therapy for adenocarcinoma of the rectum. *Brit. J. Surg.* 1986; **73:** 332–8.
31. Bown S.G., Barr H., Matthewson K., *et al.* Endoscopic treatment of inoperable colorectal cancers with the Nd YAG laser. *Brit. J. Surg.* 1986; **73:** 949–52.
32. Berry A.R., Souter R.G., Campbell W.B., Mortensen N.J.McC., Kettlewell M.G.W. Endoscopic transanal resection of rectal tumours—preliminary report of its use in 67 patients. *Brit. J. Surg.* 1990; **77:** 134–137.
33. Williams N.S., Jass J.R., Hardcastle J.D. Clinicopathological assessment and staging of colorectal cancer. *Brit. J. Surg.* 1988; **75:** 649–52.
34. Hardcastle J.D., Armitage N.C., Chamberlain J., Amar S.S., James P.D., Balfour T.W. Faecal occult blood screening for colorectal cancer in the general population: results of a controlled trial. *Cancer.* 1986; **58:** 397–403.

10

Familial adenomatous polyposis

James P.S. Thomson, DM, MS, FRCS

Polyposis is a term used to describe a condition with an unspecified number of polyps in the large intestine.[1] The word *polyp* does not specify a pathological diagnosis. Similarly the term *polyposis* is not enough to convey a diagnosis as there are many different varieties of polyposis. Histopathological examination of a sample of the polyps is essential, and the variety of polyposis may be classified according to whether the polyps are neoplastic, hamartomatous, inflammatory or members of a miscellaneous group (Table 10.1).

Familial adenomatous polyposis, defined as more than 100 adenomata in the large intestine (Fig. 10.1), is the most important variety. This is not only because of its more frequent occurrence (nearly 90 per cent of all polyposis patients in the St Mark's Hospital Polyposis Register) and its dominant inheritance, but also because, untreated, all patients will eventually develop carcinoma of the large bowel.[2] Furthermore, it is now realized that this disorder may affect the whole gastrointestinal tract, and not just the colon and rectum and different tissues at other sites.

Table 10.1 Types of polyposis

Category of polyp	Type of polyposis
Neoplastic	FAMILIAL ADENOMATOUS POLYPOSIS
	Recessive adenomatous polyposis
	Lymphosarcomatous polyposis
	Leukaemic polyposis
Hamartomatous	Peutz–Jeghers syndrome
	Juvenile polyposis
	Neurofibromatous polyposis
	Lipomatous polyposis
Inflammatory	Non-specific inflammatory bowel disease
	Pseudopolyps
	Postinflammatory polyps
	Bilharzial polyposis
	Lymphoid polyposis
Miscellaneous	Metaplastic polyposis
	Cronkite–Canada syndrome
	Pneumatosis cystoides intestinalis
	Cowden disease

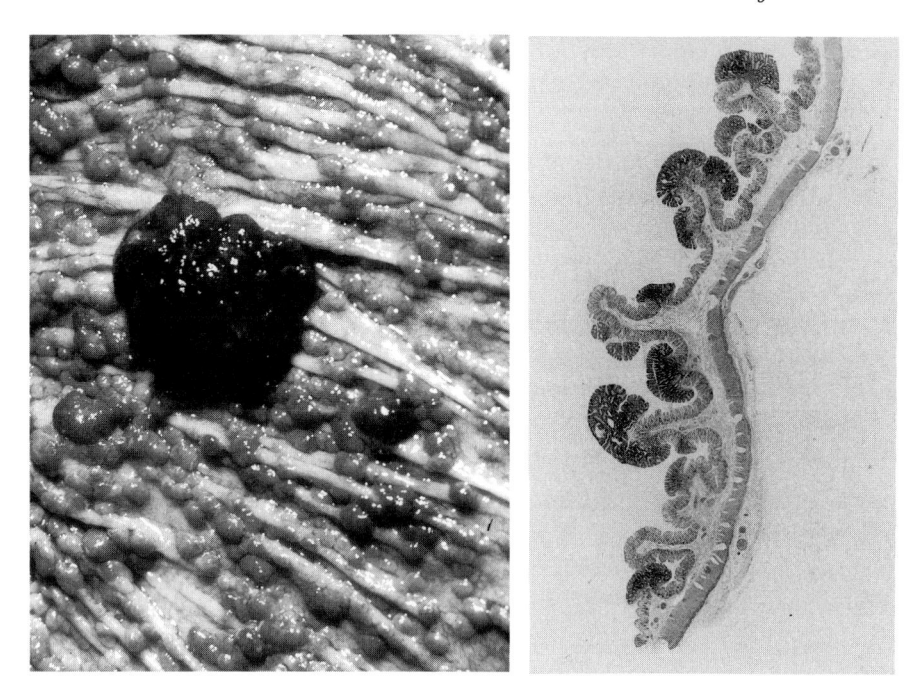

Fig. 10.1 Familial adenomatous polyposis: (a) macroscopic; (b) microscopic)

Dominant inheritance and incidence

Familial adenomatous polyposis (FAP) is a dominantly inherited disorder, implying that the offspring of affected patients will have a 50 per cent chance of developing the disease. The genetic abnormality has recently been identified as occurring on chromosome 5, and this abnormality in genetically informative families may be identified by using gene probes.[3] At present it is only in a small proportion of families that laboratory testing can assist in the diagnosis of affected individuals. However, such is the pace of genetic research that in the near future it should become possible for a relatively simple test to establish the diagnosis prenatally as well as postnatally. On occasions there may be no history of other family members being involved. In these patients it is presumed that a mutation has occurred.

It has been estimated that the frequency of FAP in the general population of the UK is 1 in 23 790.[4] However, in Sweden, Alun and Licznerski[5] have suggested a greater frequency of 1 in 7646.

Clinical features

For a long time it was considered that FAP only affected the large intestine. Indeed the old term, 'polyposis coli', now one hopes abandoned, apart from not describing the pathological type of polyp, also implied that only the colon was affected. It is now appreciated that the whole of the gastrointestinal tract may be the site of adenomata and adenocarcinomata. In addition abnormalities of the skin, connective tissue, teeth, bone, central nervous system, thyroid gland, eye and liver may occur (Table 10.2).

In 1951 Gardner† first described some of the extraintestinal manifestations of familial adenomatous polyposis.[6] The presence of multiple sebaceous cysts and osteomata of the mandible together with multiple large bowel adenomata came to be known as Gardner's syndrome. However, it is now realized that most patients, if not all, are at risk from one or more of these associated lesions, suggesting that Gardner's syndrome is not in fact a separate condition. The term is now being dropped.

Table 10.2 Manifestations of familial adenomatous polyposis

Tissue	Disorder
Gastrointestinal tract	Adenoma and adenocarcinoma
Skin	Epidermoid cyst (sebaceous)
Connective tissue	Desmoid tumour (fibromatosis)
Teeth	Supernumerary teeth
	Impacted teeth
	Odontoma
Bone	Osteoma
(Central nervous system)	(Medulloblastoma, glioma)
Thyroid gland	Papillary adenocarcinoma
Eye	Congenital hypertrophy of retinal pigment epithelium
Liver	Hepatoblastoma

Large intestine

By definition all patients with FAP have large intestinal adenomata. The number of polyps is variable and some patients will have in excess of 5000. Individual polyps, showing the typical features of an adenoma, are usually small (less than 5 mm in diameter). Occasionally larger polyps will occur. Whilst it is known that untreated patients will develop adenocarcinoma,[2] the majority of patients will be diagnosed before malignancy occurs (see below).

Adenomata are present throughout the large intestine but there is usually a preponderance in the left colon and rectum. In our experience at St Mark's Hospital it is almost unknown for there to be no polyps in the rectum; this implies that the diagnosis can always be made on sigmoidoscopy. Others, however, have reported a high incidence of rectal sparing.[9] Whether or not these patients have FAP must be a matter for speculation.

Upper gastrointestinal tract

Adenomata may be present in the stomach, duodenum, jejunum and ileum in as many as 80 per cent of patients at one or more of these sites. Most lesions

†Dr Eldon J. Gardner, Geneticist, Johns Hopkins University School of Medicine (died 1989).

are small and occur in the duodenum (Fig. 10.2), but sometimes large sessile adenomata occur. However, malignancy may occur (4.5 per cent of patients), and it is in the duodenum where malignant change seems most frequent (63 per cent of all upper gastrointestinal malignancies).[7] Within the duodenum the second part is most vulnerable, especially at the site of the ampulla of Vater.

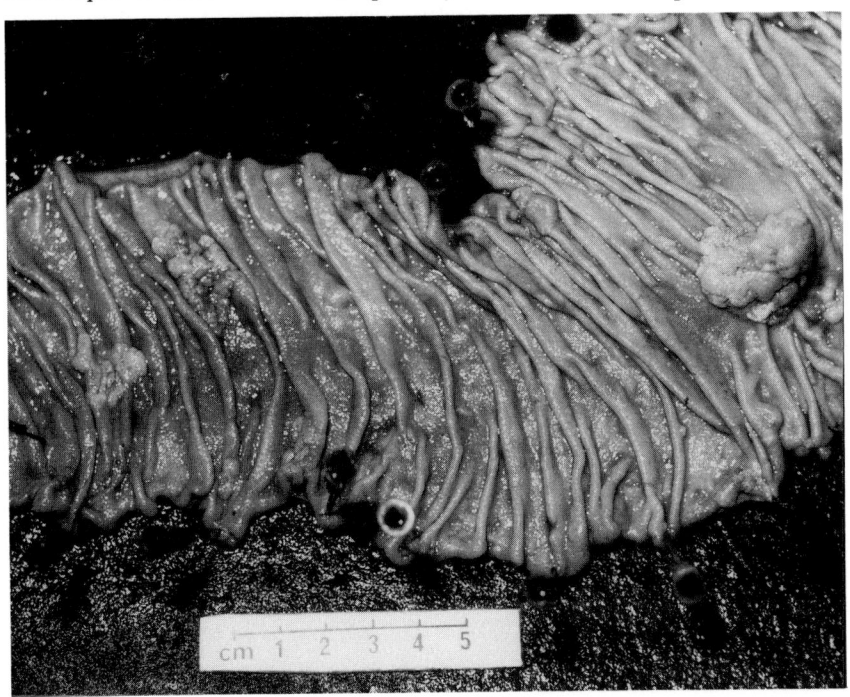

Fig. 10.2 Duodenal adenomata.

Skin

Epidermoid cysts, a variety of sebaceous cysts (the others being pilar cysts and steatocytoma multiplex), although present in perhaps 50 per cent of patients with FAP, are also very common in the general population.[8] They are rare before puberty. Their presence before the teens may therefore be a pointer to FAP and is an indication for sigmoidoscopic assessment, especially if the patient is not known to be of a polyposis family.

Connective tissue

Desmoid disease (or fibromatosis) is a disorder of fibrous tissue characterized by the development of non-metastasizing, locally invasive tumours. These lesions, which occur in approximately 10 per cent of FAP patients may arise *de novo*, but more usually occur after operation (80 per cent).

These tumours, which are often painful, may occur in the anterior abdominal

132 *Familial adenomatous polyposis*

wall, the abdominal cavity or both (Fig. 10.3). The importance of those within the abdominal cavity is that they may produce obstruction to hollow structures such as the ureters and the gut.

Treatment by surgical excision may be helpful for anterior abdominal wall tumours, although there is a high recurrence rate. Intra-abdominal lesions are basically inoperable because of their infiltrative nature and vascularity. Anti-oestrogens and prostaglandin inhibitors such as Clinoril have been reported anecdotally to have some benefit, but this role is unclear as is the use of radiotherapy and cytotoxic agents.[10]

Teeth

Supernumerary teeth, impacted teeth and odontomata probably occur in about 10 per cent of patients with FAP and may require treatment by a dental surgeon.

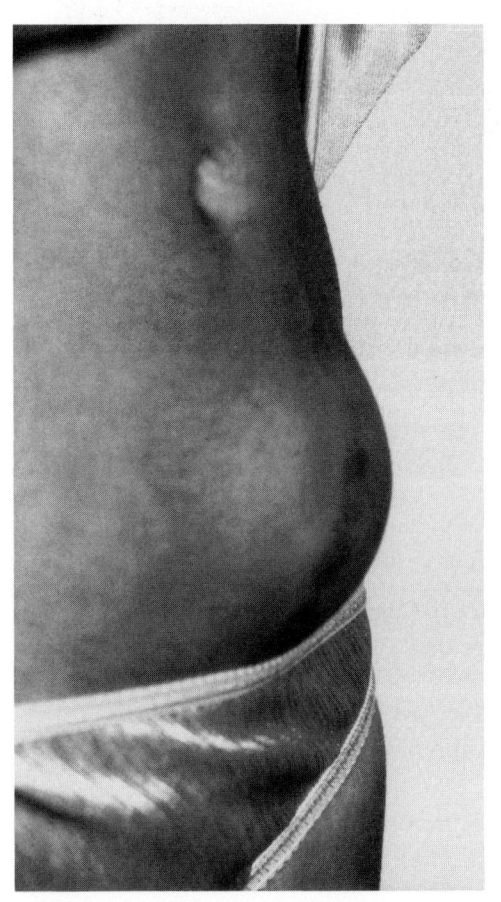

Fig. 10.3 Desmoid tumour: (a) anterior abdominal wall; (b) CT scan of intra-abdominal desmoid tumour displacing contrast-filled loops of small intestine.

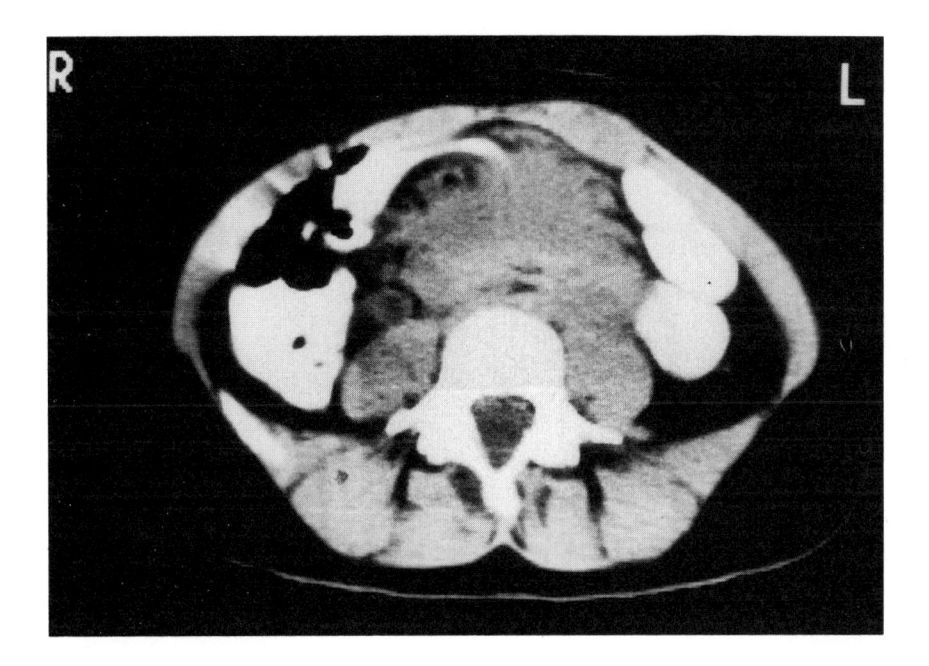

Bone

Radio-opacities seen in panoramic radiographs of the mandible were described by Utsunomiya and Nakamura in 1975.[11] These were present in over 90 per cent of their patients. Their occurrence in the maxilla was less than 10 per cent. Osteomata may also occur and these are usually in the mandible (Fig. 10.4), although the other bones of the skull may be involved. They are probably best left untreated unless they become large and unsightly as, being ivory osteomata, their removal might result in fracture of the parent bone.

Central nervous system

There is a reported association between tumours of the central nervous system and FAP. Often referred to as Turcot's syndrome, these tumours are pathologically medulloblastomata or gliomata.[12] This rare association has a low incidence and only 50 patients have so far been reported.[13]

Thyroid gland

There now seems to be unequivocal evidence that papillary adenocarcinoma of the thyroid gland is more common in these patients than in the general population. The incidence has recently been estimated as approximately 160 times that of normal individuals.[14] Whilst this means that patients with FAP should have their thyroid gland examined as part of their regular assessment, it also suggests that patients with papillary adenocarcinoma of the thyroid gland

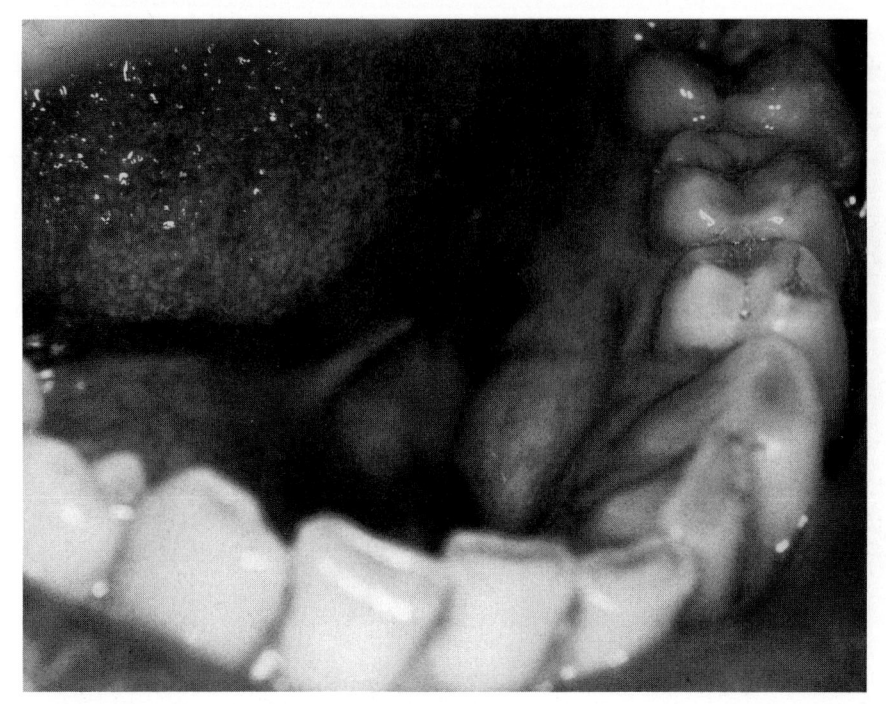

Fig. 10.4 Osteoma of the inner aspect of the mandible.

should have a bowel history taken and a sigmoidoscopy performed. At present there are no data as to the frequency of FAP in this latter group of patients.

The eyes

Congenital hypertrophy of the retinal pigment epithelium (CHRPE) probably occurs in the majority of patients with FAP. Discrete, darkly pigmented, round, oval or kidney-shaped lesions, between 0.1 and 1.0 cm in diameter, are found on ophthalmoscopy.

First described in 1980 by Blair and Trempe,[16] several reports have now appeared. The most recent report is from Chapman *et al.*[17] of the Northern Region Polyposis Register, who observed a highly significant difference between controls who never had more than two areas of pigmentation in both eyes and those with FAP who never had less than a total of two lesions. These lesions are asymptomatic but are probably an important marker of this disease, especially as these lesions occur in most patients at an earlier age than the polyps (Fig. 10.5). No progression to melanoma has been recorded.

Liver

Since 1925 there has been an association between FAP and hepatoblastoma, a rare embryonic tumour, in nine children in the UK and the USA. This is considerably in excess of the predicted number and suggests a genetic relationship.[15]

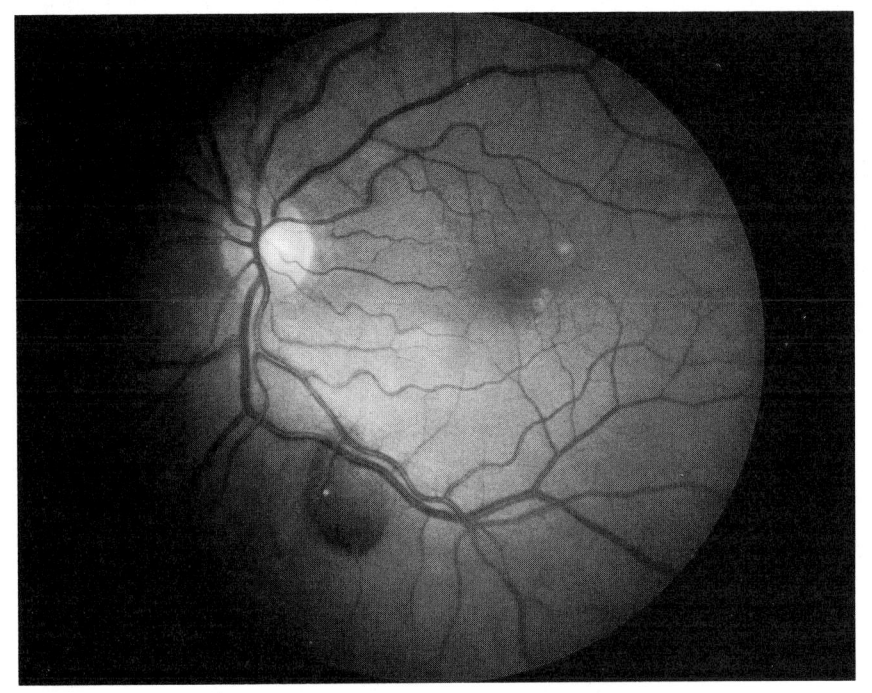

Fig. 10.5 An example of congenital hypertrophy of the retinal pigment epithelium. (Professor Barrie Jay's photograph)

Diagnosis

Some patients with familial adenomatous polyposis will be diagnosed as the result of presenting with symptoms such as alteration in bowel habit and bleeding. However, the majority of patients will be asymptomatic and will be diagnosed as the result of screening those at risk.

In a large series of patients reported from St Mark's Hospital, it is interesting to note that the incidence of large bowel carcinoma at the time of diagnosis in the patients presenting with symptoms was 20.3 per cent. In those patients diagnosed as the result of screening it was only 5.2 per cent.[18] This emphasizes the importance of screening in large bowel cancer prevention.

The diagnosis is made by finding multiple polyps on sigmoidoscopy and establishing that they are adenomata by one or more biopsies. The whole colon ought to be examined in those with symptoms, and in those over 20 years of age without symptoms, to determine whether or not a carcinoma is present (carcinoma of the large bowel under the age of 20 is very unusual). This may be done by a double-contrast barium enema or a colonoscopy. In the latter procedure the presence of multiple small polyps may be detected by employing

136 *Familial adenomatous polyposis*

the dye-spray technique; the small pink elevations become more apparent when surrounded by dye-filled interconnecting groves.[19] Multiple biopsies may be taken.

Differential diagnosis

It might be though that the detection of multiple polyps in the rectum on sigmoidoscopy would never present a problem. However, a large sessile adenoma, inflammatory bowel disease and haemangioma need to be considered in the differential diagnosis. With the exception of haemangioma (because of the bleeding it would produce), biopsy should provide the correct diagnosis. Furthermore, *familial* adenomatous polyposis must be distinguished from other forms of polyposis by histopathological analysis of a sample of the polyps.

Screening

Once a diagnosis of FAP has been made, a family history must be taken and a family pedigree diagram constructed. An example is shown in Fig. 10.6. Reference to this diagram will assist in assuring that all those at risk will be seen. New information may be added as it is acquired. The diagram provides an excellent clinical summary of a given family.

All those people who are shown to be at risk—that is, those in former generations, the same generation and subsequent generations—should be assessed by taking a history of any symptoms and by sigmoidoscopy. It is probably not necessary to screen children before 13–14 years unless there are symptoms. This is because it is almost unknown for malignancy to occur before 20 years of age. However, in a few families (10 per cent) genetic testing may be employed, and in the future this may become the standard investigation (see above). This may, in time, avoid the need for sigmoidoscopic examination in

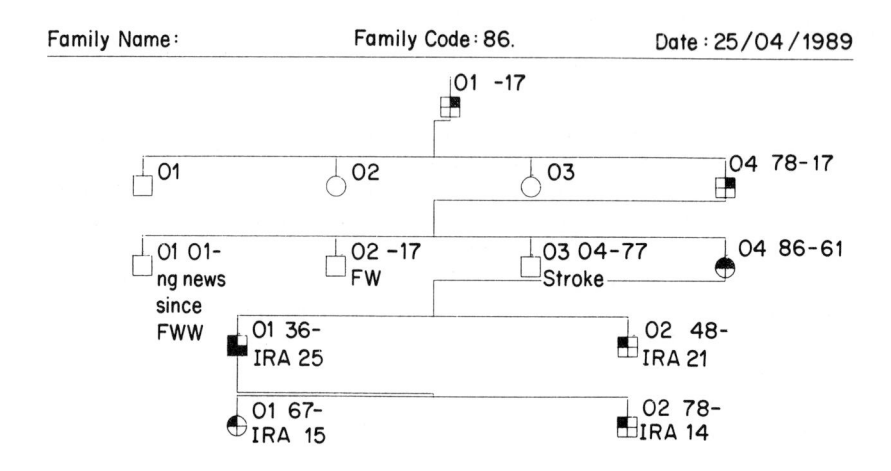

Fig. 10.6 An example of a computerized family pedigree.

many young people. In addition, ophthalmic examination for CHRPE may also become a valuable screening aid.

When an at-risk relative is examined and found to be normal, should further examinations be carried out in the future? As these people grow older the risk of FAP certainly diminishes. Two-thirds of a small group of patients who were normal when first examined but who subsequently developed FAP were shown to have the disorder by the time they were 20 years old. Thus only a relatively small group were left who developed the disorder after this age. It is therefore advisable to examine those at risk at yearly intervals until they are 20 and then at less frequent intervals. It would be appropriate to warn those being screened to seek advice should they ever have a change in bowel habit or develop anorectal bleeding.

Management of the large intestine

For years the primary concern in the management of patients with familial adenomatous polyposis has been the prevention of the development of large bowel carcinoma. It is now, of course, appreciated that there may be many more aspects to the management of these patients. However, the main thrust of management is still towards the prevention of large bowel carcinoma, and this will be covered in the remainder of this chapter.

Large bowel carcinoma may be prevented by early diagnosis and the removal of all, or the greater part, of the large intestine.

Proctocolectomy

Originally a proctocolectomy was standard treatment; this was logical as all the large intestine was removed. However, the price for protection from large bowel carcinoma was a permanent stoma, and rectal excision, with its possible nerve damage affecting bladder and sexual function and a perineal wound.

Colectomy with ileorectal anastomosis

At St Mark's Hospital and elsewhere the standard procedure became total colectomy with an ileorectal anastomosis. (The late O.V. Lloyd-Davies performed the first such operation at St Mark's Hospital on 8 December 1948.) This operation has the advantage of avoiding a permanent stoma and rectal excision with its potential problems. However, the patient must expect to have an increase in bowel frequency (usually three to four per 24 hours) and accept the need for regular surveillance of the rectal stump (the anastomosis ought to be at approximately 15 cm from the anus) as the rectum is still at risk from adenomata and malignancy.

Restorative proctocolectomy

With the advent of restorative proctocolectomy several surgeons have regarded this operation as the treatment of choice in patients with FAP[20] as well as those with ulcerative colitis. The advantages are that all the large bowel mucosa is removed, and there is no perineal dissection. However, it is now realized that adenomata can occur in the small intestine. The effect of creating a pouch from small intestine (which becomes the *neorectum*) on adenoma growth and the adenoma–adenocarcinoma sequence remains unknown. This means that regular surveillance of the pouch is probably required.

The postoperative course may be more prolonged and complicated than after a colectomy with ileorectal anastomosis, and is usually accompanied by a temporary ileostomy. When closed the patients must expect an increase in bowel frequency, although Everett reports in a small series a bowel frequency less than that after colectomy with ileorectal anastomosis.[20]

Which operation is most appropriate?

The interrelationship between the aforementioned three operations is shown in Fig. 10.7. Based on information from nine polyposis registries with reports on 960 patients undergoing primary treatment throughout the world, colectomy with ileorectal anastomosis (55.8 per cent) is the most frequently performed procedure.[10] Restorative proctocolectomy, a much newer procedure, has only been performed in 10 per cent of these patients.

Most surgeons would agree that, provided the pathology allows, total colectomy with ileorectal anastomosis is the treatment of choice, as this is the

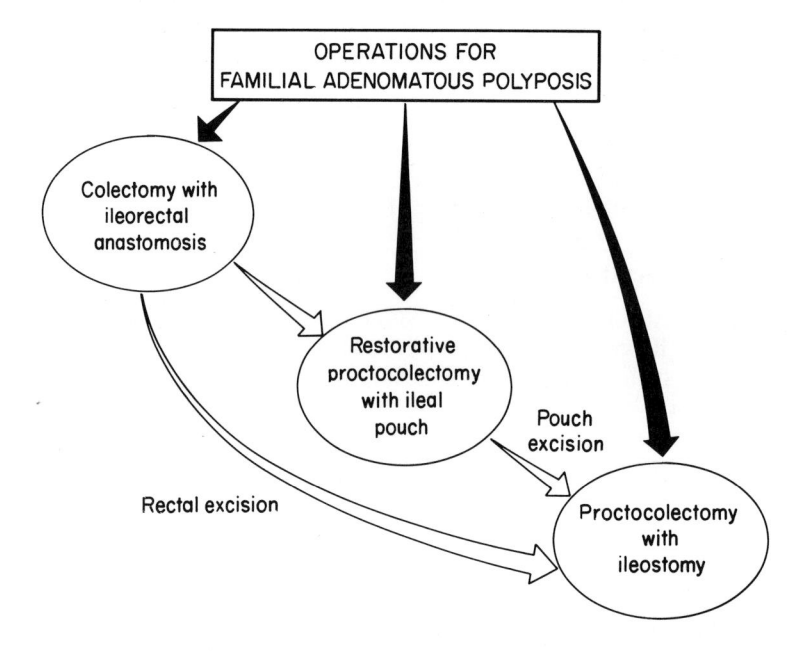

Fig. 10.7 Operations on the large bowel employed in the management of familiar adenomatous polyposis.

simplest operation with a low complication rate and satisfactory postoperative function. A restorative proctocolectomy should be considered in those patients with dense polyp formation or with large sessile polyps in the rectum which could not be controlled locally, or in whom there is a small carcinoma in the mid or upper rectum. The only indication for proctocolectomy as a primary therapy now would be in patients with a carcinoma in the rectum for which it was not felt appropriate to perform a restorative proctocolectomy.

Total colectomy with ileorectal anastomosis

Some are hesitant about performing this operation. It is, though, an established procedure and used not only in patients with familial adenomatous polyposis but also in those with inflammatory bowel disease, constipation, and some patients with other neoplastic conditions of the large bowel (especially obstructing left-sided carcinomata). Technically an ileorectal anastomosis is straightforward, and it is nearly always possible to perform an end-to-end anastomosis as the upper rectum and terminal ileum match for size very well. It is advisable to remove any polyps in the region of the divided rectum so that they are not incorporated in the suture line. It is important, though, to make certain there is good haemostasis at the site of such polyp removal.

In the early years the rectum was cleared of polyps before carrying out this procedure. More recently this has not been done as several surgeons have observed some polyp regression after colectomy with ileorectal anastomosis (although this is difficult to measure), and there is now less desire to remove all the polyps.

Postoperative mortality and morbidity

This operation has a low mortality and morbidity. In a large series of 197 patients operated on at St Mark's Hospital between 1948 and 1987, for example, only one patient died (in 1953) as the result of haemorrhage. Of the remaining 196 patients, 176 had an uneventful postoperative course and only 20 had complications. In five patients there was an anastomotic breakdown and in 13 patients prolonged ileus or obstruction, necessitating reoperation in four patients. There was one patient with a subphrenic abscess and a further patient with intestinal haemorrhage.[21]

It is therefore apparent that colectomy with ileorectal anastomosis is a safe operation which can be recommended with confidence to asymptomatic patients for cancer prophylaxis.

Functional outcome

It has been estimated that an average of three to four bowel movements in every 24 hours is usual after total colectomy. The use of codeine phosphate, loperamide or diphenoxylate may be helpful in reducing bowel frequency.

Management of the rectum

The rectum needs to be assessed at least every six months and more frequently if there are adenomata larger than 2 mm in diameter or if there is any doubt about the appearances of the rectal mucosa (see *infra*). To obtain the best view on sigmoidoscopy the rectum requires preparation, and this can be achieved by giving two phosphate enemas (400 ml) slowly. Examining the patient in the jackknife or knee–elbow position allows any remaining intestinal effluent to fall to the distal ileum, and if the effluent is excessive it may be removed by employing low-pressure suction. As the rectal stump is approximately 15 cm long a 20 cm sigmoidoscope is adequate, and a better view will be obtained with a broader instrument.

The appearance of the rectal mucosa may be simple or difficult to interpret. Discrete polyps or an ulcerating carcinoma should not present any difficulty. However, the change may be less clear-cut and consist of loss of vascular pattern or a granular mucosa with contact bleeding. Such appearances may be due to a slow adenomatous change over a wide area, or to scarring following the use of diathermy to control previous adenomata. Other changes which might be of more significance are flat, elevated plaques. With the end of the sigmoidoscope they can be probed. If there is any induration then malignancy must be suspected, although the area of malignant change might be quite small (Fig. 10.8). Adenomata probably ought to be treated if they are in excess of 5 mm in size, and this may be done using biopsy forceps, submucosal excision or diathermy fulguration. With the former two techniques a sample may be obtained for histopathological diagnosis. Diathermy fulguration is quicker and should be done in an inert atmosphere (carbon dioxide). Fulguration carries a definite risk of reactionary haemorrhage of about 2 per cent, and it is inadvisable to undertake this therapy if the patient is to go on a significant journey during the subsequent 10–14 days.

Incidence of rectal carcinoma

Despite this programme of follow-up assessment and the treatment of any polyps, there is in most people's experience an incidence of carcinoma in the rectal stump. Reference to Fig. 10.9 will indicate the cumulative risk of developing carcinoma in the St Mark's series, and it will be noted that at 25 years after the colectomy with ileorectal anastomosis the risk is approximately 10 per cent. After that time there is a sharp increase in the incidence, but this is based on a smaller total number of patients, and as this follow-up continues the curve should become somewhat flatter.

It was noteworthy in this series that even with good follow-up compliance the carcinomata were not necessarily diagnosed at an early stage. Eight of the 14 were Dukes B or C. This may represent the difficulty in interpreting the findings on sigmoidoscopy. It is the author's opinion that as screening of the rectum may be difficult these patients are probably best seen at specifically dedicated sessions, and if at all possible by the same clinician. Whilst these clinics should be held every three months, many patients would only need to attend twice a year. Not only are these attendances important for the follow-up of the patients,

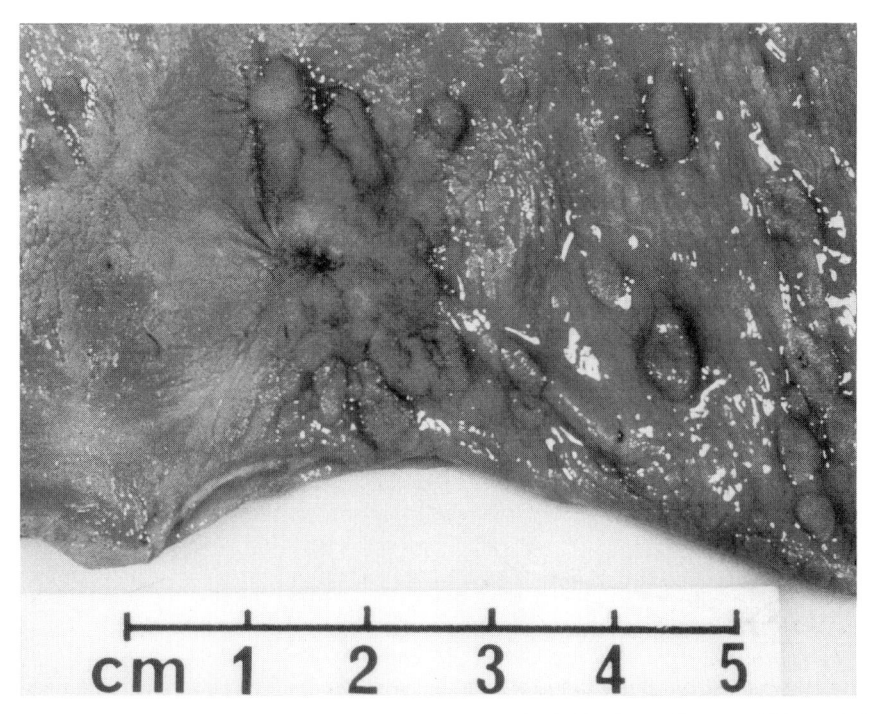

Fig. 10.8 A sessile adenoma with a small area of ulceration indicating malignancy. This might be difficult to detect on signoidoscopy; there would probably be bleeding and the area would feel hard when touched with the sigmoidscope.

but they also enable the review of families and provide facilities for assessing those at risk. There would seem to be no place for a clinician only seeing the occasional patient with this disease.

The detection of a rectal carcinoma probably necessitates excision of the rectum with the construction of an ileostomy. Restorative proctocolectomy might be an alternative with a small carcinoma in the upper rectum.

Rectal excision

There have been in the St Mark's series other reasons for rectal excision in addition to carcinoma. These included uncontrollable adenomata, sessile adenomata, patient insistence and occasionally haemorrhage following fulguration. In all, by the end of 1987, 25 rectal excisions have been performed, 14 being for carcinoma and 11 for other reasons.

Follow-up

All patients, whichever operation they have had to prevent large bowel carcinoma, should be followed regularly. Although this will be mainly for the examination of the rectal stump in those who had a colectomy with

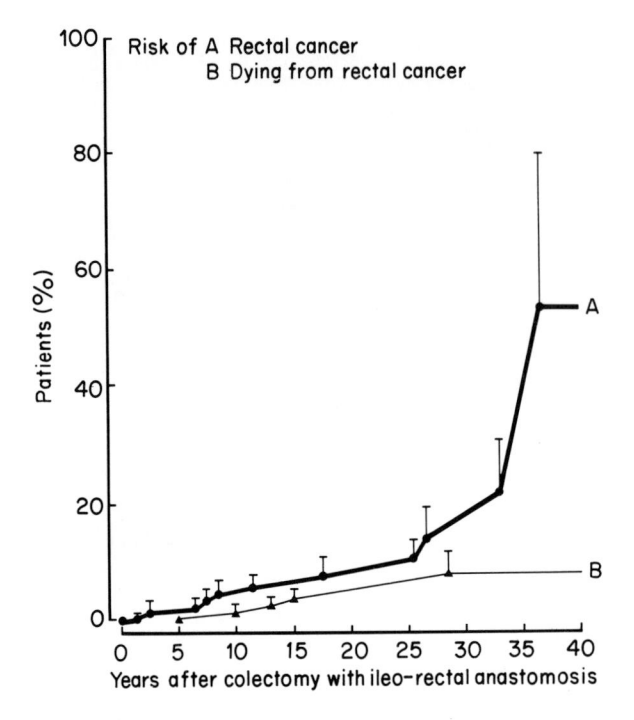

Fig. 10.9 Line A: the cumulative risk of developing rectal carcinoma in 196 patients following colectomy with ileal rectal anastomosis (St. Mark's Hospital series 1948–87). Line B: the cumulative risk of dying from rectal carcinoma.

ileorectal anastomosis, assessment should be made at regular intervals for the development of upper gastrointestinal lesions, although at the present time the management of adenomata at this site is undetermined. Clearly if an adenoma in the duodenum is sessile and repeated biopsy at one- or two-year intervals suggests increasing severity of dysplasia, or if the lesion is causing anaemia through bleeding, or if it is frankly malignant, then some form of operative treatment may be required. Whilst conservative operations such as a transduodenal submucosal excision may be appropriate for duodenal adenomata, more major procedures such as pancreaticoduodenectomy may be required. However, such a procedure must have clear indications and not be done prophylactically. Patients will need to be examined for other associated lesions, especially desmoid tumours and thyroid swellings.

A polyposis registry

A registry is essential for the satisfactory management of polyposis patients and their families. Not only is a registry an essential repository for all clinical and research data, and for the family pedigrees which are constantly requiring to be updated, but the registry staff can assist in the organizing of patient care by

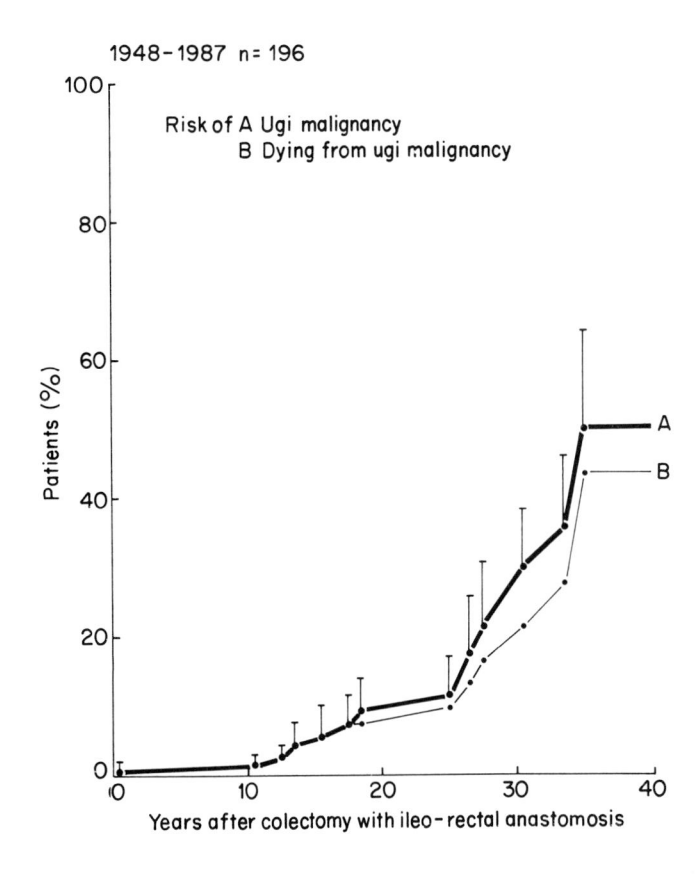

Fig. 10.10 Line A: the cumulative risk of developing an upper gastrointestinal malignancy in 196 patients following colectomy with ileal rectal anastomosis (St Mark's Hospital series 1948–87). Line B: the cumulative risk of dying from upper gastrointestinal malignancy.

keeping in contact with those who require follow-up examinations or screening. Furthermore, a registry ensures an accurate database which is essential for any clinical or laboratory research.

The St Mark's Polyposis Registry houses a register which is now 65 years old. This is an informal registry. However, regional registries are now being started in other centres, and in the UK two regional registries, the Northern[17] and West Midlands, have recently been established.

Conclusions

It is clear that familial adenomatous polyposis is a disorder which is now attracting considerably more interest than it has in the past. All medical students know it to be an important example of a dominantly inherited condition and a disease in which cancer prophylaxis can be practised, screening those at risk and removing vulnerable large intestine. The additional interest is being generated by the genetic developments and by the realization that this disease is a systemic problem with many extracolonic manifestations. Other forms of polyposis will also attract interest as more is understood about them.

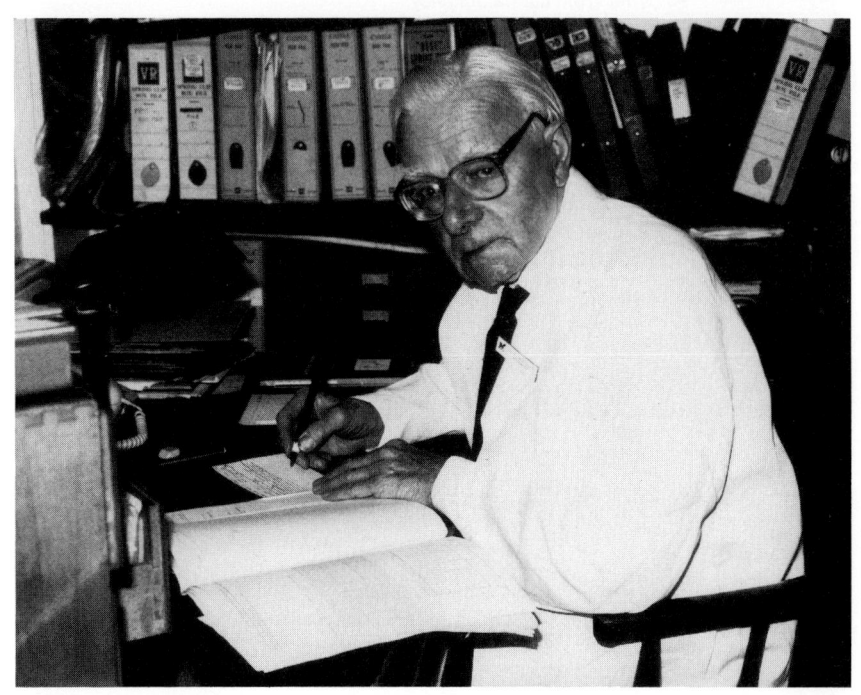

Fig. 10.11 Dr H.J.R. Bussey, OBE, who was one of the co-founders of the St Mark's Polyposis Register with the late J.P. Lockhart-Mummery and the late Cuthbert Dukes in 1924, at his desk in 1989. The author wishes to acknowledge the considerable assistance he has received from Dr Bussey at all times and, in particular, in the preparation of data for this chapter.

References

1. Bussey H.J.R. *Familial Polyposis Coli*. Baltimore: Johns Hopkins University Press, 1975.
2. Morson B.C., Dawson I.M.P. In: *Gastrointestinal Pathology*. 2nd edn. Oxford: Blackwell Scientific, 1979.
3. Bodmer W.F., Bailey C.J., Bodmer J., Bussey H.J.R., Ellis A., Gorman P., Lucibello F.C., Murday V.A., Rider S.H., Scambler P. Localization of the gene for familial adenomatous polyposis on chromosome 5. *Nature*. 1987; **328:** 614–16.
4. Veale A.M.O. *Intestinal Polyposis*. (Eugenics Laboratory Memoirs Series 40). Cambridge University Press, 1965.
5. Alm T., Licznerski G. The intestinal polyposes. *Clin. Gastroenterol*. 1973; **2:** 577–602.
6. Gardner E.J. A genetic and clinical study of intestinal polyposis a predisposing factor for carcinoma of the colon and rectum. *Amer. J. Human Gen*. 1951; **3:** 167–76.
7. Jagelman D.G., Decosse J.J., Bussey H.J.R. Uppergastrointestinal cancer in familial adenomatous polyposis. *Lancet*. 1988; **1:** 1149–51.
8. Leppard B.J., Bussey H.J.R. Epidermoid cysts, polyposis coli and Gardner's syndrome. *Brit. J. Surg*. 1975; **62:** 387–93.

9. Bess M.A., Adson M.A., Elveback L.R., Moertez C.G. Rectal cancer following colectomy for polyposis. *Arch. Surg.* 1980; **115:** 460–7.
10. Thomson J.P.S. The Leeds Castle Polyposis Group meeting. *Dis. Colon Rect.* 1988; **31:** 613–16.
11. Utsunomiya J., Nakamura T. The occult osteomatous change in the mandible of patients with familial polyposis coli. *Brit. J. Surg.* 1975; **62:** 45–51.
12. Turcot J., Despres J.-P., St Pierre F. Malignant tumours of the central nervous system associated with familial polyposis of the colon. *Dis. Colon Rect.* 1959; **2:** 565–8.
13. Jarvis L., Bathurst N., Mohan D., Beckely D. Turcot's Syndrome: a review. *Dis. Colon Rect.* 1988; **31:** 907–14.
14. Plail R.A., Bussey H.J.R., Glazer G., Thomson J.P.S. Adenomatous polyposis: an association with carcinoma of the thyroid. *Brit. J. Surg.* 1987; **74:** 377–80.
15. Kingston J.E., Krush A.J. Association of hepatoblastoma and polyposis coli. *Brit. J. Surg.* 1985; **72:** S138.
16. Blair N.P., Trempe C.L. Hypertrophy of the retinal pigment epithelium associated with Gardner's Syndrome. *Amer. J. Ophthal.* 1980; **80:** 661–7.
17. Chapman P.D., Church W., Burn J., Gunn A. Congenital hypertrophy of retinal pigment epithelium: a sign of familial adenomatous polyposis. *Brit. Med. J.* 1989; **298:** 353–4.
18. Bussey H.J.R., Eyres A.A., Ritchie S.M., Thomson J.P.S. The rectum in adenomatous polyposis: the St Mark's policy. *Brit. J. Surg.* 1985; **72:** 529–31.
19. Cotton P.B., Williams C.B. In: *Practical Gastrointestinal Endoscopy.* Oxford: Blackwell Scientific, 1989.
20. Everett W.G., Forty J. The functional result of pelvic ileal reservoir in 10 patients with familial adenomatous polyposis. *Ann. R. Coll. Surg.* 1989; **71:** 28–30.
21. Thomson J.P.S., Bussey H.J.R., Ritchie S., Neale K. Colectomy with ileorectal anastomosis—40 years experience in the management of familial adenomatous polyposis (previously unpublished).

11

Hydatid disease of the liver

J. Miles Little, MD, MS, FRACS, FACS

Those who work in hydatid endemic areas are used to dealing with the surgical problems of hydatid cysts. Those who work in the many parts of the world where it is rare find their occasional encounters with the disease stressful and puzzling. In these days of rapid and frequent international travel, it is essential that every general surgeon knows enough about the disease and its treatment to be able to cope at short notice with chance encounters with the disease.

This chapter is, therefore, designed to be a practical guide to the surgeon who may be unfamiliar with the disease. It is not for the expert, who will find little that is new and practically no help with the problems that he finds taxing.

A practical approach to the parasite's life cycle

It may seem odd to review yet again the familiar life cycle of *Echinococcus granulosus*, and there is a not unnatural feeling that it is a subject of 'academic' interest only. This is not quite true.[1-4]

Basically, in most countries, the domestic dog contracts the cestode *Taenia echinoccocus* and a grazing animal—commonly the sheep — develops the cystic phase of the parasite, usually in the liver but potentially anywhere in the body. The sheep never contracts the worm, and the dog never develops a cyst. Man accidentally replaces the sheep by ingesting ova from the dog's faeces. The infestation in man is usually acquired in childhood, the time when there develops the closest possible relationship with the dog and the most distant relationship with hygiene. Ova ingested by the intermediate host, be that host sheep or man, hatch in the upper gastrointestinal tract and migrate through the portal radicals to the liver. It is possible that some migrate through the liver to metastasize elsewhere (the lungs most commonly, but anywhere in the body). Some ova may make their way into the lacteals and thence into the thoracic duct, bypassing the liver filter altogether.

It is important to understand this life cycle. It must be clearly understood that a patient with a hydatid cyst is not infective to other members of the family. It is surprising how frequently a person with hydatid disease is segregated by his or her relatives. There is no logic in this, but much more logic in encouraging hygiene and a visit to the veterinary surgeon by the family dog.

E. multilocularis is a much less common variant of the parasite, which uses the fox as its usual definitive host and a rodent such as a vole or lemming as the intermediate host.[5-7] In the intermediate host, including man, this form of the parasite behaves much more like a malignancy, producing a honeycomb of cystic spaces filled with a glairy material. It infiltrates and at times metastasizes. I do not propose to deal with this form of the parasite, which is most commonly encountered in central Europe, in some parts of Russia, particularly Siberia, in Alaska and Northern Canada and in Japan. It is rare outside these areas, and only about six cases have been encountered in Australia, where *E. granulosus* remains relatively common.

Structure of the cyst of *Echinococcus granulosus*[1-4]

The hydatid cyst in the intermediate host has three layers. The outermost layer is the adventitia, and belongs to the host organ. It consists in essence of compressed native tissue and dense scar tissue which forms in reaction to the physical and chemical presence of the parasite. In the liver, the adventitia is thick, well-developed and incorporates the biliary and vascular structures. In the lung, the adventitia is much less developed. Surgery carried out in the plane outside the adventitia is made somewhat difficult by the presence of large blood vessels and bile ducts. It is this plane which is used in the operation of cystopericystectomy.

Inside the adventitia is the extraordinary laminated membrane. In a viable cyst, this is a white, gelatinous layer which is readily detached from the adventitia. It is acellular, but appears to have remarkable metabolic properties which include the ability to transport essential nutrients into the cyst, while keeping out harmful substances such as antibodies. Because the laminated membrane detaches so readily from the adventitia, the standard operation for removal of a hydatid cyst concentrates on detaching and removing the laminated membrane.

Lining the inner surface of the laminated membrane is the all-important germinal epithelium. It is at this point that we reach the infective part of the cyst—the part which can become a worm in the primary host and the part which can cause further cysts if spillage occurs as a result of surgery or rupture.

From the germinal epithelium there bud out brood capsules, small vesicles containing the so-called protoscolices which are recognizable microscopically as worm heads. Normally, these worm heads are inverted, and will not evert and become mature worms unless they are exposed to appropriate bile. Human bile will not cause eversion, whereas dog bile will.

Inside the cyst is the cyst fluid. This is crystal-clear in a viable cyst, milky and turbid or bile-stained in a degenerating cyst, and toothpaste-like in consistency in a dead cyst. In a viable cyst, the fluid contains the so-called hydatid sand, which consists of brood capsules, protoscolices and the degenerated hooklets from dead protoscolices.

Germinal epithelium, brood capsules, scolices and the cyst fluid containing all of these structures are infective. Spillage of any of these materials at the time of operation exposes the patient to the hazard of cyst dissemination.

Natural history in the human

When the six-hooked embryo first makes its way through the portal circulation to the liver, it lodges in a terminal portal radical and begins to excite a granulomatous reaction. After a few weeks, the centre of the granuloma develops a cavity, and a cyst develops, usually quite deep within the parenchyma of the liver. As the cyst enlarges, it does so towards areas of lower pressure.[1] For this reason, it usually makes its way towards the capsule of the liver on its peritoneal or extraperitoneal surface. It may also make its way to the bile ducts, eroding the walls and allowing extrusion of laminated membrane and germinal epithelium into the ducts. When bile leaks into the cyst, it commonly produces death of the main mother cyst, but endogenous daughter cysts are not necessarily affected. Less commonly, the cyst will make its way through the diaphragm into the thoracic cavity, where it may communicate with the bronchi.[8-11] On occasions, the cyst may erode the portal vein or hepatic vein. If laminated membrane secures access to the hepatic vein, the patient will develop multiple pulmonary emboli of obscure origin.

It was pointed out many years ago by Dew[1] that minor trauma is part of the growth and development of a hydatid cyst. As the cyst grows, the laminated membrane becomes less stable. The minor traumas of day-to-day living will cause detachment of laminated membrane carrying germinal epithelium. This appears to act as a stimulus to the formation of endogenous daughter cysts—that is, cysts consisting of laminated membrane lined by germinal epithelium but without adventitia, which float in the cyst fluid of the mother cyst. Sometimes, splitting of the adventitia will allow extrusion of laminated membrane with the formation of exogenous daughter cysts. It is very easy to miss these at the time of operation, and to leave a viable cyst behind when surgery is carried out in the plane of the laminated membrane.

A knowledge of the natural history of the hydatid is essential. At surgery, it is necessary to look at other peritoneal and retroperitoneal sites, since a cyst extruding to the surface of the liver may easily leak into the peritoneum or retroperitoneal space, and distant cysts may be found in virtually any abdominal or retroperitoneal site. When mobilizing a cyst in the commonest site—that is, the right lobe of the liver in segments VII and VIII—great care must be taken lest the cyst is protruding through the diaphragm. It is imperative to search all the recesses of the cyst for endogenous daughter cysts, and to account for any extruded daughter cysts that are identified by ultrasound or CT scanning. Bile leaks are common. If a significant bile leak is found, there is an appreciable chance that laminated membrane can be recovered from the main bile duct, and cholangiography is therefore mandatory.[3,4]

Diagnosis

Immunodiagnosis has a limited value outside endemic areas. There are many tests available,[12-21] including intradermal tests, indirect haemagglutination tests, complement fixation tests, latex agglutination tests, bentonite floculation tests, indirect fluorescent antibody tests, immunoelectrophoresis, counter-immunoelectrophoresis, double diffusion tests, enzyme-linked immunosorbent assay and radio-allergosorbent tests. A short review of these investigations will be found in Little and Deane.[4]

Organ imaging by ultrasound (Fig. 11.1) and CT scanning (Fig. 11.2) have demonstrated great usefulness in the diagnosis of hydatid disease.[22-26] The appearance with both modes of investigation is frequently characteristic, although confusion can arise with multiseptate simple cysts. Ultrasonography is about as powerful in diagnosis, but the scan appearances are less easy for a surgeon to interpret. Ultrasound is of particular value in following patients postoperatively, since no radiation exposure is involved.

It is possible with either mode of imaging to determine the anatomical distribution of cysts, and it is possible to detect cysts of 2 cm or more elsewhere in the peritoneal cavity or retroperitoneum. Confusion can obviously arise with simple cysts in the kidney, but it is usually possible to resolve this confusion at operation. Further detail may be sought from angiography and ERCP (Fig. 11.3),[27] particularly in complicated cases where cystopericystectomy or hepatic resection are planned. They reach their greatest use in planning the treatment of recurrent hydatids that have required several previous procedures.

Planned surgery

When a hydatid cyst has been diagnosed preoperatively, surgery must be carefully planned. The disease needs to be 'staged' as if it were a malignancy, and a careful search

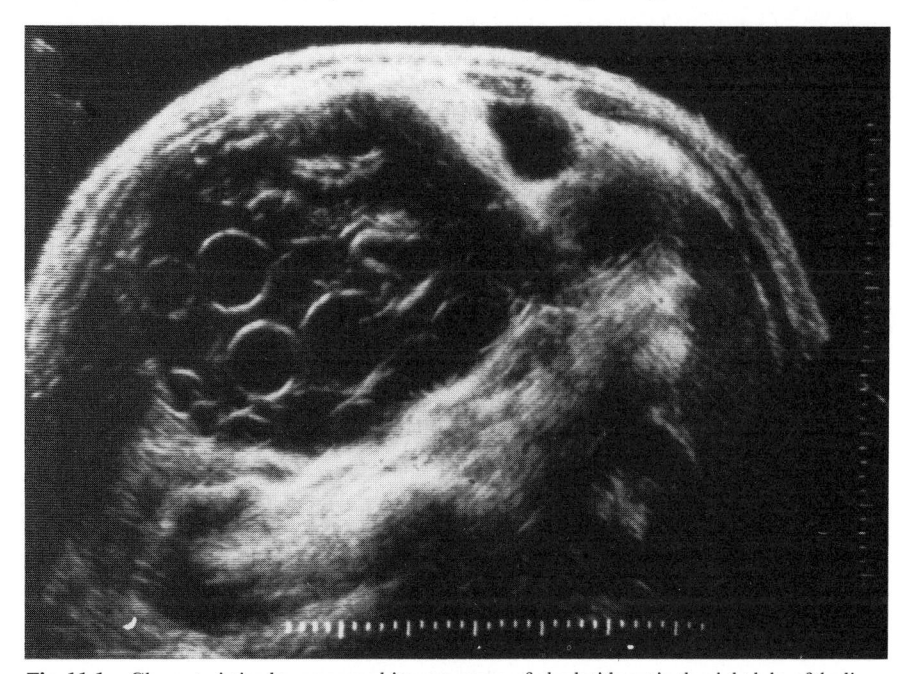

Fig. 11.1 Characteristic ultrasonographic appearance of a hydatid cyst in the right lobe of the liver. Daughter cysts can be clearly seen within the mother cyst. (Reproduced from reference 4 with the kind permission of Churchill Livingstone)

150 *Hydatid disease of the liver*

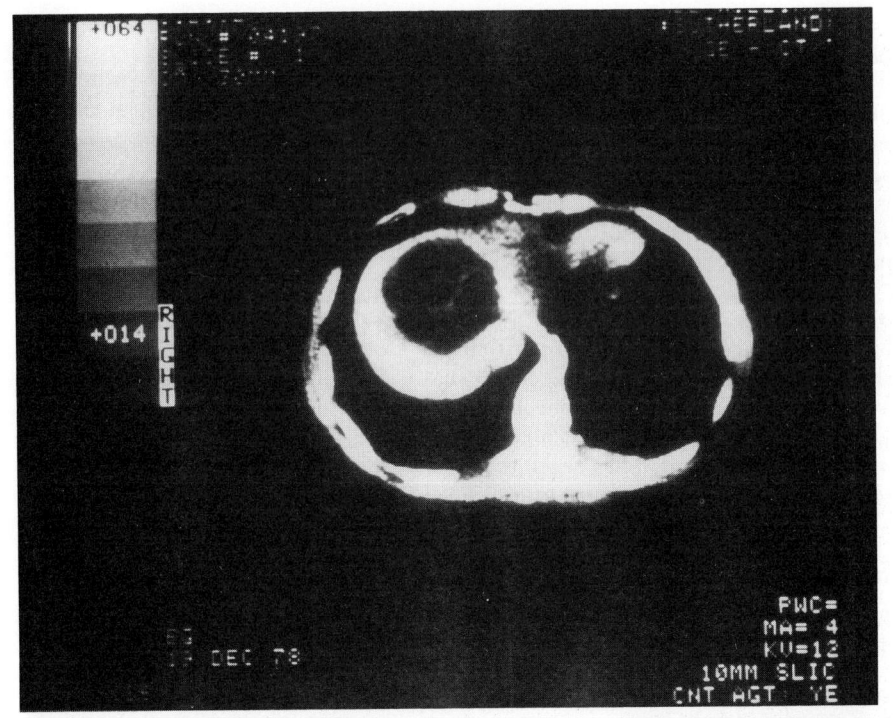

Fig. 11.2 Computerized tomographic appearance of a hydatid cyst in the dome of the right lobe of the liver. Once again, daughter cysts can be seen within the main cyst. (Reproduced from reference 4 with the kind permission of Churchill Livingstone)

made for other possible sites of involvement. In hydatid disease complicated by jaundice, recurrence or infection, ERCP and angiography should be carried out.

The anaesthetist should be warned of the diagnosis. Although anaphylactic reactions are rare,[28] they are catastrophic when they occur, and adrenalin and steroids should be on hand.

Exposure should be wide and generous (Fig. 11.4).[3,4,29] It is essential to remember that complete control of the operative field must be secured early and maintained throughout the procedure. If the surgery can be accomplished through the abdomen, it is best to avoid opening the chest. Most abdominal hydatids can be safely dealt with through the abdomen, without exposing the patient to the discomforts of a thoracoabdominal incision and the hazards of intrathoracic dissemination of the disease. A long transverse bilateral subcostal incision with vertical extension allows excellent exposure. Some form of fixed retraction can be used to elevate the costal margin, and in most instances this will give excellent exposure to the dome of the right lobe of the liver. Mobilization of the liver is essential, but must be carried out with great care. The cyst tends to protrude through the capsule of the liver, and its attachment to the diaphragm may be dense and difficult to dissect. It is possible to enter the cyst inadvertently during mobilization.

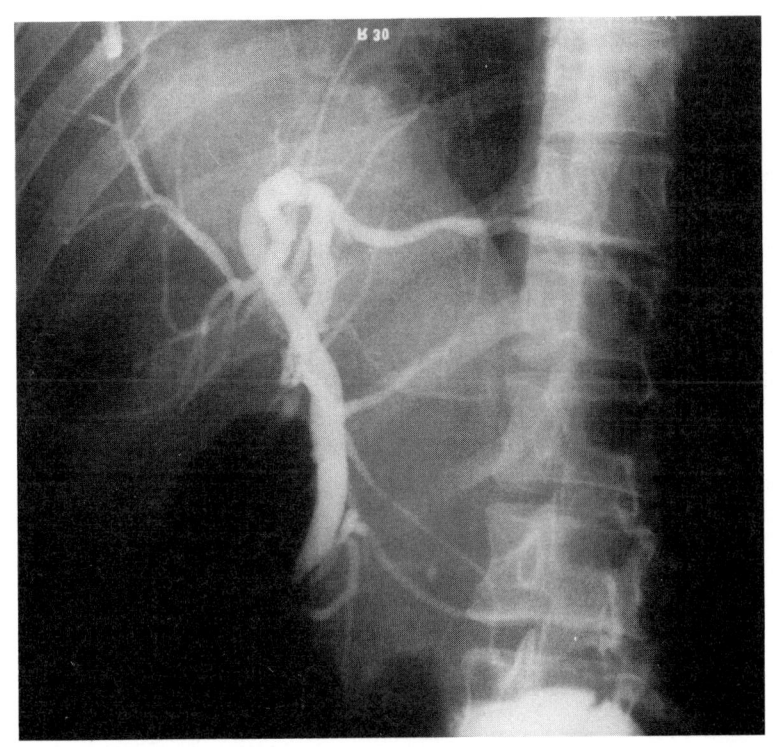

Fig. 11.3 ERCP appearance in a complex case of recurrent hydatid disease affecting the right lobe of the liver. Most of the right lobe has been destroyed, and there is hypertrophy of the left lobe.

When mobilization is complete, the next step is isolation by packing. It is our practice to soak sponges used for packing in 3 per cent saline,[3,4] and to avoid other scolicides on the sponges. Packs should be placed all around the operative field and over the skin edges, but must allow good, controlled access to the presenting portion of the white, thick adventitia protruding through the liver capsule.

It is essential to have three high-pressure suckers throughout the operation.[3,4] Wall suction is frequently inadequate, and pump suction is preferable. Large suction tubing is essential, since laminated membrane is gelatinous and will repeatedly block standard suction tubing. We use uterine evacuation tubing connected to mobile suckers.

The next step involves relieving the pressure within the cyst. A viable cyst contains fluid under considerable tension, and any loss of control will result in profuse spillage of infective fluid. Aspiration with a wide-bore aspirating needle connected by a three-way tap to a 50 ml syringe will frequently help to control the pressure (Fig. 11.5). It may only be possible to aspirate 20–50 ml of fluid if there are many daughter cysts or if the laminated membrane has already begun to fragment. Even this, however, will produce a significant drop in the cyst pressure.[29]

The cyst should be emptied as far as possible with the aspirating needle and syringe. There is some dispute about the value of using scolicidal agents. 2 per cent formalin, hypertonic saline, cetrimide and immune serum have been advocated

152 *Hydatid disease of the liver*

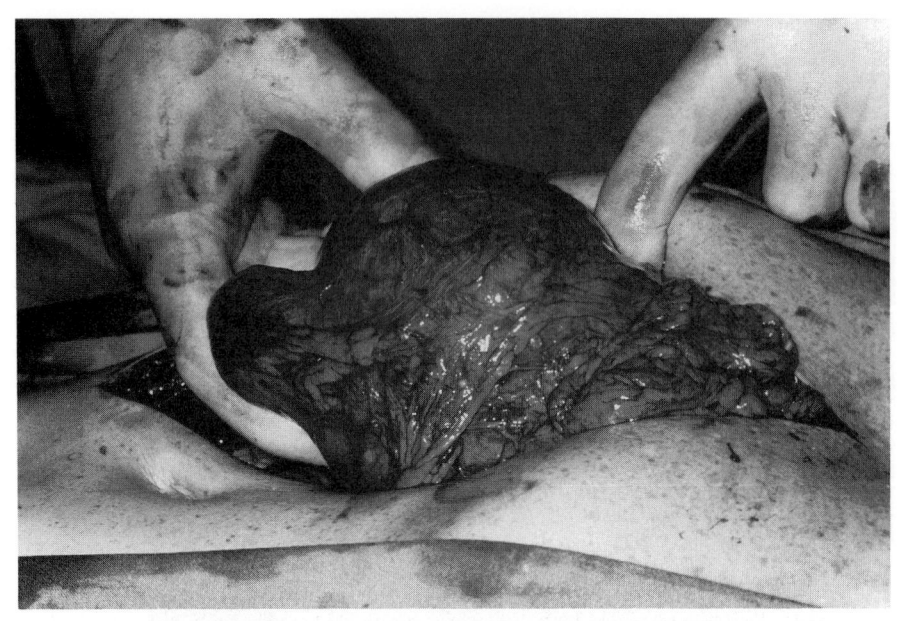

Fig. 11.4 Initial wide exposure of a right lobar hydatid cyst. (Reproduced from reference 43 with the kind permission of Romaine Pierson Publrs Inc., Port Washington)

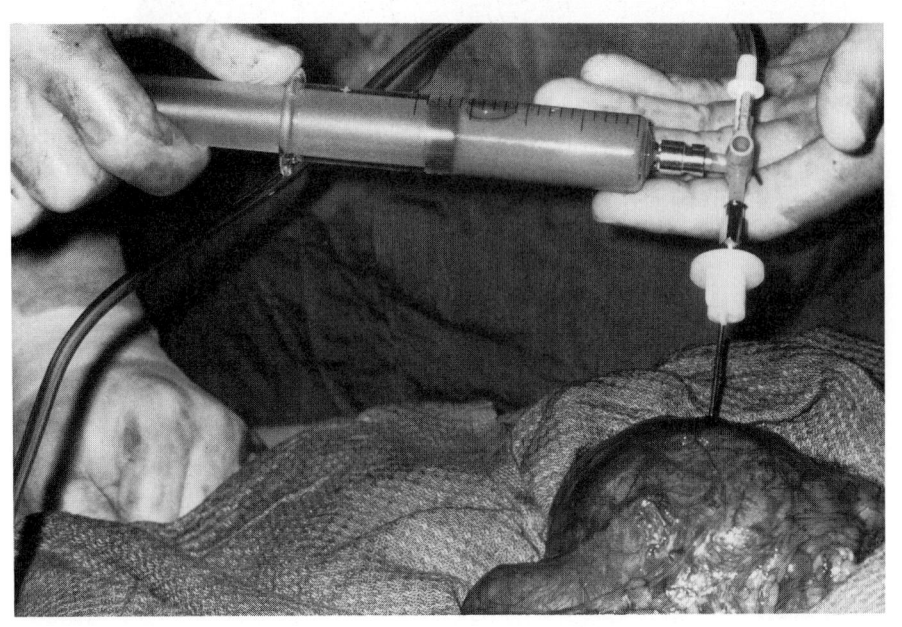

Fig. 11.5 Aspiration of the contents of the cyst. In this case, the fluid is turbid and bile stained, suggesting a biliary leak into the cyst. Scolicides should not be used under these circumstances. (Reproduced from reference 43 with the kind permission of Romaine Pierson Publrs Inc.)

as scolicides. There is, however, little evidence for their effectiveness, and there is considerable dispute about their value. Relieving the intracyst tension is more important. Scolicides will not penetrate viable daughter cysts, which will remain potentially infective. In addition, there is the risk that the scolicides will gain access to the biliary tree. Formalin has been associated with both acute toxicity[30] and with sclerosing cholangitis[31] in the long term, and its use should be avoided. It is probably wise to avoid any form of scolicide if the aspirate from the cyst is bile stained.

The cyst should next be opened in a controlled fashion. Stay sutures are inserted to maintain control of the cyst wall. Isolation cones may be of value. These are of two patterns. The Saidi cone[32] is frozen on to the wall of the cyst, whereas the simpler Aarons cone (Fig. 11.6)[30] has a suction groove in the base which allows the cone to be held in place by the negative pressure of the theatre suction. The cone is not essential for successful surgery. We find the Aarons cone moderately useful at times, but it suffers from the problem of losing grip on the cyst as the adventitial wall collapses.

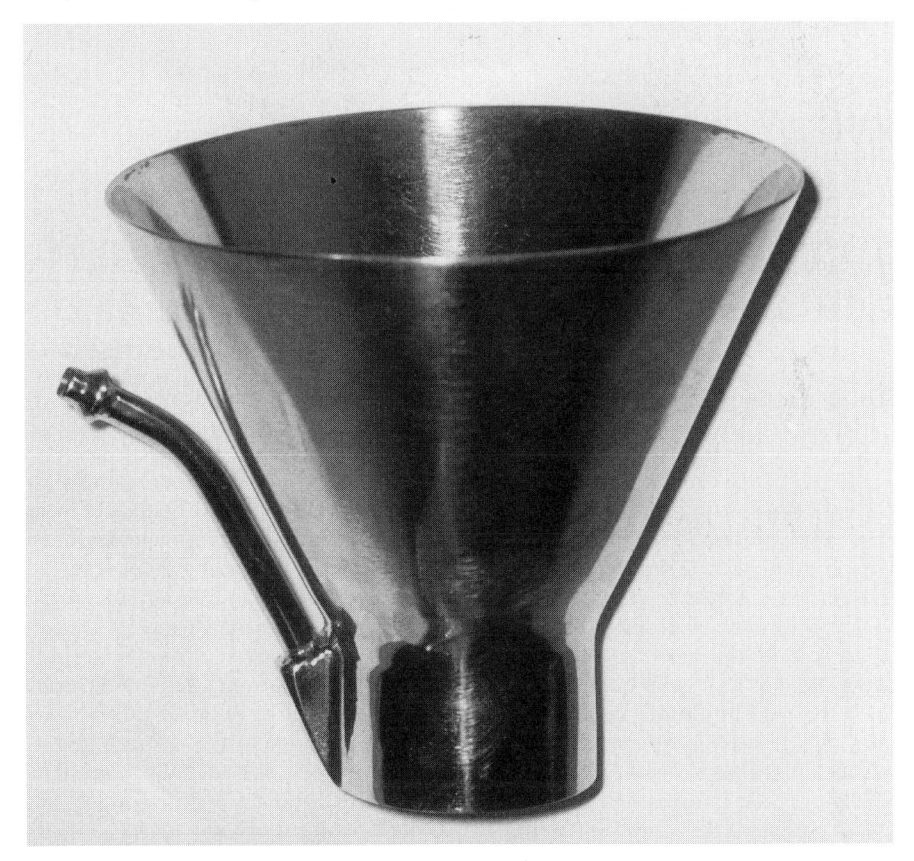

Fig. 11.6 The Aarons cone. There is a groove beneath the inferior margin, which communicates with the suction nozzle to the left-hand side of the cone. High-pressure suction attached to the nozzle creates a partial vacuum in the groove, which in turn fastens on to the cyst wall.

154 Hydatid disease of the liver

An opening is made in the wall of the cyst with the diathermy, and the three suction tubes already set up are now used to suck away both the fluid contents and the laminated membrane (Fig. 11.7), which falls away from the adventitia as the supporting fluid in the cyst is removed. The laminated membrane will block the tubing, and must be broken up by repeatedly squeezing the membrane within the tubing with large artery forceps.

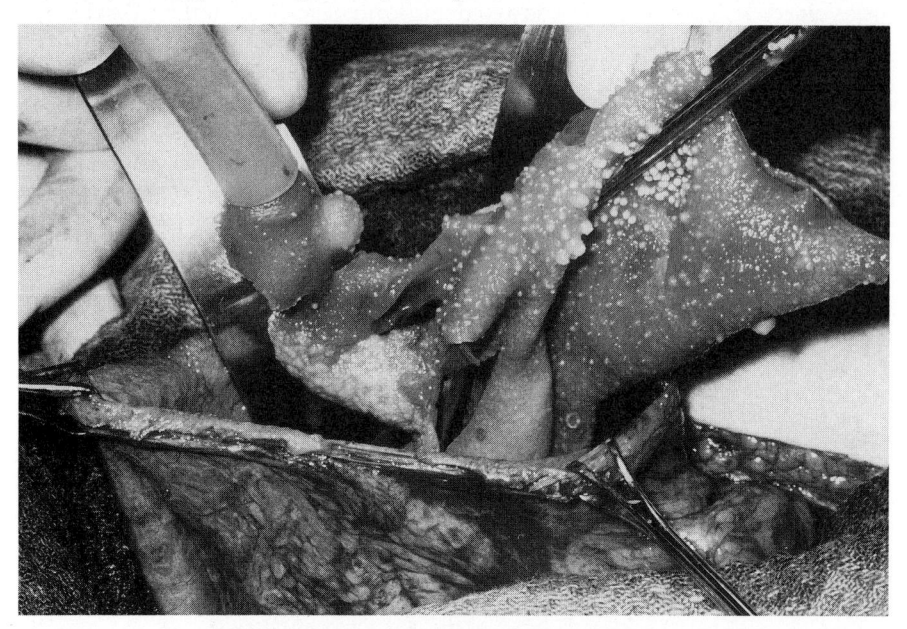

Fig. 11.7 Laminated membrane being removed from the main cyst. The suction tubing is perhaps the most important instrument during this phase of the operation. (Reproduced from reference 43 with the kind permission of Romaine Pierson Publrs Inc.)

Once the laminated membrane has been completely removed with suction, sponge-holding forceps and swabs held in forceps, a careful search must be made for endogenous daughter cysts in the recesses of the mother cyst. Daughter cysts are easily missed (Fig. 11.8). If exogenous daughter cysts have been identified on the preoperative imaging, a systematic search must also be made for these.

When all viable hydatid material has been removed, the free surface of the cyst is removed as far as viable liver will allow. This will usually leave a saucer-shaped defect of variable size (Fig. 11.9). This in turn must now be carefully searched for any evidence of bile leaks. We have not found cholangiography to be helpful in identifying bile leaks, nor the injection of dyes into the biliary tree. It has been more useful to place a clean, dry sponge against what remains of the adventitia, to compress the liver nearby and to search for bile staining on the sponge. It is our practice to close bile leaks carefully, since prolonged bile leakage is a potent source of morbidity, particularly if the adventitia is calcified.

It is usually prudent to carry out an operative cholangiogram, and the gall bladder can be used if it is still present. The presence of laminated membrane in the bile duct will dictate an exploration of the bile duct using standard techniques.

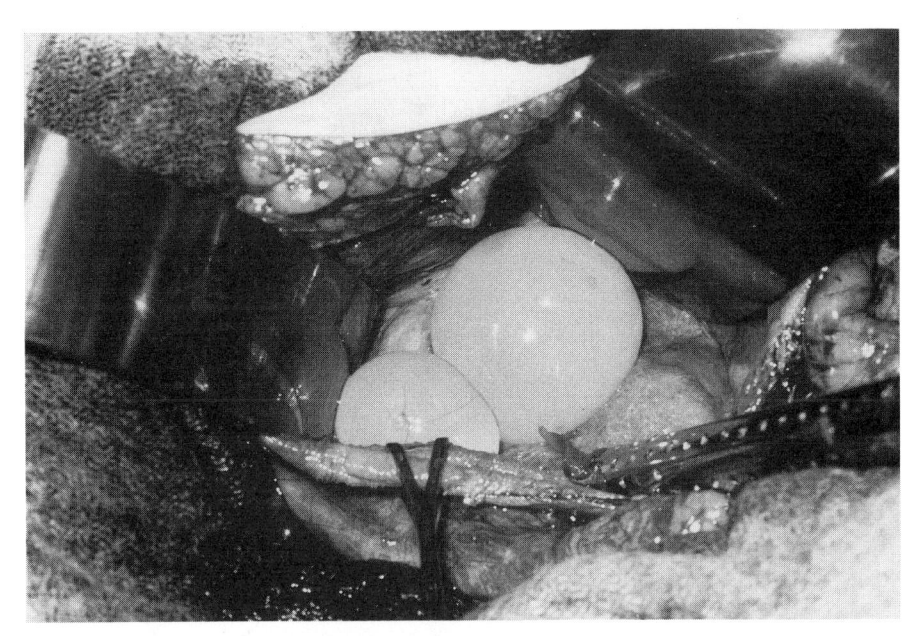

Fig. 11.8 Daughter cysts in the depths of the main cyst. In this particular case, the lining of the main cyst was calcified and was presumably not viable. These daughter cysts are viable. (Reproduced from reference 43 with the kind permission of Romain Pierson Publrs Inc.)

With the cyst largely removed, a significant dead space will be created in and around what remains of the liver. There are various techniques for dealing with this, such as capitonage, which involves infolding of the margins of the residual cyst. The cyst can be simply left open into the peritoneal cavity. Marsupialization of the cyst is no longer an acceptable technique.[33] Perhaps the best available method for dealing with this problem is to carry out an omentoplasty.[33] This will involve a variable amount of freeing of the omentum from the transverse colon, and at times the creation of a pedicle of omentum by division of one gastroepoploic artery—usually the left—in order to secure an adequate bulk of omental tissue to provide a complete lining for the residual cyst wall (Fig. 11.10). Omentoplasty has provided a significant reduction in the occurrence of subphrenic collection and prolonged biliary leakage.[3,4,33]

It is our practice to provide short-term sump drainage after hydatid surgery, since a small amount of bile leakage is common. We prefer to remove drains as soon as they have ceased to do their job—usually at about 48 to 72 hours.

There are other operations which can be used at times. The first of these is *cystopericystectomy*.[34] In this very useful procedure, dissection proceeds outside the adventitia with the idea of removing the adventitia completely. This is particularly useful for dealing with calcified cysts, and is made much easier by the use of a Cavitron ultrasonic dissection device. The advantages cited for the procedure are that bile leakage is prevented, since bile ducts are ligated as they are encountered; and that there is no significant problem in closing the cavity postoperatively, since the walls are so pliable. It must be realized,

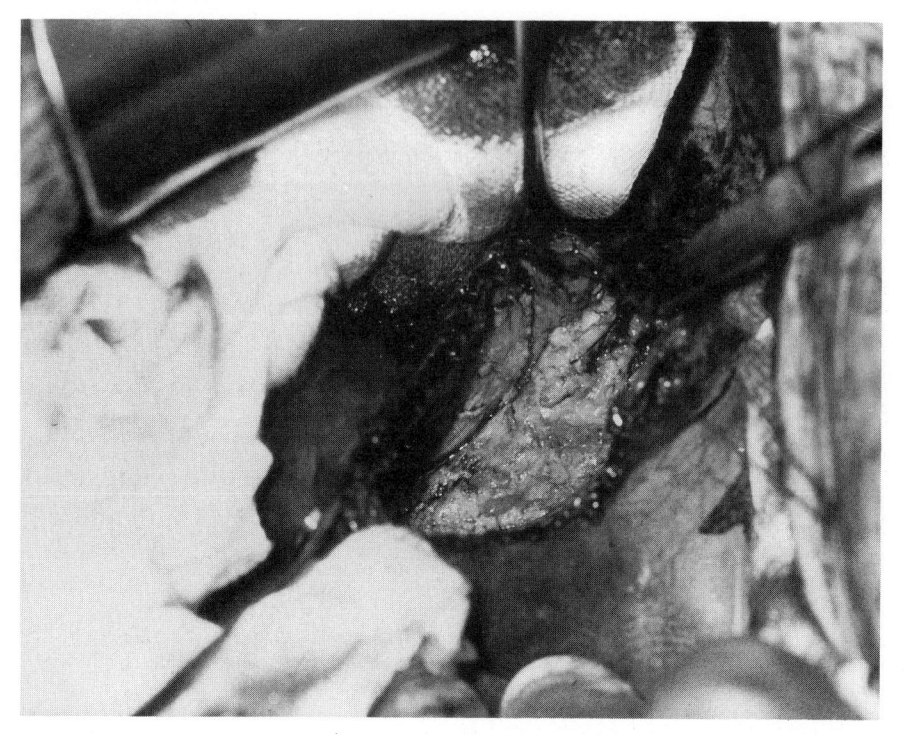

Fig. 11.9 The cavity left in the liver after removal of excess cyst wall. (Reproduced from reference 4 with the kind permission of Churchill Livingstone)

however, that massive cysts cannot be dealt with completely in this way, since the medial wall of a huge right lobar cyst invariably contains the inferior vena cava and dissection in this region would be very hazardous.

The second procedure which finds a place with complicated hydatid disease, and particularly for recurrent disease, is hepatic resection. It should probably not be regarded as a general first-line method of treatment, but is certainly justified for recurrent disease or for disease which has caused atrophy of a segment of liver.

Chance encounters with hepatic hydatids

From time to time, a surgeon will encounter a hydatid unexpectedly when operating for some other cause. With the frequent use of ultrasound, such chance encounters are less common than they were. The decision about appropriate action must be based first on the surgeon's experience with the disease, and second on the operating conditions. An experienced surgeon operating in a clean abdomen can safely and justifiably carry out one or other definitive procedure for the cyst. In a contaminated field, even an experienced surgeon should think twice, and would need pressing indications to remove the cyst. An inexperienced surgeon with neither the experience nor the facilities would be well advised to leave such a

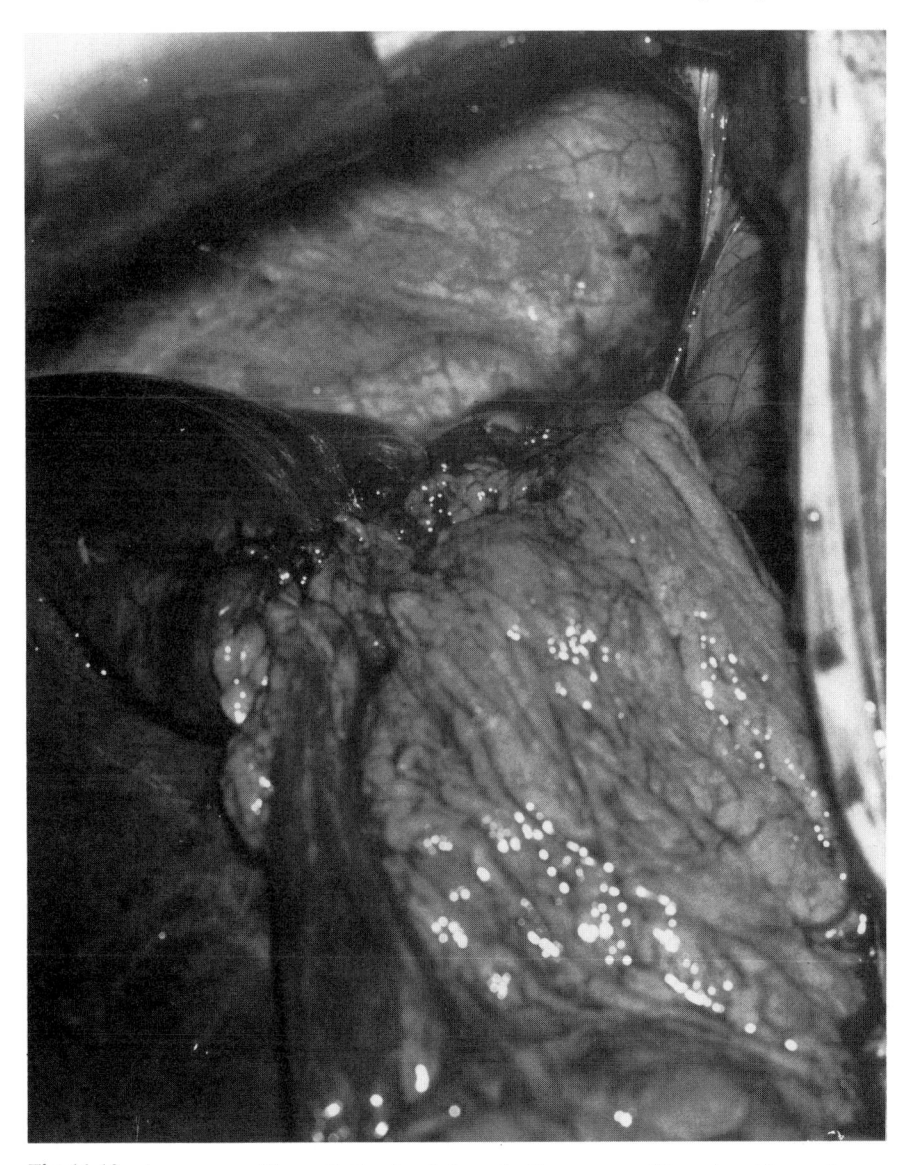

Fig. 11.10 Appearance of the cavity lined and plugged with omentum. (Reproduced from reference 4 with the kind permission of Churchill Livingstone)

patient strictly alone. We have had one patient, whose hydatid was removed by an inexperienced surgeon, and who developed a fistula between the transverse colon and the remnant of the cyst. He died ultimately of gas forming infection in the right side of the liver.

If the decision is made not to operate but to refer the patient elsewhere, it is better to avoid further dissection, which will make the subsequent surgery more difficult.

When to leave a hydatid cyst alone

Not all cysts require surgery. During their growth phase, cysts have a tendency to rupture into the retroperitoneum or peritoneal cavity, to make their way into the bile ducts, the hepatic veins or through the diaphragm. During the phase when they become effete and start to die, they commonly cause symptoms of severe pain. Infection in a cyst is not uncommon, and between 10 and 15 per cent of our patients have had evidence of infection in their cysts at operation.[3,4] On the other hand, many cysts are never recognized by the patient, but simply go on to die and calcify. While it is true that calcification in the wall of a cyst does not mean that the cyst is dead, a heavily calcified cyst without translucent areas in its centre is almost certainly dead and can be left alone, particularly in the asymptomatic and elderly patient. It is also reasonable to manage small, deeply intraparenchymal cysts conservatively. Their surgery would involve searching through the parenchyma of the liver, preferably with an operative ultrasound. As Saidi[29] has pointed out, these small intraparenchymal cysts can be followed by serial ultrasound. If they do not enlarge, they can be left alone. If they enlarge to reach the capsule of the liver, surgery is needed.

Follow-up

Our own experience suggests that a patient with operated hydatid disease should be followed for a minimum of two and a half years, with six-monthly ultrasound examinations.[35] Although further hydatid disease at the original site was uncommon in our study, the development of hydatid disease elsewhere during the period of follow-up was alarmingly common. The cumulative recurrence rate at 30 months was 22 per cent. No recurrences have been seen after that time. It must be stressed that recurrence is only common amongst patients who have evidence of disease dissemination at the time of the original surgery, with multiple cysts or evidence of extruded laminated membrane in the bile duct or peritoneal cavity.

It is not uncommon to see cystic areas on the ultrasound, particularly in relation to the omentoplasty after successful surgery.[36] A diagnosis of recurrence should not be made unless the cystic area is seen to be growing in size and developing daughter cysts. In the early years of our study, we explored several patients with apparent recurrence not fulfilling the criteria of growth and daughter cyst development, only to find small biliary collections of no clinical significance.

Medical therapy

Although the drug mebendazole did not appear to be particularly successful,[37–40] we have been impressed with recent experience of the drug Albendazole.[41] Albendazole appears to be better absorbed, and to reach a more effective concentration within viable cysts. At the moment, in Australia, Albendazole is restricted for use in recurrent disease, disseminated disease, inaccessible disease and in medically compromised patients for whom surgery is out of the question.

The most widely used dose regimen is 10 mg/kg per day in two divided doses. This usually means a dose of 400 mg twice a day. The drug is given for four weeks, then stopped for two. At the end of the two weeks, a full blood count and liver function tests are carried out. It is common to find a modest rise of gamma GT and ALT, without clinical symptoms. Ultrasounds are repeated at six-weekly intervals at the same time as the haematological and biochemical tests. So far, all four patients under treatment have tolerated the drug well and all have shown either disappearance of their cysts or striking reduction in size (more than 50 per cent). It is recommended by the marketing company that a full course should consist of no more than eight cycles.

The future

Hydatid disease can be abolished by veterinary and public health measures.[42] It was once common in Iceland, New Zealand and Tasmania, but has virtually disappeared from those places. In the state of New South Wales, preventive programmes have had little impact and the incidence remains much the same as it was 20 years ago. Eradication measures consist of controlled disposal of sheep offal, regular screening of dogs for the ova of *Taenia echinococcus*, and the vigorous treatment of infected dogs until their faeces are clear of ova.

While Albendazole appears promising as a medical alternative to surgery, surgery remains the standard against which all other methods of treatment must be compared.

References

1. Dew H. *Hydatid Disease: Its Pathology, Diagnosis and Treatment*. Sydney: Australian Medical Publishing Company, 1928.
2. Braithwaite P.A. Hydatid disease: epidemiology and pathology. *Aust. NZ J. Surg.* 1983; **53:** 203–9.
3. Little J.M., Deane S.A. Hydatid disease. In: Bengmark S., Blumgart L.H. (eds.): *Liver Surgery*. Edinburgh: Churchill Livingstone, 1986: 118–29.
4. Little J.M., Deane S.A. Hydatid disease. In: Blumgart L.H. (ed.): *Surgery of the Liver and Biliary Tract*. Edinburgh: Churchill Livingstone, 1988: 955–66.
5. West J.T., Hillman F.J., Rausch R.L. Alveolar hydatid disease of the liver: rationale and technics of surgical treatment. *Ann. Surg.* 1963; **157:** 548–59.
6. Samuels S., Formoe R. Alveolar hydatid disease with involvement of the inferior vena cava. *Amer. Surg.* 1970: 698–701.
7. Kasai Y., Sasaki E., Koshino I., Kawanishi N., Kumagai M. Operative treatment of alveolar echinococcosis of the liver. *Jap. J. Surg.* 1978; **8:** 28–33.
8. Alestig K., Holm C., Nystrom G., Schersten T. Biliobronchial fistula secondary to echinococcal abscess of the liver. *Acta Chir. Scand.* 1972; **138:** 90–4.
9. Amir-Jahed A.K., Sadrieh M., Farpour A., Azar H., Namdaran F. Thoracobilia: a surgical complication of hepatic echinococcosis and amebiasis. *Ann. Thor. Surg.* 1972; **14:** 198–205.
10. Yacoubian H.D. Thoracic problems associated with hydatid cyst of the dome of the liver. *Surgery*. 1976; **79:** 544–8.
11. Reventos J., Nogueras F.M., Rius X., Lorenzo T. Hydatid disease of the liver with thoracic involvement. *Surg. Gyn. Obst.* 1976; **143:** 570–4.
12. Kagan I.G. A review of serological tests for the diagnosis of hydatid disease. *Bull. WHO*. 1968; **39:** 25–37.
13. Lass N., Laver Z., Lengy J. The immunodiagnosis of hydatid disease: postoperative evaluation of the skin test and four serological tests. *Ann. Allergy*. 1973; **31:** 430–6.

14. Farag H., Bout D., Capron A. Specific immunodiagnosis of human hydatidosis by the Enzyme Linked Immunosorbent Assay (ELISA). *Biomedicine.* 1975; **23:** 276–8.
15. Varela-Diaz V.M., Coltorti E.A., Prezioso U., Lopez-Lemes M.H., Guisantes J.A., Yarzabal L.A. Evaluation of three immunodiagnostic tests for human hydatid disease. *Amer. J. Trop. Med. Hyg.* 1975; **24:** 312–19.
16. Matossian R.M. The immunological diagnosis of human hydatid disease. *Trans. R. Soc. Trop. Med. Hyg.* 1977; **71:** 101–4.
17. Ito K., Horiuchi Y., Kumagai M., Ueda M., Nakamura R., Kawanishi N., Kasai Y. Evaluation of RAST as an immunological method for diagnosis of multilocular echinococcosis. *Clin. Exper. Immunol.* 1977; **28:** 407–12.
18. Coltorti E.A., Varela-Diaz V.M. Detection of antibodies against *Echinococcus granulosus* Arc 5 antigens by double diffusion test. *Trans. R. Soc. Trop. Med. Hyg.* 1978; **72:** 226–9.
19. Sorice F., Delia S., Vullo V., Aceti A., Ferone V. Sensitivity and specificity of the RAST (radioalergosorbent test) in biological diagnosis of hydatidosis. *Ann. Sclavo.* 1979; **21:** 800–15.
20. Matossian R.M., McLaren M.I., Draper C.C., Bradstreet C.M.P., Dighero M.W., Kane G.J., MacKinlay L.M., Rickard M.D. The serodiagnosis of human hydatid disease. 2: Additional studies on selected sera using indirect haemagglutination (IHA), enzyme-linked immunosorbent assay (ELISA) and defined antigen substrate spheres (DASS). *J. Helminthol.* 1979; **53:** 287–91.
21. Guisantes J.A., Rubio M.F., Diaz R. Application of an Enzyme Linked Immunosorbent Assay (ELISA) method to the diagnosis of human hydatidosis. *Bull. Pan-Amer. Health Org.* 1981; **15:** 260–6.
22. Vicary F.R., Cusick G., Shirley I.M., Blackwell R.J. Ultrasound and abdominal hydatid disease. *Trans. R. Soc. Trop. Med. Hyg.* 1977; **71:** 29–31.
23. Scherer U., Weinzierl M., Sturm R., Schildberg F.W., Zrenner M., Lissner J. Computed tomography in hydatid disease of the liver: a report on 13 cases. *J. Comp. Assist. Tomog.* 1978; **2:** 612–17.
24. Niron A., Ozer H. Ultrasound appearances of liver hydatid disease. *Brit. J. Radiol.* 1981; **54:** 335–8.
25. de Diego Choliz J., Lecumberri Olaverri F.J., Franquet Casas T., Ostiz Zubieta S. Computed tomography in hepatic echinococcosis. *Amer. J. Radiol.* 1982; **139:** 699–702.
26. MacPherson C.N., Romig T., Zeyhle E., Rees P.H., Were J.B. Portable ultrasound scanner versus serology in screening for hydatid cysts in a nomadic population. *Lancet.* 1987; **2:** 259–61.
27. Cottone M., Amuso M., Cotton P. Endoscopic retrograde cholangiography in hepatic hydatid disease. *Brit. J. Surg.* 1978; **65:** 107–8.
28. Jakubowski M.S., Barnard D.E. Anaphylactic shock during operation for hydatid disease. *Anesthesiology.* 1971; **34:** 197–9.
29. Saidi F. In: Calne R.Y. (ed.): *Liver Surgery.* Padua: Piccin Medical Books, 1982; 61–74.
30. Aggerwal A.R., Garg R.L. Formalin toxicity in hydatid liver disease. *Anaesthesia.* 1983; **38:** 662–5.
31. Khodadadi D.J., Kurgan A., Schmidt B. Sclerosing cholangitis following the treatment of echinoccocosis of the liver. *Int. Surg.* 1981; **66:** 361–2.
32. Aarons B.G., Kune G.A. A suction cone to prevent spillage during hydatid surgery. *Aust. NZ J. Surg.* 1983; **53:** 471–2.
33. Papadimitriou J., Mandrekas A. The surgical treatment of hydatid disease of the liver. *Brit. J. Surg.* 1970; **57:** 431–3.
34. Belli L., Del Favero E., Marni A., Romani F. Resection versus pericystostomy in the treatment of hydatidosis of the liver. *Amer. J. Surg.* 1983; **145:** 234–42.
35. Little J.M., Hollands M.J., Ekberg H. Recurrence of hydatid disease. *World J. Surg.* 1988; **12:** 700–4.
36. Chaimoff C., Lubin E., Dintsman M. The postoperative appearance of the liver on scanning following omentopexy of the hydatid cyst. *Int. Surg.* 1980; **65:** 331–3.
37. Bekhti A., Schaaps J.P., Capron M., Dessaint J.P. Treatment of hepatic hydatid disease with mebendazole: preliminary results in four cases. *Brit. Med. J.* 1977; **2:** 1356.
38. Wilson J.F., Davidson M., Rausch R.L. A clinical trial of mebendazole in the treatment of alveolar hydatid disease. *Amer. Rev. Resp. Dis.* 1978; **118:** 747–57.
39. Braithwaite P.A. Long-term high-dose mebendazole for cystic hydatid disease of the liver: failure in two cases. *Aust. NZ J. Surg.* 1981; **51:** 23–7.

40. Morris D.L., Gould S. Serum and cyst levels of mebendazole and flubendazole in hydatid disease. *Brit. Med. J.* 1982; **285:** 175.
41. Saimot A.G., Meulemans A., Cremieux A.C., Giovananceli M.D., Hay J.M., Delaitre B., Coulaudi J.P. Albendazole as a potential treatment for human hydatidosis. *Lancet.* 1983; **2:** 652–6.
42. Christie M., Beard T.C., Nicholas W.L. The control of hydatid disease and ovine cysticaroses in the Australian Capital Territory and Southern New South Wales. *Med. J. Aust.* 1977; **1:** 773–5.
43. Little J.M. The management of multiple hydatids in the peritoneal cavity with a report of a case. *Surgical Rounds.* 1980; **3:** 22–30.

12

Prostatic carcinoma

David Kirk, DM, FRCS

Until some fifteen years ago the choice of treatment for men with adenocarcinoma of the prostate appeared to raise few difficulties. It seemed that radical prostatectomy, although not generally practised in the United Kingdom, could cure many of the small percentage of tumours presenting at an early stage,[1] while hormonal treatment provided an effective method of controlling more advanced disease and was considered to prolong the patient's life.[2] Recently, the whole role of aggressive treatment of the localized primary tumour has been questioned,[3] and hormonal therapy, far from being the universal treatment it once was, is being used more selectively.[4] It is instructive to examine the reasons for these changes in attitude.

Natural history of prostatic carcinoma

It is well-known that postmortem examination of the prostates of elderly men will demonstrate histological foci of tumour in a percentage increasing with age and with an overall prevalence of 30 per cent in those over 50 years old.[5] McNeal has demonstrated the progression of these foci to overt carcinomata[6] which tend to become histologically less well differentiated as they grow. He has suggested that tumour aggression may be proportional to its size, with a tumour of volume less than 1 ml being incapable of metastasizing, and one over 4 ml likely already to have done so.[7]

The typical patient presenting with carcinoma of the prostate is elderly, will therefore have a comparatively short expectation of life and may well suffer from additional life-threatening disease. It is no surprise that of those patients who died during the course of the Veterans Administration Cooperative Urological Research Group (VACURG) studies the majority did so from other conditions.[8] This has important implications. If a patient is destined to die from other causes, treatment of his prostatic carcinoma will not affect his life expectation. Thus treatment of those who are at risk will be at the expense of subjecting others who will not benefit to the treatment and its possible side-effects. Even where treatment does improve survival, for an elderly man the achievement of a few months extra life might be of less significance than for a young woman with family responsibilities suffering from cancer of the breast.

This creates a number of paradoxes, recognition of which is essential for the realistic management of prostatic carcinoma. At one extreme, the small localized tumour which might be amenable to surgical cure would, untreated, be likely to progress over a time course longer than many patients' life expectation. At the other, advanced prostatic cancer, while being an incurable fatal disease, is one from which only a proportion of sufferers will die.

Treatment of early prostatic carcinoma

Is earlier diagnosis of prostatic carcinoma now possible?

Unless there are dramatic developments in cytotoxic chemotherapy, a reduction in the mortality from prostatic cancer can come only from early diagnosis and treatment of lesions before local or distant spread has occurred. Clinical digital examination is a crude method of assessing the prostate, and tumours so detectable already are fairly advanced. The advent of transrectal ultrasonography and the development of prostate-specific antigen assays may have altered the prospects for early diagnosis.

Ultrasonography

Assessment of localized prostatic cancer by digital palpation is notoriously inaccurate.[9] Transrectal ultrasonography[10] provides a method of accurate imaging, valuable not only in assessing the clinically obvious tumour, but also with the potential of detecting tumours too small to be felt on rectal examination (Fig. 12.1), albeit with a significant false-positive rate.[11] However, routine screening by this method alone would be expensive and time-consuming, and many men might find it unacceptable. Could a smaller population particularly at risk be identified?

Prostate-specific antigen

Besides being a useful histochemical marker of prostatic tissue,[12] prostate-specific antigen (PSA) is found in increased levels in the serum of patients with prostatic carcinoma.[13] It is a more sensitive indicator of prostatic carcinoma than prostatic acid phosphatase (PAP), although mild elevations occurring in benign prostatic hypertrophy reduce its specificity.

PSA falls in response to successful treatment, and appears to be the first marker to rise as an indication of relapse after hormonal treatment,[14] although the current lack of effective treatment for such relapsed patients reduces the value of this observation. PSA undoubtedly is a significant advance in the management of the disease, but its final role perhaps has yet to be determined.

Possibly one such role is screening. PAP is elevated only in advanced carcinoma; indeed elevation of PAP is an accepted indicator of likely metastatic disease. Thus it is not a test which will identify potentially curable disease. On the other hand, the sensitivity of PSA might identify a group of men, a significant proportion of whom could have prostatic carcinoma and on whom transrectal ultrasonography should be performed.

Even then there is a problem. The wholesale extirpation of prostate glands containing small foci of tumour picked up by ultrasonography but undetectable

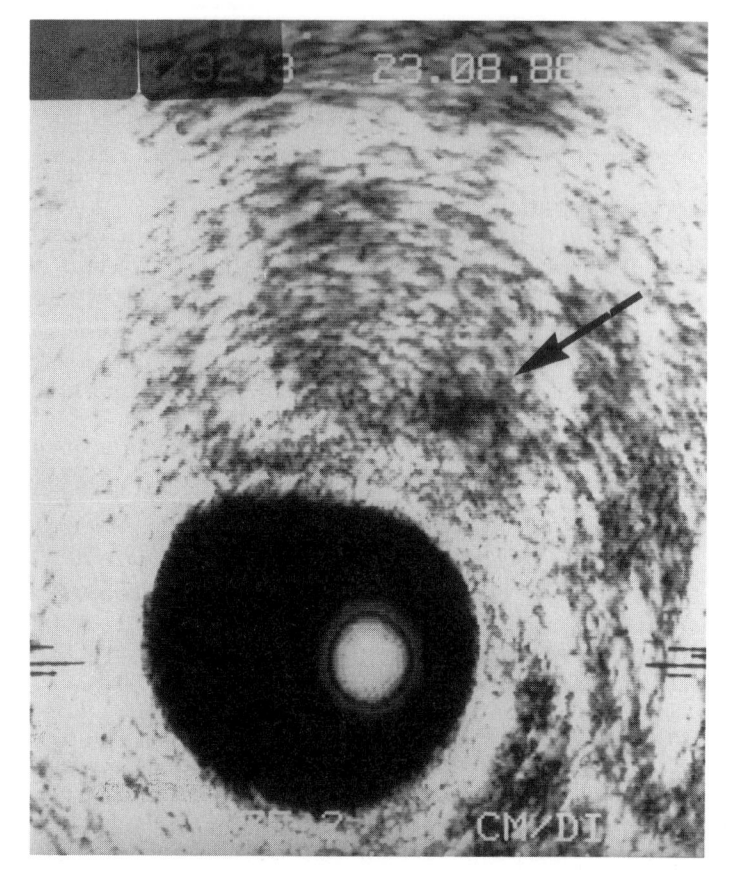

Fig. 12.1 Transrectal ultrasound scan of clinically benign prostate containing small hypoechoic tumour (arrowed). (Courtesy of Mr Brian Peeling)

clinically seems difficult to justify, since we would expect many men over 50 to have such lesions, most of whom are unlikely to develop clinical prostatic carcinoma. Despite this, it is reasonable to suppose that many men presenting today with advanced prostatic cancer will at some time in the past have had such a potentially curable lesion. Once more there seems to be a paradox, and we need to be able to decide which of the lesions diagnosable on ultrasonography should be treated.

If McNeal's views are correct, and the patient with a clinically occult focus, or even a small palpable nodule, of less than 1 ml volume is not in immediate danger of developing metastases[7] and if the rate of growth of his tumour is uncertain, a strong case could be made for initial observation, treating the tumour only when its growth approaches this size. Using transrectal ultrasound to assess objectively alterations in tumour size,[15] deferred management of small tumours may be a practical possibility. Transrectal ultrasonography becomes the key to the management of early disease, perhaps providing a route towards reducing the mortality from prostatic cancer. Unfortunately most

British urologists, even in centres with an interest in prostatic cancer, do not have access to this facility. Yet this must be one of the challenges to modern urologists, and it is to be hoped that they can be provided with the tools to deal with it.

Methods of treating localized tumours

Accepting that the need for treatment of some early or localized tumours still is a subject of debate, treatment itself provides a number of options. While radical prostatectomy will appeal to the surgeon, and perhaps is more reassuring to the patient in 'removing' his tumour, radiotherapy might be a more viable proposition in some situations.

Radical prostatectomy

In Britain the value of radical prostatectomy has been questioned on the grounds that it was applicable to few patients, that it had serious side-effects (universal impotence and frequent incontinence), and that its benefits were dubious. This raised wrath from across the Atlantic[16] where the operation has been seen as a cornerstone of the management of prostatic carcinoma. Currently the position is more complicated. In the early part of this decade, there seemed to be a reappraisal of the value of the operation by some American urologists,[3] while in the UK in the last few years a small number of urologists, likely to increase, is performing radical prostatectomies, and the active treatment of early disease is very much on the agenda at urological meetings.[17] Perhaps a transatlantic consensus on this issue is in sight.

Certainly, many of the objections no longer apply. In the USA, far more men now present with localized tumours amenable to local treatment,[18] a trend likely to be seen here, particularly if the issue of screening is taken up. The perineal operation of Young and Jewett almost invariably produced impotence, and incontinence was a frequent complication.[19] Patrick Walsh, after studying the relationship of the pelvic nerves to the prostate, devised a nerve-sparing technique which enables retropubic radical prostatectomy to be performed without interfering with potency.[20] As damage to the distal bladder sphincter mechanism now is more readily avoided, these two major complications no longer have to be weighed so strongly against the possible benefits of radical prostatectomy.[21]

Perhaps it is only in the area of potential benefit that doubt remains. Certainly reported series give good results, but are these a tribute to the treatment or a reflection of the inherent good prognosis of the tumour diagnosed early enough for radical surgery? Indeed, is there evidence that early local treatment improves survival? Unfortunately there is a lack of adequate controlled trials assessing the true value of radical local treatment. The study of radical prostatectomy by the Veterans Administration[22] only recruited a small number of patients with a 22 per cent exclusion rate for protocol violation. They found no difference in survival attributable to radical prostatectomy, and although there was a greater progression rate in unoperated patients, it was not statistically significant. However, the trial is open to criticism[23] and may well not be relevant to the 1990s. Paulson's study comparing radiotherapy with radical prostatectomy favoured the latter, but disease progression rather than survival was taken as the end-point, with a comparatively short follow-up period.[24] Unequivocal evidence that immediate aggressive local treatment reduces mortality has yet to be obtained, and those of us unhappy about how to treat these patients would appreciate a well-conducted large-scale controlled study.

However, if this *is* the correct way to treat early prostatic tumours, and if more early tumours can be identified, the British man should not be denied this treatment. If the expertise to treat prostatic tumours surgically has to be acquired specially, and if as a result it is necessary for the management of at least some prostatic tumours to be centralized, so be it. Extracorporeal lithotripsy for stone disease has taught us that not every advance in urology can be available in every unit, and British urologists may well have to come to terms with the need to refer patients to specialized centres for other conditions, of which prostatic cancer may be one.

Alternatives to radical surgery

Irradiation has been accepted as effective treatment for localized disease[25] and is the method of local treatment most widely practised in the UK.[26] External-beam irradiation has a significant complication rate,[27] and most published series contain patients with complications of a catastrophic nature—for example, fistulae requiring bowel and urinary diversion. The prognosis depends on the tumour grade,[28] indicating that the biology of the patient's disease may have as great a bearing on the outcome as how he is treated. Interstitial radiotherapy, implanting radio-isotope seeds through needles placed in the prostate, originally required an open retropubic operation.[29] It now can be done as a semi-closed procedure, ^{125}I seeds being introduced through needles inserted via the perineum, under guidance of a rectal ultrasound probe.[30] Long-term results are available for the open technique,[31] but those for whom the technique is recommended have in any case a good prognosis.

Attempts to eradicate the tumour by cryosurgery[32] and more recently by laser destruction of the tissue remaining after an aggressive TUR[33] have been described, but until the real role of radical surgery and radiotherapy is clear, other therapies perhaps merely cloud the issue.

Treatment of advanced localized disease

Attempts at *curing* clinically evident prostatic carcinoma are directed largely at small tumours classified under UICC criteria as T1[34] and in the USA as stage B1.[35] Many patients with more advanced tumours will have no evidence of metastatic disease. It is attractive to consider that such men are still curable by eradicating their local disease—or at least that disease progression can be delayed—and that this will improve survival. Even if these objectives are not realized, treatment might prevent local progression which can cause recurrent urinary symptoms, retention, or ureteric obstruction.

There is little general agreement on how these patients should be managed. Radical prostatectomy is not impossible,[36] although adequate excision of the tumour will preclude the nerve-sparing technique and continence must be at greater risk. Radiotherapy is perhaps more appropriate than surgery for these more advanced tumours,[37] but many British urologists employ hormonal treatment even where metastatic disease appears absent.[26] Since the prognosis of men with negative bone scans, as far as death from prostatic cancer is concerned, is relatively good,[38] a case can also be made for deferring any treatment. Patients so managed may require a further TUR if local symptoms recur,[39] which might then become an indication either for radiotherapy or hormonal treatment.

There is some sense in this expectant approach, provided the urologist is alert to the needs of the occasional patient whose disease progresses rapidly, but it is difficult to adjudicate between these various options.

The case for radiotherapy in *advanced* localized disease has perhaps not been helped by considering it able to 'cure' such tumours.[25] This in my opinion is an unrealistic aim, since many patients with negative bone scans will have lymph node metastases[40] and probably microscopic bone involvement. On the other hand, the prognosis of patients without positive bone scans *is* relatively good, and all urologists will have many patients with advanced localized disease who have survived many years from diagnosis. Thus good survival figures from anecdotal series of patients receiving radiotherapy have little meaning. Unfortunately if the aim is cure, there will be a temptation to maximize the dose of radiation, with an increase in complications. Unrealistic claims for a therapy seen to have unpleasant complications will not endear it to sceptics.

On the other hand, it is more logical to treat or prevent local complications of the primary tumour with radiotherapy rather than with systemic hormonal treatment. Re-obstruction with the need for repeated TURs is a significant problem in advanced prostatic cancer,[39] and an increase in the use of radiotherapy simply to prevent this could well be justified. More modest aims for radiotherapy with a dose aimed at palliation would be less likely to produce complications. More patients could be considered for such treatment, and not only those without metastases. For men who have relapsed after hormonal therapy, recurring episodes of obstruction can be an additional source of misery, for which a palliative dose of radiotherapy often is the best solution.[41] The concept of curative therapy which associates prostatic irradiation only with non-metastatic disease is to the detriment of this important group of patients.

Hormonal therapy

Androgen withdrawal was, when it was introduced,[42] and remains[43] the only effective treatment once metastases have occurred. Although in use for 40 years it is as much a source of controversy now as ever before. When Nesbit and Baum[2] reviewed 1818 patients treated in the USA up to 1950, they found a marked improvement in survival compared with patients treated in the pre-hormone period.[44] These misleadingly were called a 'control group'. The difference was ascribed to the beneficial effect of hormonal treatment, and soon any patient even suspected of having prostatic carcinoma was treated, usually with diethylstilboesterol (DES) which was prescribed in increasingly large doses.

168 Prostatic carcinoma

In 1950 the need for controlled trials and the danger of historical controls perhaps was not recognized. Between 1940 and 1950 many other developments in medicine, not least the discovery of antibiotics, had considerably altered the prospects of survival for men in this age group. It perhaps is surprising (but fortunate) that the Veterans Administration should feel able to include a placebo-treated control arm in their studies.[8] They were surprised to find that initial placebo treatment was not associated with poorer survival. The trial protocol allowed a change in treatment on progression. Thus placebo-treated patients could then be, and usually were, started on hormonal therapy. Since the survival rate of these men was comparable to the survival rate of those treated from diagnosis, it was inferred that hormonal therapy was as effective in terms of survival even if delayed until progression occurred and the idea of deferring treatment, briefly practised by some in the 1940s,[2] was revived.

Timing of hormonal therapy

Where there are symptomatic metastases, there can be little argument against immediate hormonal treatment which will benefit perhaps 80 per cent of patients (Fig. 12.2).[45] Where there are no symptoms, to some the VACURG reports are sufficient to justify deferring therapy until symptoms occur.[46] However, while the results of the VACURG studies did stimulate interest in deferring treatment, the studies were not actually designed to investigate timing of treatment. In particular, there were no specific indications laid down for when and how patients should be treated on progression. Also, veterans are a selected group,[47] and even for men with prostatic cancer the average age of the VACURG patients was high. Although one recently reported retrospective review could not show any disadvantage from delaying treatment,[48] experience in Newcastle where deferred treatment has been standard practice for some

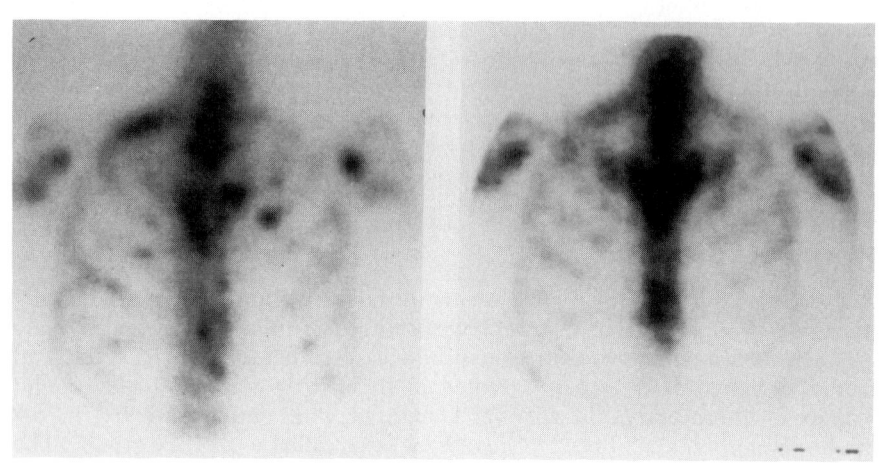

Fig. 12.2 Response of bony metastases to hormonal therapy: ^{99}Tc bone scan prior to therapy (left) with dark areas of increased uptake due to tumour deposits. On right, scan six months after subcapsular orchiectomy shows almost complete resolution.

years has highlighted possible disadvantages, in particular the risk of rapid progression occurring before treatment can be started.[39]

Not until now has the question been directly tested. The Medical Research Council currently is comparing immediate and deferred treatment in patients with advanced prostatic cancer.[49] This study is recognized to be dealing with the central question related to hormonal treatment of prostatic carcinoma.[43] It should be noted that the arguments to be addressed are more complicated simply than whether early treatment improves survival, although even on this point the data from the VACURG study are inconclusive.[50] The question of survival can only be determined by a prospective controlled study specifically devised to test this question. This is a major undertaking since to compensate for the expected high death rate from other causes, a very large trial entry will be needed, and this study is unlikely to produce a meaningful result for some years.

Quality of life

Any improvement in survival from early treatment is likely to be small. In the context of the life expectation of most men with prostatic cancer, many urologists now feel that treatment should be aimed as much at avoiding complications and symptoms as at prolonging survival. A number of factors can affect the quality of life of men with prostatic cancer.[51]

Local progression

There is little doubt that a significant number of patients develop further outflow obstruction requiring a second TUR[39] due to tumour progression which might be prevented or slowed down by early hormonal treatment. Whether this is sufficiently common to warrant early *systemic* treatment in all patients is less certain, and indeed in patients without metastases radiotherapy might be the more logical method of controlling the primary tumour. The need for repeated TUR for tumour recurrence could be considered an indication for therapy, and it provides an excellent opportunity to perform an orchiectomy if this is the treatment indicated.

General ill-health

In the absence of specific symptoms such as back pain, more subtle effects (e.g. weight loss, anaemia), resulting from the presence of an uncontrolled tumour, and unrecognized by the patient or his doctor, might respond to early treatment with an improvement in general well-being. This is certainly true in some patients, and general malaise in itself sometimes may justify abandoning deferred treatment. However, a lot of men with untreated prostatic cancer remain in excellent health. Early treatment of *all* patients on these grounds may not be justified, but regular clinical assessment and monitoring weight, haemoglobin etc. are essential if hormonal treatment is deferred.

Avoidance of catastrophes

The risk of a pathological fracture or paraplegia occurring suddenly in the untreated patient causes justifiable concern and certainly demands careful follow-up so that prompt treatment can be given as soon as premonitory symptoms occur.

Side-effects of treatment

Any benefits of early treatment have to be balanced against its potential side-effects, from which no method of androgen deprivation — be it orchiectomy, oestrogens, antiandrogens or LH-RH analogues—is free. Their significance depends on the patient. An 80-year-old widower may tolerate impotence better than a married man of 60. Supporters of deferred treatment will point out that these side-effects will be better accepted by the patient who has had symptoms before treatment is started, and avoided by those who die from other causes before an indication for treatment occurs.

The arguments are finely balanced. The MRC trial is collecting data to monitor all these possibilities. It may resolve the issue, but until then this will continue to be a topic hotly argued by urologists. It should be noted that deferred treatment, like surveillance of patients with stage I testicular teratoma, is *not* an easy option. Some urologists discharge patients who have received hormonal treatment; deferring treatment prohibits this luxury, and it should only be practised where the urologist can keep the patient under close review, and both patient and his doctor are aware of the need to promptly report any change in his condition.

Choice of hormonal therapy

The hormonal regulation of the prostate (Fig. 12.3) provides a number of possible methods of androgen deprivation. In practical terms, currently we can offer a patient an orchiectomy, oestrogen therapy, an antiandrogen or a luteinizing hormone releasing hormone (LH-RH) analogue. The evidence from the many clinical trials comparing these agents is that, in strictly therapeutic terms, all are broadly similar, their merits being argued in terms of side-effects, convenience and expense. The latter is an important consideration; to the user it may be a factor militating against a particular agent, to the manufacturer it reflects the high cost incurred in development, a cost he would hope to recoup from sales of the drug. Some patients may require treatment for a number of years and in budget-conscious times expense cannot be ignored.

Orchiectomy remains the standard against which other treatments are compared and still appears to be the choice of many urologists. It has clear advantages. The patient, who may be elderly and may be on a number of other medications, is saved the need to remember his treatment, and once performed compliance ceases to be a problem. Hot flushes are a frequent and sometimes troublesome complication;[52] otherwise orchiectomy in the long term creates few problems. However, it is easy to underestimate the disadvantages. Minor though the operation is to the surgeon, any operation is a significant

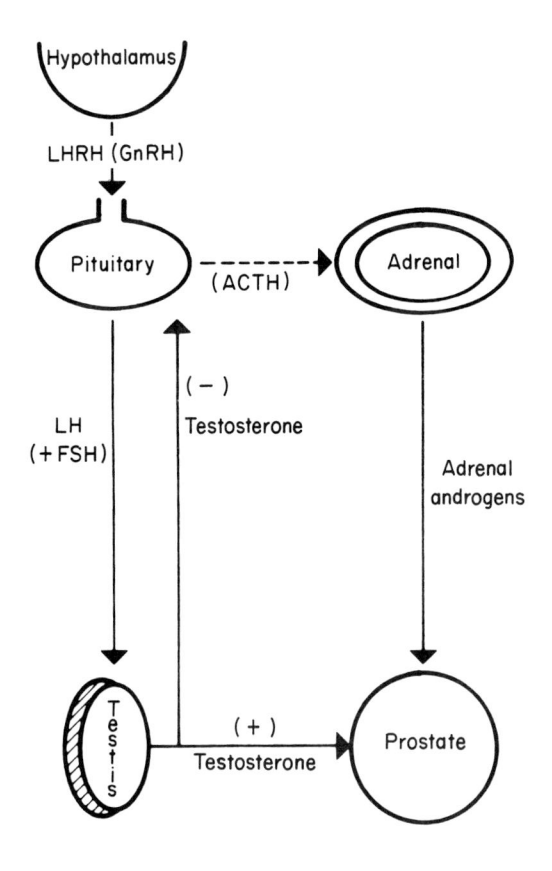

[Figure: Hormonal regulation diagram showing Hypothalamus → LHRH (GnRH) → Pituitary, with ACTH to Adrenal; LH (+FSH) to Testis; Testosterone feedback (−) to Pituitary; Testosterone (+) from Testis to Prostate; Adrenal androgens to Prostate]

Fig. 12.3 Hormonal regulation of the prostate. (Reproduced from reference 77 with the kind permission of the Medical Tribune Group, London)

imposition on the patient. Lesser complications such as haematomata are not uncommon. It is a moot point as to how significant are psychological problems after orchiectomy.[53,54] The stigma of 'castration' associated with orchiectomy is avoidable when the subcapsular operation is performed with adequate explanation; that is, an explanation to the effect that the operation removes that part of the testis which is inactivated by the alternative medical treatments.

What is the current role of oestrogens in prostatic cancer? Because of the risks of cardiovascular disease uncovered by the VACURG studies,[8] many might say 'none'. Indeed, it is unfortunately true that some men are still being subjected to the risk of inappropriately high doses of oestrogens. However, cardiovascular complications are dose-related, and a recent study indicated that DES 1 mg daily was as effective and as safe as other forms of treatment.[55] This was in fact the dose originally proposed by Huggins[42] in the 1940s.[56] This simple daily regimen is much the cheapest option. I would hesitate still to use even this low dose in someone with known cardiovascular disease, and really there can *never* be any justification for doses higher than the more conventional dose of 3 mg per day.

The newest of the alternatives to orchiectomy are the long-acting preparations of the LH-RH analogues (e.g. Zoladex, ICI).[57] The monthly injection is a minor inconvenience, and the fact it is an injection helps with compliance. The treatment is expensive, although the true cost of orchiectomy is difficult to determine for comparison. The position of these drugs now is well established, although there is some lack of agreement as to the importance of the temporary rise in testosterone levels which occur during the first few days of treatment. Adverse effects of the resulting tumour flare have been reported,[58] and can be prevented by temporary use of an antiandrogen; but this is not universal practice.

Antiandrogen drugs fall into two classes. The steroid cyproterone acetate (Cyprostat, Schering) is a progesterone, and thus, while it is an antiandrogen, it also inhibits LH secretion centrally.[59] Non-steroidal pure antiandrogens do not have this action. They have the theoretical disadvantage of not only acting peripherally to block testosterone stimulation at the prostate, but of also blocking the negative feedback.[60] Thus, during use as monotherapy, a rise in LH and testosterone occurs, since LH secretion is preserved. Whether this is sufficient to overcome the blockade and reverse the therapeutic effect is less clear, and the main disadvantage of these drugs is their toxicity compared with other methods of androgen withdrawal.[61] ICI is developing an antiandrogen which in animal models appeared to have a selective peripheral effect, thus avoiding risk from rebound stimulation.[62] Unfortunately early human studies show that some testosterone stimulation does occur,[63] but it may be less toxic than other antiandrogens. One advantage of pure antiandrogens is the relative sparing of sexual function compared with other methods of androgen withdrawal.[64] In practical terms, cyproterone acetate is the antiandrogen used for primary hormonal treatment, and is a useful alternative to orchiectomy where oral treatment is desired, although its price is similar to Zoladex.

Where hormonal therapy is indicated a useful range of options is now available. If orchiectomy is inappropriate, the patient can be offered the choice of oral therapy with cyproterone acetate (or perhaps low-dose oestrogen), or a monthly injection of Zoladex. Where there are contraindications to, or side-effects from, one therapy, there are now sufficient alternatives to ensure that effective androgen depletion can be obtained with the minimum disadvantage. It is clear that no one treatment is the 'best' and the ideal for each patient will depend on his circumstances.

Total androgen ablation

If adrenal androgens (Fig. 12.3) were a significant component of the hormonal drive to a prostatic tumour, an antiandrogen prescribed in addition to conventional hormonal therapy might increase its effect.[65] Labrie and his colleagues have reported substantial series of patients managed by total androgen ablation, with response rates and survival figures far better than those to be expected from conventional therapy.[66] Since these comparisons were from uncontrolled data, the judgement of most of us has been suspended until the results of randomized controlled trials are available. A Canadian trial comparing orchiectomy alone with orchiectomy combined with the non-steroidal Anandron (Roussel) shows improvements in response rates and early survival which reach statistically significant levels, but at the expense of side-effects which have to be balanced against what are, in fact, quite small benefits for the patients.[67] It seems unlikely, even if there are improvements resulting from total androgen ablation, that they will be as dramatic as those postulated by its early proponents.

Other methods of hormone manipulation

The antifungal drug ketoconazole in large dosage blocks androgen synthesis both in testis and adrenal. Not only is it active in prostatic cancer; it also effectively provides single-agent total androgen ablation. Indeed its greatest promise seemed to lie in management after hormone relapse. However, in the dose necessary for androgen suppression it is unacceptably toxic,[68] and it has been withdrawn, even for trial purposes, as a treatment for prostatic carcinoma. The progestogen megestrol acetate may be a safe and inexpensive form of treatment[69] but is not widely used. Estramustine phosphate, a combination of oestrogen and a nitrogen mustard, is especially popular in Scandinavia for primary treatment, although elsewhere more usually considered as an option in relapsed patients.[70]

In the prostate cell, androgens are reduced to dihydrotestosterone which is the active form of the hormone. The enzyme involved is 5 α-reductase, an inhibitor of which is under very early clinical investigation.[71] This might have a very selective action, perhaps avoiding many of the side-effects of other hormone therapies.

Treatment after relapse from hormonal therapy

A proportion of men with prostatic cancer will not respond to hormonal therapy. Those who do inevitably will relapse, usually within two years in those with metastases. How these patients should be managed is one of the major unresolved problems in prostatic carcinoma. In the space available in this review I do not wish to pursue the question of modifying the disease process by second-line hormonal therapy[14] or cytotoxic drugs[72] in detail. Currently these are disappointing and it is skilled palliation which at present has most to offer these men.

Many men may not live long once relapse occurs,[73] but some can survive for considerable periods, and although little is available to slow the course of their disease, much can be done to mitigate its effects. Bone pain is the major symptom, for which radiotherapy is the tested remedy. All too often, local radiotherapy is followed by development of pain elsewhere, and perhaps half-body irradiation[74] should be used more frequently. Possibly the most encouraging development in the treatment of prostatic cancer recently has been of the use of ^{89}Sr injections in patients with bone pain.[75] Handled like calcium, it is taken up into the active bone at the site of osteoblastic metastases.

So good have responses been in those relapsing after external radiotherapy that its use at an earlier stage seems justifiable, and in Scotland we are conducting a randomized study comparing ^{89}Sr treatment with radiotherapy in patients with painful metastases.

If pain can be relieved, many of these patients will have a period of relative good health. Others, however, are more debilitated, often requiring blood transfusion for anaemia. Conventional bone scans only demonstrate metastases in cortical bone. ^{99}Tc-labelled nanocolloid is taken up by reticuloendothelial cells, including those in bone marrow. Preliminary studies[76] have enabled us to demonstrate the central bone marrow destruction in the anaemic patients (Fig. 12.4), and this investigation may be a useful addition to the tools available for managing these patients.

The management of men in the terminal stages of prostatic cancer is one of the most challenging aspects of urological practice. Particularly if a good working relationship can be developed with a sensible radiotherapist, pain clinic and hospice, it can also be one of the most rewarding.

Conclusions

It could be questioned whether much progress has been made in managing prostatic cancer in recent decades. If now we know our limitations better, if treatment is used selectively, and more importantly, if men are not subjected to unnecessary treatment, this *is* progress of a sort. Certainly, we must look more positively at early disease, and if we do have the means of earlier diagnosis, this might lead to a reduction in the mortality from prostatic cancer.

The situation of the patient with more advanced disease is less certain. Ultimately an improved outlook for these patients will depend on the type of dramatic developments in chemotherapy that have occurred with testicular tumours. Until then, we have much we can do to alleviate the disease. There is a school of thought which advocates 'an orchiectomy and then discharge the patient'. Sometimes this might indeed be the right course of action. What is clear to me is that the individual problems of each patient with prostatic cancer are so different that general pronouncements on therapy are impossible. Perhaps here lies the true challenge of prostatic cancer.

References

1. Jewett H.J. The case for radical prostatectomy. *J. Urol.* 1970; **103:** 195–9.
2. Nesbit R.M., Baum W.C. Endocrine control of prostatic cancer: clinical survey of 1818 cases. *J. Amer. Med. Ass.* 1950; **143:** 1317–20.
3. Stamey T.A. Cancer of the prostate: an analysis of some important contributions and dilemmas. *Monogr. Urol.* 1982; **3:** 65–96.
4. Catalona W.J., Scott W.W. Carcinoma of the prostate. In: Walsh P.C., Gittes R.E., Perlmutter A.D., Stamey T.A. (ed.): *Campbell's Urology,* Philadelphia: W.B. Saunders, 1986: 1463–534.
5. Franks L.M. Latent carcinoma of the prostate. *J. Path. Bacteriol.* 1954; **68:** 603–16.
6. McNeal J.E. Origin and development of carcinoma in the prostate. *Cancer.* 1969; **23:** 24–34.
7. McNeal J.E., Bostwick D.G. Kindrachuck R.A., Redwine E.A., Freiha F.S., Stamey T.A. Patterns of progression in prostate cancer. *Lancet.* 1986; **i:** 60–3.

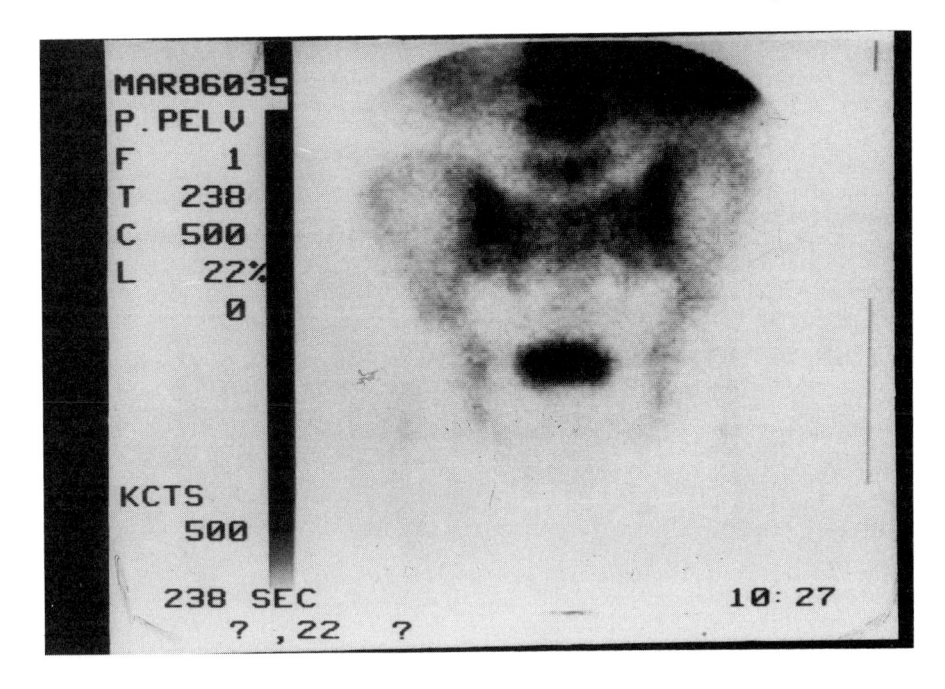

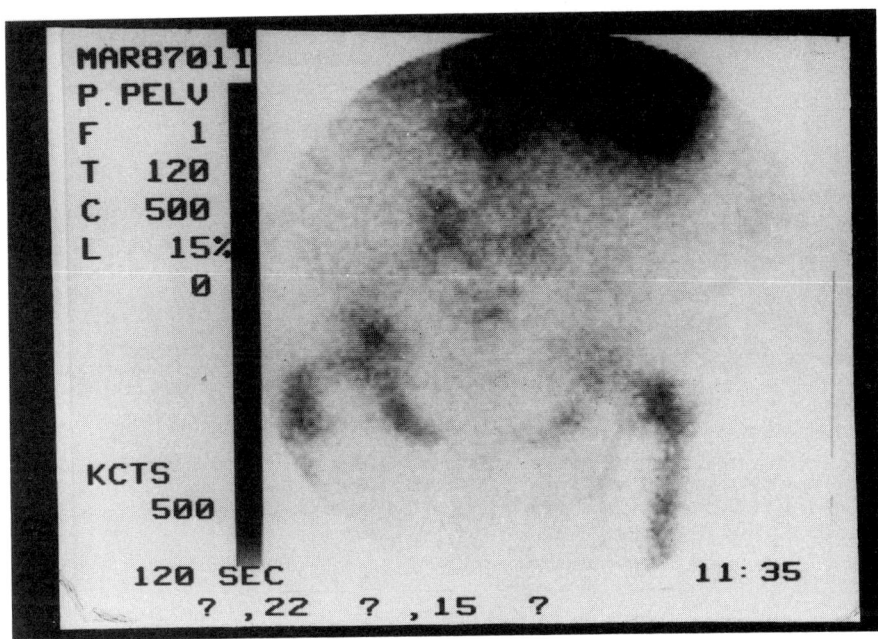

Fig. 12.4 (a) Normal bone marrow scan using ^{99}Tc-labelled nanocolloid. Note the activity mainly in the marrow of the lumbar spine and sacrum. (b) Bone marrow scan in man with advanced prostate cancer. Note the reduction of uptake in the spine and the abnormal extension of active marrow into the shaft of femur. (Scans by courtesy of Dr H.W. Gray)

8. Byar D.P. The Veterans Administration Cooperative Research Group's studies of cancer of the prostate. *Cancer.* 1973; **32:** 1126–30.
9. Grayhack J.T., Bockrath J.M. Diagnosis of carcinoma of the prostate. *Urology.* 1981; **17** (Suppl. 1): 54–60.
10. Resnick M.I. Ultrasound in evaluating prostatic cancer. *J. Urol.* 1985; **134:** 314.
11. Chodak G.W., Wald V., Parmer E., Watanabe H., One H., Saitoh M. Comparison of digital examination and transrectal ultrasound for the diagnosis of prostatic cancer. *J. Urol.* 1986; **135:** 951–4.
12. Ford T.F., Butcher D.N., Masters J.R.W., Parkinson M.C. Immunocytochemical localization of prostate-specific antigen: specificity and application to clinical practice. *Brit. J. Urol.* 1985; **57:** 50–5.
13. Ferro M.A., Barnes I., Roberts J.B.M., Smith P.J.B. Tumour markers in prostatic carcinoma: a comparison of prostate-specific antigen with acid phosphatase. *Brit. J. Urol.* 1987; **60:** 69–73.
14. Killian C.S., Yang N., Emrich L.J., Vargas F.P., Kuriyama M., Wang M.C., Slack N.H., Papsidero L.D., Murphy G.P., Chu T.M., and the Investigators of the National Prostatic Research Project. Prognostic importance of prostate-specific antigen for monitoring patients with stages B_2 to D_1 prostate cancer. *Cancer Res.* 1985; **45:** 886–91.
15. Brooman P.J.C., Peeling W.B., Griffiths G.J., Roberts E., Evans K. A comparison between digital examination and per rectal ultrasound in the evaluation of the prostate. *Brit. J. Urol.* 1981; **53:** 617–20.
16. Moon T. Prostatic carcinoma. *Brit. Med. J.* 1985; **290:** 1824.
17. O'Donoghue E.P.N., McNicholas T.A., Sibley G.N.A., Carter S.St.C., Charig C. Radical local therapy in the management of early prostatic carcinoma. Paper read at the Annual Meeting of the British Association of Urological Surgeons, Buxton, 22 June 1988.
18. Schmidt J.D., Mettlin C.J., Nachimuthu N., Peace B.B., Beart R.W., Winchester D.P., Murphy G.P. Trends in patterns of care for prostatic carcinoma 1974–83: results of surveys by the American College of Surgeons. *J. Urol.* 1986; **136:** 416–21.
19. Schmidt J.D. Indications and surgical approaches for prostatic cancer. *Urology.* 1981; **17** (Suppl. 2): 4–6.
20. Walsh P.C., Lepor H., Eggleston J.C. Radical prostatectomy with preservation of sexual function: anatomical and pathological considerations. *The Prostate.* 1983; **4:** 473–85.
21. Walsh P.C. Radical retropubic prostatectomy. In: Walsh P.C., Gittes R.E., Perlmutter A.D., Stamey T.A. (ed.): *Campbell's Urology.* Philadelphia: W.B. Saunders, 1986: 2754–75.
22. Byar D.P., Corle D.K. VACURG randomised trial of radical prostatectomy for stages I and II. *Urology.* 1981; **17** (Suppl.2): 7–11.
23. Walsh P.C. Randomised study of prostatic cancer. *Urology.* 1981; **18:** 291.
24. Paulson D.F., Lin G.H., Hinshaw W., Stephani S., and the Uro-Oncology Research Group. Radical surgery versus radiotherapy for adenocarcinoma of the prostate. *J. Urol.* 1982; **128:** 502–4.
25. Bagshaw M.A., Ray G.R., Cox R.S. Radiotherapy of prostatic cancer: long or short term efficacy. *Urology.* 1985; **25** (Suppl.): 17–23.
26. Tolley D.A., Robinson S.M. Attitudes towards the management of prostatic cancer—results of a postal survey. Paper read at the Annual Meeting of the British Association of Urological Surgeons, Dublin, 13 July 1984.
27. Lindholt J., Hansen P.T. Prostatic carcinoma: complications of megavoltage radiation therapy. *Brit. J. Urol.* 1986; **58:** 52–4.
28. Ritchie A.W.S., Smith G., Preston C., Beynon L.L., Duncan W., Chisholm G.D. Prediction of response to radiotherapy for localised prostatic cancer. *Brit. J. Urol.* 1985; **57:** 729–32.
29. Herr H.H. Iodine-125 implantation in the management of localised prostatic carcinoma. *Urol. Clin. N. Amer.* 1980; **7:** 605–13.
30. Holm H.H., Juul N., Pedersen J.F., Hansen H., Strøyer I. Transperineal ^{125}iodine seed implantation in prostatic cancer guided by transrectal ultrasonography. *J. Urol.* 1983; **130:** 283–6.
31. Grossman H.B., Batata M., Hilaris B., Whitmore W.F. ^{125}I implantation for carcinoma of prostate: further follow-up of first 100 cases. *Urology.* 1982; **20:** 591–8.
32. Loening S., Bonney W., Fallon B., Gerber W., Hawtrey C., Lubaroff D., Narayana A., Culp D. Perineal cryosurgery of prostate cancer. *Urology.* 1981; **17** (Suppl. 2): 12–14.
33. McNicholas T.A., Carter S.St.C., Wickham J.E.A., O'Donoghue E.P.N. YAG laser treatment of early carcinoma of the prostate. *Brit. J. Urol.* 1988; **61:** 239–43.

34. Wallace D.M., Chisholm G.D., Hendry W.F. TNM classification for urological tumours (UICC)—1974. *Brit. J. Urol.* 1975; **47:** 1–12.
35. Jewett H.J. The present status of radical prostatectomy for stages A and B prostatic cancer. *Urol. Clin. N. Amer.* 1975; **2:** 105–24.
36. Zincke H., Utz D.C., Benson R.C., Patterson D.E. Bilateral lymphadenectomy and radical retropubic prostatectomy for stage C carcinoma of prostate. *Urology.* 1984; **24:** 532–9.
37. Walsh P.C., Lepor H.L. The role of radical prostatectomy in the management of prostatic cancer. *Cancer.* 1987; **60:** 526–37.
38. Lund F., Smith P.H., Suchu S., and the EORTC Urological Group. Do bone scans predict prognosis in prostatic cancer? A report of the EORTC protocol 30762. *Brit. J. Urol.* 1984; **56:** 58–63.
39. Handley R., Carr T.W., Travis D., Powell P.H., Hall R.R. Deferred treatment for prostate cancer. *Brit. J. Urol.* 1988; **62:** 249–53.
40. Prout G.R., Griffen P.P., Daly J.J., Shipley W.U. Nodal involvement as prognostic indicator in prostatic carcinoma. *Urology.* 1981; **17** (Suppl.1): 72–9.
41. Kynaston H.G., Keen C.W., Matthews P.N. Palliative radiotherapy for symptomatic relief in locally advanced prostatic carcinoma. Paper read at Edinburgh Urological Festival British Prostate Group Meeting, Edinburgh, 18 August 1988.
42. Huggins C., Hodges C.V. Studies on prostate cancer. 1: The effect of castration of oestrogen and of androgen injection on serum phosphatases in metastatic carcinoma of the prostate. *Cancer Res.* 1941; **1:** 293–7.
43. Editorial: Dilemmas in the management of prostatic carcinoma. *Lancet.* 1985; **ii:** 1219–20.
44. Nesbit R.M., Plumb R.T. Prostatic carcinoma: a follow-up on 795 patients treated prior to the endocrine era and a comparison of survival rates between these and patients treated by endocrine therapy. *Surgery.* 1946; **20:** 263–72.
45. Resnick M.I., Grayhack J.T. Treatment of stage IV carcinoma of the prostate. *Urol. Clin. N. Amer.* 1975; **2:** 141–61.
46. Fraser K.S. Prostatic carcinoma. *Brit. Med. J.* 1985; **290:** 1824.
47. Stamey T.A. Editorial. *Monogr. Urol.* 1985; **6:** 105.
48. Parker M.C., Cook A., Riddle P.R., Fryatt I., O'Sullivan J., Shearer R.J. Is delayed treatment justified in carcinoma of the prostate? *Brit. J. Urol.* 1985; **57:** 724–8.
49. Kirk D. Prostatic carcinoma. *Brit. Med. J.* 1985; **290:** 875–6.
50. Kirk D. Trials and tribulations in prostatic cancer. *Brit. J. Urol.* 1987; **59:** 375–9.
51. Kirk D. Principles of patient management: immediate or deferred treatment. *Brit. J. Clin. Pract.* 1987; **41** (Suppl. 48): 84–7.
52. Charig C.R., Rundle J.S. Flushing: a long term side-effect of orchiectomy in the treatment of carcinoma of the prostate. Paper read at the Annual Meeting of the British Association of Urological Surgeons, Buxton, 22 June 1988.
53. Parmar H., Edwards L., Phillips R.H., Allen L., Lightman S.L. Orchiectomy versus long-acting D-Trp-6-LHRH in advanced prostatic cancer. *Brit. J. Urol.* 1987; **59:** 248–54.
54. Kirk D. Orchiectomy has its advantages. *Hosp. Doctor.* 1987; 16 April: 12.
55. Robinson M.R.C. EORTC protocol 30805: a phase III trial comparing orchiectomy versus orchiectomy and cyproterone acetate and low-dose stilboestrol in the management of metastatic carcinoma of the prostate. In: Smith P.H., Pavone-Macaluso M. (eds.): *Management of Advanced Cancer of Prostate and Bladder.* New York: Alan R. Liss Inc., 1988: 101–10.
56. Smith P.H. Medical management of prostatic cancer: single or combination therapy? *Brit. J. Clin. Pract.* 1987; **41** (Suppl. 48): 105–11.
57. Beacock C.J., Buck A.C., Zwinck R., Peeling W.B., Rees R.W.M., Turkes A., Walker K., Griffiths K. The treatment of metastatic prostatic cancer with the slow-release LH-RH analogue Zoladex ICI 118630. *Brit. J. Urol.* 1987; **59:** 436–42.
58. Waxman J.H., Man A., Hendry W.F., Whitfield H.N., Besser G.M., Tiptaft R.C., Paris A.M., Oliver R.T.D. Importance of early tumour exacerbation in patients treated with long-acting analogues of gonadotrophin releasing hormone for advanced prostatic cancer. *Brit. Med. J.* 1985; **291:** 1387–8.
59. Neumann F., Schenck B. Pharmacological principles and rationale of the various methods of endocrine therapy. In: Klosterhalfen H. (ed.): *The Therapy of Advanced Carcinoma of the Prostate.* West Germany: Schering AG, 1984: 15–23.
60. Neumann F. Different principles of androgen deprivation for palliative treatment of prostatic

cancer. In: Schroeder F. (ed.): *Androgens and Anti-androgens*. Weesp: Schering, 1983: 97–114.
61. Lund F., Rasmussen F. Flutamide versus stilboesterol in the management of advanced prostatic cancer: a controlled prospective study. *Brit. J. Urol.* 1988; **61:** 140–2.
62. Furr B.J.A. ICI 176,334: a novel non-steroidal, peripherally selective antiandrogen. In: Smith P.H., Pavone-Macaluso M. (eds.): *Management of Advanced Cancer of Prostate and Bladder*. New York: Alan R. Liss Inc., 1988: 13–26.
63. Milstead R.A.V. ICI 176,334: a new non-steroidal anti-androgen in prostate cancer. Paper read at the Edinburgh Urological Festival British Prostate Group Meeting, Edinburgh, 18 August 1988.
64. Lundgren R. Flutamide as primary treatment for metastatic prostatic cancer. *Brit. J. Urol.* 1983; **59:** 156–8.
65. Labrie F., Dupont A., Belanger A., Lacoursiere Y., Raynaud J.P., Husson J.M., Gareau J., Fazekas A.T.A., Sandow J., Monfette G., Girard J.G., Emond J., Houle J.G. New approach in the treatment of prostate cancer: complete instead of partial withdrawal of androgens. *The Prostate*. 1983; **4:** 579–94.
66. Labrie F., Belanger A., Dupont A., Emond J., Lacoursiere Y., Monfette G. Combined treatment with LHRH agonist and pure antiandrogen in advanced carcinoma of prostate. *Lancet*. 1984; **ii:** 1090.
67. Beland G., Elhilalli M.M., Fradet V., Laroche B., Ramsey E.W., Trachtenberg J., Venner P.N. Complete androgen blockade for metastatic prostate cancer: results of the Canadian trial. Paper read at the Edinburgh Urological Festival British Prostate Group Meeting, Edinburgh, 18 August 1988.
68. Moffatt L.E.F., Kirk D., Tolley D.A., Smith M.F., Beastall G. Ketoconazole as primary treatment of prostatic cancer. *Brit. J. Urol.* 1988; **61:** 439–40.
69. Geller J., Albert J., Yen S.S.C. Treatment of advanced prostate cancer with megestrol acetate. *Urology*. 1979; **12:** 537–41.
70. Walzer Y., Oswalt J., Soloway M.S. Estramustine phosphate—hormone, chemotherapeutic agent, or both? *Urology*. 1984; **24:** 53–8.
71. Moncloa F., Stoner E. The treatment of prostatic diseases with a 5α-reductase inhibitor (MK-906). Paper read at the Edinburgh Urological Festival British Prostate Group Meeting, Edinburgh, 18 August 1988.
72. Gibbons R.P. Prostate cancer chemotherapy. *Cancer*. 1987; **60:** 586–8.
73. Beynon L.L., Chisholm G.D. The stable state is not an objective response in hormone-escaped carcinoma of the prostate. *Brit. J. Urol.* 1984; **56:** 702–5.
74. Wilkins M.F., Keen C.W. Hemi-body radiotherapy in the management of metastatic carcinoma. *Clin. Radiol.* 1987; **38:** 267–8.
75. Robinson R.G. Radionuclides for the alleviation of bone pain in advanced malignancy. *Clin. Oncol.* 1986; **5:** 39–49.
76. Haddock G., Gray H.W., McKillop J.H., Bessent R.G., Kirk D. Bone marrow imaging in advanced prostatic cancer. *Brit. J. Urol.* 1989; **63:** 497–502.
77. Kirk D. *Brit. J. Sexual Med.* 1987; **14:** 144–148.

13

Male infertility

John P. Pryor, MS, FRCS

The surgery of male infertility, like every other aspect of urology, has undergone a complete revision over the past decade. The widespread availability of hormone estimations by radio-immunoassay, the application of microsurgery, and the advent of assisted conception, have all had important consequences for the urologist.

Current management of the male partner of an infertile marriage requires proper assessment of the couple in order to establish the causative factors of the infertility and in order to establish the prognosis. Surgery has important diagnostic and therapeutic roles but, in a book of surgery in general, a most important aspect is the prevention of male infertility in surgical procedures.

Surgery and the prevention of infertility

Testicular maldescent and inguinal surgery

The failure of the maldescended testis to produce spermatozoa has been known for centuries, and surgical intervention is recommended at an increasingly early age in an attempt to permit the development of normal spermatogenesis. The pitfalls in making a diagnosis are well-recognized. Mobile testes often cause a problem, as do testes secondarily ascended from the scrotum as the result of fibrous tissue contracture following inguinal surgery. The phenomenon of the retractile testis must also be borne in mind. Some children have deficiency of gonadotrophic hormones and treatment with LH-RH analogues may bring about testicular descent in 40–80 per cent of children.[1]

The operation of orchidopexy is often difficult and many a surgeon in training has damaged the vas deferens by resection, division or ischaemia. The risks of vasal damage are even greater in very young children, and the same considerations apply to herniotomy operations. Such damage may not be evident until many years later when the patient presents for the investigation of infertility.

Testicular torsion and epididymitis

The prompt recognition of these conditions is essential if infertility is to be prevented in these patients who are often young. Once the patient reaches hospital, delay in operating rarely occurs, but the importance of fixing the contralateral testis, without damaging the epididymis, must be stressed. There has been a suggestion that the failure to remove a partially ischaemic testis may result in immunological damage to the contralateral testis. There is no good evidence to show that this occurs in man, and prospective study has shown that there are often histological abnormalities of both testes at the time of the original torsion.[2]

The prompt recognition of acute epididymitis is important if testicular infarction (rare) or epididymal obstruction (common) are to be avoided. In many patients the infection is sexually transmitted, but in others it is important to exclude an underlying congenital abnormality of the urinary tract.

Vasectomy

This simple operation, performed under local anaesthetic, should be carried out in such a manner as to prevent recanalization and yet facilitate reversal. There is no necessity to remove a long length of vas, or indeed any at all, provided that the ends are placed in separate fascial planes. It is also important to divide the vas well away from the convoluted distal part near the epididymis.

Pelvic surgery and salazopyrine

The adverse effects of salazopyrine on spermatogenesis and fertility have been well publicized, but the damage is temporary and reverses in two months.[3] The adverse, and variable, effect of radical surgery on erectile and ejaculatory function is well-known, and these functions should not be damaged whilst resecting the rectum of patients with benign disorders. Nerve-sparing operations may also be considered for cancers of the rectum, bowel and prostate.

Aortoiliac disease and retroperitoneal surgery

In 1971, Sabri and Cotton stressed the importance of preserving the pelvic sympathetic nerves during aortoiliac surgery. Unfortunately, some surgeons continue to disregard this and occasional patients seek financial recompense for postoperative ejaculatory failure. Damage to the sympathetic fibres during retroperitoneal node resection for testicular tumours was considered inevitable, but improvements in the survival of such patients has led to a reappraisal of the operation. It is now considered important to try to conserve the sympathetic ganglia in these patients and maintain ejaculatory function and fertility.

Testicular tumours

These tumours often occur in young men who have yet to father a child. At the time of presentation it may be possible to collect semen samples for storage by cryopreservation. Many patients have semen of a poor quality at the time of presentation, but following the orchidectomy the quality may improve. For this reason a preoperative and a postoperative sample should be obtained and evaluated, and those of better quality preserved. It is important to consider the contralateral testis in those patients who are treated with retroperitoneal irradiation. Lead shielding of the testis protects spermatogenesis, but about 10 per cent of these patients will subsequently develop a second testicular tumour. Evidence of such a tumour at an early stage may be sought by biopsying the contralateral testis at the time of orchidectomy. Ultrasound examination of the contralateral testis may also be useful in this context.

Bladder neck surgery

Resection of the bladder neck may cause retrograde ejaculation and an angry patient. It is essential that all patients undergoing prostatectomy should be warned of the risks of retrograde ejaculation, as even octogenarians may have young wives. However, it is in the younger age group that the greatest care should be taken. The hypertrophied bladder neck is rarely a cause of obstruction in boys with urethral valves, and even in young men with proven bladder neck obstruction it is safer to incise rather than resect the bladder neck and even then once their family is complete. The indications for a Y–V-plasty of the bladder neck are now rare and this cause for retrograde ejaculation should not be a problem in the future.

Surgery in the diagnosis of male infertility

If the ejaculate contains no sperms (azoospermia), and either the testes are small (less than 4.0 cm long or 15 ml in volume), or FSH levels are grossly elevated (greater than twice the upper limit of normal), testicular biopsy is unnecessary because it can be reliably predicted to show testicular failure (Tables 13.1 and 13.2). If, however, the sperm count is appreciable though subnormal (consistently less than 10 million sperms per ejaculate: oligozoospermia), and the testes are greater than 4 cm long while the FSH levels are not grossly elevated, testicular biopsy is valuable in diagnosis.

There are many causes of oligozoospermia, ranging from hormonal deficiency of the testis, and including obstruction in the epididymis or vas (Table 13.3). Therefore it is important not only to biopsy the testis, but also to demonstrate the level of any obstruction by inspection of the epididymis and by vasography. There is no indication for the traditional limited testicular biopsy via a small nick in the skin and tunica vaginalis.

Testicular exploration is performed through a midline incision under general anaesthesia. The tunica vaginalis is incised, the testes are delivered from the wound, and the epididymes inspected for evidence of obstruction. This may be in the form of multiple small congenital cysts in the caput epididymis, or it may be possible to see the distended proximal part of the epididymis containing sperm-filled ducts in contrast to the collapsed distal part of the epididymis. Of particular interest is the association between an obstruction in the caput epididymis and bronchiectasis (Young's syndrome). The nature of this association remains obscure and it may be no more than a congenital malunion between the collecting tubules of the testis and the Wolffian duct system occurring in a population with a high incidence of chest disorders.

A vasal obstruction is diagnosed by vasography, and in such patients the

182 *Male infertility*

epididymes may look remarkably normal. Vasography is performed at the time of scrotal exploration and may conveniently be carried out by direct puncture of the lumen with a 19-gauge hypodermic needle (Fig. 13.1). Two to three millilitres of a 45% hypaque solution are injected, and the patient may either be screened or isolated radiographs taken. The normal vasogram is characterized by the absence of any ductal dilatation, the symmetrical filling of each vas deferens and seminal vesicle, and free efflux of contrast into the bladder. Much has been written about minor abnormalities seen on vasography, and Boreau produced a beautiful encyclopaedia of the various appearances. Unfortunately, these do not always seem to correlate with the observed pathology, and the clinical significance of minor changes is doubtful.

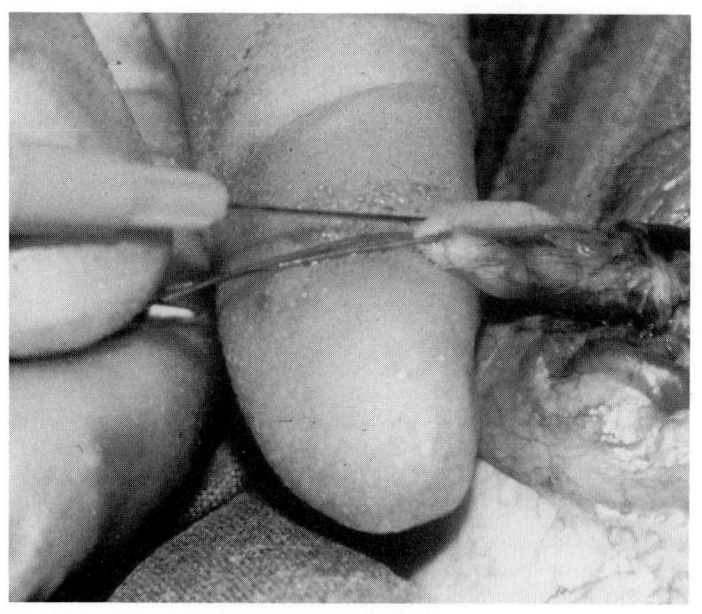

Fig. 13.1 The technique of vasography. The sling around the vas deferens facilitates puncturing the lumen by permitting the needle to be correctly aligned.

It has been stated that vasography may damage the vas and cause obstruction. At King's College Hospital we found no evidence of this in a series of 154 oligozoospermic men who underwent vasography at the time of testicular exploration. It has also been stated that it is sufficient to ensure the free injection of saline along the vas, but this technique fails to diagnose congenital Wolffian or Mullerian duct anomalies which may cause infertility (see 'Ejaculatory duct Obstruction' below). In general an abnormality on vasography is found in about 4 per cent of oligozoospermic men and in 10 per cent of azoospermic men. It is convenient to biopsy the testis whilst waiting for the vasograms to be developed, and it is essential to ensure that the specimens are placed into a suitable preservative. The standard solution of formol saline should never be used as it causes shrinkage of the seminiferous tubules and makes an accurate histological assessment of spermatogenesis difficult or impossible. Bouins, a yellow solution, is used in many centres.

Table 13.1 Correlation between testicular size and spermatogenesis in 261 azoospermic men (398 testicular biopsies)

Testicular		Biopsies (number and %)	Mean Johnsen score* (number and %)		
Length (cm)	Volume (ml)		≤ 2.0	2.1–7.9	≥ 8.0
2	3	11 (100)	11 (100)		
3	8	71 (100)	36 (51)	34 (48)	1 (1)
4	15	118 (100)	39 (33)	35 (30)	44 (37)
5	30	198 (100)	11 (6)	35 (18)	152 (77)

* Johnsen described a method of scoring the stage of spermatogenesis in seminiferous tubules according to the presence of: Sertoli cells (step 2); spermatogonia (step 3); spermatocytes (steps 4 and 5); spermatids (steps 6 and 7); spermatozoa (steps 8, 9 and 10).

Table 13.2 Correlation between plasma follicle stimulating hormone levels and spermatogenesis in 214 azoospermic men

		Mean Johnsen score (number and %)		
FSH level*	Number	≤ 2.0	2.1–7.9	≥ 8.0
Normal	123		42 (33)	82 (67)
Mild elevation	29		18 (58)	11 (42)
Gross elevation	25	1	16 (64)	8 (32)

* The normal range varies in different laboratories and a gross elevation is more than twice the upper limit of the normal range.

Table 13.3 Causes of obstructive oligozoospermia

Site of obstruction	Causes
Intratesticular	Congenital
	Immunological
	Infective
	Hypercurvature
Epididymal	Congenital dysplasia
	Infective
	Immunological
Vasal	Infective
	Adynamic
Ejaculatory duct	Congenital anomalies
	Infective
	Adynamic

Many techniques have been described for assessing spermatogenesis, and it is useful for the surgeon to have both a description and semi-quantitative analysis. In the Johnsen technique, spermatogenesis is graded from one to

184 *Male infertility*

ten and the proportion of seminiferous tubules showing Sertoli cells (step 2), spermatogonia (step 3), spermatocytes (steps 4 and 5), spermatids (steps 6 and 7), or spermatozoa (steps 8, 9 and 10) are counted. In addition to this the Leydig cell numbers are assessed and the presence of inflammatory cells noted.

Carcinoma-in-situ of the testis is apparent in the testicular biopsy of approximately 0.05 per cent of infertile men and almost always progresses to a germ cell tumour of the testis. Patients with carcinoma-in-situ of the testis require careful surveillance, orchidectomy when unilateral and in an atrophic testis, or treatment by low-dose radiation.

The correlation between the obstructed appearance of the epididymis and testicular histology is shown in Table 13.4. The macroscopic appearance of the epididymis is usually sufficient to determine the presence of spermatozoa; but, if there is any doubt, microscopic inspection of the epididymal fluid should be carried out in the operating theatre. In those patients with a normal epididymis the obstruction is assumed to be within the testis and in some patients is amenable to treatment with low-dose steroids.

Table 13.4 Correlation between the macroscopic appearance of the epididymes and the histological appearance of the testes*

Epididymes	Number	Mean Johnsen score (number and %)		
		≤ 2.0	2.1–7.9	≥ 8.0
Normal	116	20 (17)	56 (48)	40 (35)
Dilated tubules	258			258 (100)

* All patients had plasma FSH levels less than twice the upper limit of normal.

Endoscopic assessment

This rarely contributes to the diagnosis of male infertility but may be important in the assessment of men with retrograde ejaculation or when abnormalities of the ejaculatory ducts have been found on vasography. On one occasion, an unsuspected urethral stricture was found following vasography in an infertile man.

Surgery in the treatment of male infertility

Reconstructive procedures for obstruction

An obstructive lesion was found in 65 per cent of 494 men undergoing testicular exploration for azoospermia. The level of obstruction is shown in Table 13.5, and each of these sites will be considered although no surgical procedure is indicated in those men with an intratesticular obstruction. The reconstructive procedure is attempted at the time of the initial operation in all but a few patients where it is necessary to await the testicular histology before proceeding. These patients usually appear to have an obstructive lesion on the side of the testis which is assumed to have normal spermatogenesis and no extratesticular evidence of obstruction on the other side.

Table 13.5 Level of obstruction in 321 azoospermic men

Site of obstruction	Number (%)
Intratesticular	47 (16)
Epididymal	163 (51)
Bilateral vasa aplasia	58 (18)
Unilateral vasa aplasia and another obstruction	11 (3)
Vasal	39 (12)
Ejaculatory duct	3 (1)

Epididymal obstruction

An obstructive lesion in the epididymis may be overcome by performing an epididymovasostomy as has been popluarized by Handley and Schoysman. In this operation a side-to-side anastomosis is performed between the vas deferens and an incision into the epididymis. The success of the procedure relies on the creation of a fistula between the divided ducts of the epididymis and the lumen of the vas deferens. The results of these procedures vary greatly and many British urologists have stated that they have never had a successful outcome. Other authors have reported patency rates of up to 70 per cent, with conception occurring in 30 per cent of the partners. In 1955, Hanley observed that patency was to be expected in 50 per cent of patients with a postgonococcal obstruction, but rarely occurred in those men with congenital obstruction. The prognosis for men with obstructive lesions as a result of chlamydial infections is extremely poor, and as such infections have become more common the overall results of surgery have declined. It is difficult to make comparisons between different centres as not only does the case mix vary but so do the 'exclusions'. Useful information can be obtained by analysing the results obtained from a single centre. In my own practice, the overall patency rate was 25 per cent with conception occurring in half of the partners.

A careful technique combined with magnification is essential for epididymal surgery. There is a growing tendency to replace optical loupes, giving a four-fold magnification, with an operating microscope, and this is essential if the lumen of the epididymis is to be anastomosed to the lumen of the vas deferens. Silber described a technique for transecting the epididymis and performing an end-to-end anastomosis using 10-0 non-absorbable sutures to fashion a tubulovasostomy between a single tubule of the epididymis and the lumen of the vas deferens. Many surgeons find it easier to perform a side-to-side tubulovasostomy and improved patency rates have been reported with both these techniques.

Lee, working in Seoul, operated on 174 patients in an 18-year period and was able to follow up 155 patients. He had used a microsurgical technique in 57 patients and he has a large experience of microsurgical vasovasostomies. He found little difference in the results of macroscopic and microsurgical techniques, with 31 and 33 per cent having sperm in the ejaculate and 12 and

21 per cent of the wives conceiving. The patency rates were 41 and 22 per cent, respectively, for non-tuberculous and tuberculous obstruction, and although the patency rates were similar for anastomoses made in the caput (35 per cent), corpus (33 per cent) or cauda (36 per cent) epididymis, the conception rates were 17, 14 and 21 per cent, respectively.

Schoysman and Bedford found a 14 per cent fertility rate in a group of 723 patients following reconstructive surgery for epididymal obstruction (using both microscopic and macroscopic techniques).[4] They studied a group of 117 men with patent anastomoses and found that fertility and motility were related to the distance of the anastomosis from the testis. Motility was usually absent in the first 8 mm of the epididymis, and the partner of only one of the 20 where the anastomosis was less than 4 mm conceived whereas five of the 20 partners conceived where the anastomosis was 4–8 mm along the epididymis. The spermatozoa were always motile when the anastomosis was beyond 8 mm, and 28 of the 55 wives conceived when the anastomosis was between 16 and 24 mm.

Vasal obstruction

Vasal obstruction may occur as a result of infection by sexually transmitted diseases or tuberculosis or as a result of surgical division—be it inadvertent or planned when performed for contraceptive purposes. Many techniques have been described for vasovasostomy, and whilst the operation may be performed using the naked eye by younger surgeons, some form of magnification is essential. The degree of magnification that is available with an operating microscope is probably unnecessary, but its use provides a ready means of maintaining the expertise that is necessary when performing a tubulovasostomy. Patency rates of 80–90 per cent have been reported using a macroscopic technique and of 90–100 per cent using microscopic surgery. Failures usually occur as a result of stenosis of the anastomosis or may be due to unrecognized epididymal obstruction (not uncommon) or a failure of spermatogenesis (rare). Pregnancy rates of between 50 and 65 per cent within two years of operation should be expected and depend upon a variety of factors, including abnormalities in the female partner. The occurrence of antisperm antibodies following vasectomy is almost inevitable, but changes in the titre of these antibodies in the blood plasma following vasectomy reversal are unpredictable. It is only when high-titre plasma titres are obtained that antisperm antibodies are found in the seminal plasma, and no conception occurred when this was greater than 1 : 8. It has been suggested that the relief of a unilateral obstruction may improve fertility by reducing the presence of antisperm antibodies, but the mechanism and evidence for this remains uncertain.

On some occasions it is not possible to reconstruct the vas as the gap between the patent ends is too long. Attempts to overcome this by the insertion of silastic tubes with long bilateral gaps have been unsuccessful, although it is occasionally possible to perform a crossed vasovasostomy or epididymovasostomy. On some occasions it is not possible to get above the obstruction on one side, and on other occasions there may be an atrophic testis on the opposite side of the obstructive vas. The results of crossed vasovasostomies or epididymovasostomies are poor.

Ejaculatory duct obstruction

Ejaculatory duct obstruction is an uncommon cause for infertility, and a classification of the causes of obstruction in 80 patients is given in Table 13.6.

The classic presentation of bilateral ejaculatory duct obstruction is of azoospermia, and the patient is found to have palpable vasa on clinical examination, a small-volume (0.5 ml) acid (pH 7.0) ejaculate which does not contain fructose. The pattern is complicated by the finding that the obstruction may be unilateral, partial or intermittent, and in some patients there is a secondary epididymal obstruction. Vasography is essential to demonstrate the abnormality and assess treatment.

Table 13.6 Causes of ejaculatory duct obstruction in 80 patients

Mullerian duct abnormalities	12
Wolffian duct abnormalities	25
Previous trauma/surgery	7
Previous infection	16
Carcinoma of prostate	2
Adynamic	7
Miscellaneous	9

Endoscopic incision of the obstructed duct system is facilitated by the injection of methylene blue at the conclusion of vasography. Incision of the duct orifice or Mullerian cyst may be performed with the Schachse knife, but when the obstruction is further from the orifice it may be necessary to resect prostatic tissue. This may be imaged with continuous transrectal ultrasound control or, with less success, radiologically. Improvement in semen quality is likely to occur with Mullerian duct cysts where they are resected, but the results are less good with other forms of obstruction; and in particular where the obstruction is the result of tuberculous infection, as in these instances the vas deferens may also be affected. The Brindley sperm reservoir may be inserted when it is not possible to rectify the ejaculatory duct obstruction (see *infra*).

Operations designed to facilitate the retrieval of sperm

In some patients it is not possible to perform a reconstructive procedure, and in such patients sperm reservoirs may be fashioned with spermatozoa aspirated from these reservoirs. These procedures were designed for patients with vasal aplasia but may also be used for men with high vasal obstruction or ejaculatory failure. Hanley achieved a single success by fashioning a pouch of human amnion which was sutured to an incision made in the epididymis. These pouches, and those constructed from the saphenous vein that Schoysman described, fibrosed. Kelami (Fig. 13.2) and Wagenknecht designed a synthetic prosthesis which was sutured on to the epididymis. Brindley (Fig. 13.3) has designed a prosthesis which could be sutured on to the vas deferens as his prosthesis was designed primarily for use in paraplegics. There has been some success with each of these prostheses, but unfortunately in many of them it

188 *Male infertility*

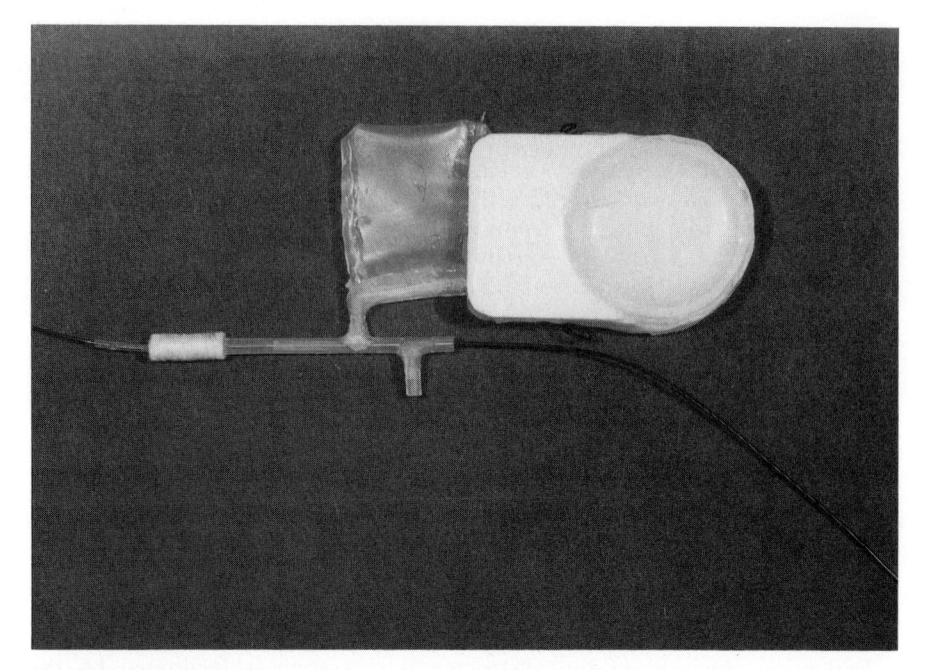

Fig. 13.2 A Kelami epididymal sperm reservoir. The brim of the round reservoir is sutured to the edges of an incision into the epididymis and the brim of the flattened reservoir is sutured to the external oblique aponeurosis in the inguinal region. Sperms may be aspirated percutaneously from the inguinal reservoir.

is not possible to aspirate sperms in the long term and many of them only yield immotile sperm. This may be due to the underlying epididymal defect, or to the anoxic conditions in the reservoir. In an attempt to overcome these problems, and with the increasingly successful techniques of monitoring and controlling ovulation, retrieval of spermatozoa at open operation has been performed. Spermatozoa obtained by this means are then used in association with *in vitro* fertilization. Some success has been achieved[5] but the overall results are disappointing (Table 13.7).

Surgery to improve fertility

Testicular transplantation

Autotransplantation of the intra-abdominal testis is a useful technique. Although heterologous transplantation has been performed by Kirpatovsky in Moscow for hypogonadism, such operations only improve fertility when carried out between identical twins.[6]

Varicocele ligation

The relationship between varicocele and infertility is the subject of much debate. Enthusiasm for the operation stems from the success of Tulloch who performed

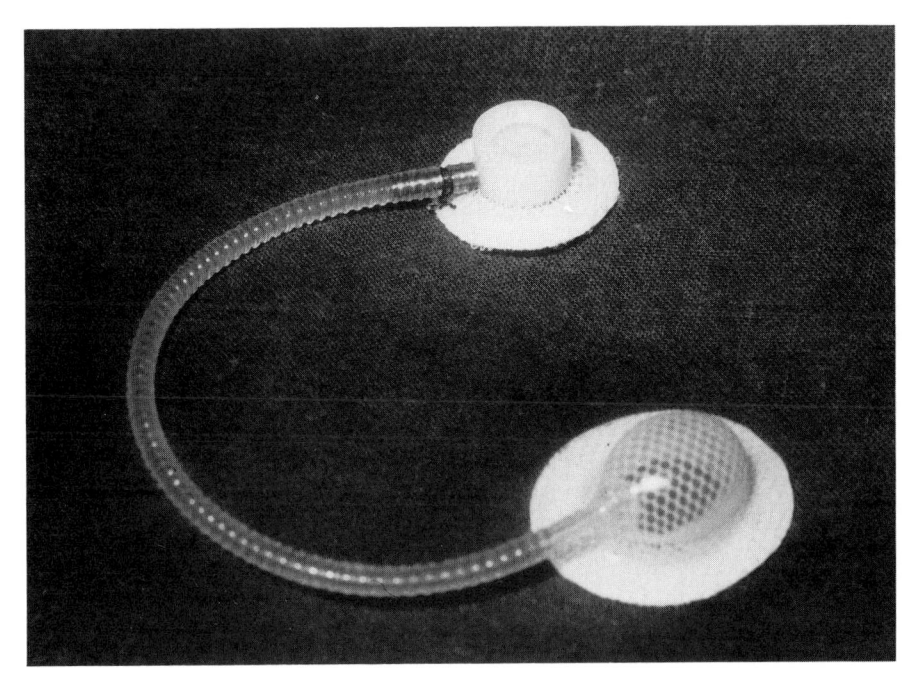

Fig. 13.3 A Brindley vasal sperm reservoir. The binding around the narrow tubing in the left of the reservoir is sutured to the wall of the vas deferens and the narrow tube is situated within the lumen of the vas. The reservoir is situated in the inguinal region and is aspirated percutaneously.

Table 13.7 Outcome of attempts at the operative retrieval of sperms and assisted conception in 34 couples (52 cycles)

Failure of egg production/collection	14
Failure to obtain motile sperm	7
Failure of fertilization	27
Failure of implantation	3
Pregnancy and spontaneous miscarriage	1

bilateral varicocele ligation in an azoospermic man and whose testicular biopsy at the time of operation showed a spermatogenic arrest. Spermatozoa appeared subsequently in the ejaculate and his wife had four children. He then requested a bilateral vasectomy and at the time of that operation a testicular biopsy confirmed the presence of normal spermatogenesis. The peak of enthusiasm for varicocele ligation followed the report of Dubin and Amelar,[7] who found that in a series of 986 operations the semen quality improved in 70 per cent of men and 53 per cent of wives conceived. Doubts about the efficacy of the operation were expressed by Nilson et al.[8] who, in a prospective trial, found no difference in the semen quality for the two groups of patients, and in fact fewer partners conceived in the operated group. Rodriguez-Rigau et al.[9] and Baker et al.,[10] in their studies of operation or no operation, were also unable to show benefit from the operation. The controversy does not rest at that stage as Okwuyama *et al.*,[11] in a series of 224 subfertile men, found a significant increase in sperm concentration ($P > 0.01$), sperm motility ($P > 0.05$) and a higher conception rate ($P > 0.05$) in the wives of those men who had been operated upon.

Infertility is multifactorial in origin, and in a study at King's College Hospital of men whose wives had not conceived following varicocele ligation we found many other factors that would have prevented conception (Table 13.8). Improvement in semen quality and conception undoubtedly follows varicocele ligation in some patients, and the operation is indicated in those men who require testicular exploration for oligozoospermia or azoospermia or in those where other causes for infertility have been excluded from both husband and wife.

Table 13.8 Adverse factors identified in 351 men whose wives failed to conceive following the ligation of a varicocele*

Azoospermia	Obstructive	25
	Deficient spermatogenesis	43
Severe oligozoospermia	Deficient spermatogenesis	42
(< 1 million sperms/ml)	Idiopathic	71
Oligozoospermia	Deficient spermatogenesis	40
(1–20 million sperms/ml)	Idiopathic	77
Poor motility	< 15%	14
	15–30%	7
Antisperm antibodies		13
Negative heterologous oocyte penetration test		21
Female factors		37

* In only 75 couples was no cause for infertility found, and multiple factors were present in 48 couples.

The choice of operation for varicocele is much easier. In those men who require a full testicular exploration and vasography, the operation may be performed through a left inguinal incision. The internal spermatic vein(s) and cremasteric veins are ligated at the internal inguinal ring, and the right testis may also be delivered through the medial end of the wound to permit the testicular exploration to be carried out. High ligation of the varicocele (Palomo operation) should be performed in those patients where the sperm concentration is adequate as there is little morbidity associated with this muscle-splitting incision. The testicular artery should not be ligated and testicular atrophy is uncommon after either of these high operations. There has been some enthusiasm for sclerotherapy of the testicular veins. This technique has a low morbidity but does not permit a testicular exploration to be performed in those men with poor-quality semen.

Surgery of erectile and ejaculatory failure

The inability to obtain intravaginal ejaculation is an uncommon cause of infertility and in some instances it is amenable to surgical treatment.

Erectile dysfunction

Gross lymphoedema of the penis may render it too large for vaginal penetration, and in these patients it is possibly to excise the lymphoedematous tissue and permit intercourse. A small penis rarely interferes with fertility, although it may be associated with testicular failure; but in those patients in whom the penis has been amputated—usually self-inflicted or because of infection—it is possible to perform a phalloplasty. The original technique described by Gillies, a multistage procedure with a high incidence of complications, has been abandoned by most surgeons in favour of local flaps or a forearm flap based on the radial artery. It is beyond the scope of this chapter to deal with those men who are unable to achieve an erection as a result of organic factors. Many arterial revascularization procedures have been described but satisfactory short-term results are only achieved in the younger age groups. Magnification to improve the technique of vascular anastomoses, anticoagulants after the operation to keep the anastomoses patent, and possibly regular intracorporeal injections of papaverine during the first three months, are all thought to be beneficial in obtaining good results.

The surgery of venous incompetence has attracted much attention in recent years, and although successful results have been obtained in some patients—particularly in young men with congenital abnormalities — overall results have been disappointing. This reflects the outcome of surgery on venous problems in general, but is also because the leakage problem may lie in the muscle of the corpora cavernosa rather than the veins that drain these bodies.

Those men with organic impotence, with the exception of a small number of men who are suitable for a reconstructive procedure or intracavernous drug therapy, are candidates for the insertion of a penile prosthesis. These prostheses—and there is a choice of malleable, self-contained or multi-part inflatable ones—restore a man's ability to have intercourse. They are particularly useful when the loss of potency is due to pelvic surgery or an accident and enable both partners to obtain sexual satisfaction and fertility. The morbidity of such operations is low except when infection occurs—as it does in about 5 per cent of patients, and is more common in diabetics and following priapism.

Finally, one should mention the Finetech–Brindley bladder controller device which is a surgically implanted stimulator for the sacral anterior roots (usually S2, S3 and S4). It is used in spinal cord damage, and its primary purposes are to improve bladder emptying and to assist defecation and to enable male patients to have a sustained full erection when they wish. The device contains no implanted power supply and is driven by electromagnetic induction at the radio frequency of 7 MHz and 9 MHz. The device enables male patients to have a sustained full erection when they wish, but many decline to do this for sexual purposes on account of associated muscle spasms at the time of stimulation.[12]

Ejaculatory failure

Ejaculatory dysfunction, with the exception of premature ejaculation which has social consequences, is only of importance when it interferes with fertility. Most patients with primary ejaculatory failure have psychological causation to their problem, and many respond to counselling or the application of vibratory stimulation to the penis. In other patients it may be necessary to stimulate the pelvic sympathetic fibres by inserting an electrode through the anus. Electroejaculation is painful in the normal subject, and anaesthesia may be required, but this is unnecessary in paraplegics. Another approach is to implant a hypogastric nerve stimulator around the sympathetic nerve fibres anterior to the sacrum which may be activated by an exterior control. Brindley has used this technique in eight men, and five of the partners have conceived.[13]

It is rarely necessary to correct retrograde ejaculation surgically. Bladder neck closure may be enhanced by sympathomimetic drugs, or spermatozoa may be collected from the bladder and used for artificial insemination. There remains a small group of patients in whom a reconstructive procedure is carried out in an attempt to improve fertility, or in some older men who are not warned about retrograde ejaculation before undergoing bladder neck surgery.

Abrahams et al.[14] described a technique of bladder neck reconstruction by excising a wedge from the anterior part of the bladder neck. Ramadan and Pryor find it more convenient to reconstruct the posterior part of the bladder neck and use a modification of the Young Dees operation for incontinence. In this operation, a 5 cm posterior flap of urethra/bladder mucosa is tubed around a 14-gauge urethral catheter and the bladder/bladder neck/prostatic capsular tissue is wrapped around this tube to make a bladder neck. Antegrade ejaculation was restored in all six patients on whom this operation was performed.[15]

Conclusions

Surgery has an important role in prevention and management of the male partner of an infertile marriage. The simple techniques of yesteryear have been replaced by those of greater sophistication which are carried out in units where consideration is given to both partners. There is no longer a role for empirical treatment and every effort should be made to diagnose the cause for infertility and offer specific therapy. On some occasions this is not possible and the couple should be counselled about artificial insemination with donor semen. The prospects for an infertile couple are now excellent.

References

1. MacKellar A. Cryptorchidism. In: Pryor J.P., Lipshultz L.I. (eds.): *Andrology*. London: Butterworths, 1987: 53–68.
2. Anderson J.B., Williamsson R.C.N. The fate of the human testes following unilateral torsion of the spermatic cord. *Brit. J. Urol*. 1986; **58:** 698–704.
3. Bonnie G.G. McLoed T.I.F., Watkinson G. Incidence of sulphasalazine induced male infertility. *Gut*. 1981; **22:** 452–5.
4. Schoysman R.S., Bedford J.M. The role of the human epididymis in sperm maturation and sperm storage as reflected in the consequences of epididymovasostomy. *Fert. Steril*. 1986: 293–9.
5. Patrizio P., Silber S., Ord T., Balmaceda J.P., Asch R.H. Two births after microsurgical sperm aspiration in congenital absence of vas deferens. *Lancet*. 1988; **2:** 1364.
6. Silber S.J. Transplantation of a human testis for anorchia. *Fert. Steril*. 1978; **30:** 181–2.

7. Dubin L., Amelar R.D. Varicocelectomy: 986 cases in a twelve year study. *Urology.* 1977; **10:** 446–9.
8. Nilsson S., Edmonsson A., Nilsson B. Improvement of semen and pregnancy rate after ligation and division of the internal spermatic vein: fact or fiction? *Brit. J. Urol.* 1979; **51:** 591–6.
9. Rodriguez-Rigau L.J., Smith K.D., Steinberger E. Relationship of varicocoele to sperm output and fertility of male partners in infertile couples. *J. Urol.* 1978; **120:** 691–4.
10. Baker H.W.G., Burger H.S., de Kretsner D.M., Hudson B., Rennie G.G., Straffon W.G.E. Testicular vein ligation and fertility in men with varicoceles. *Brit. Med. J.* 1985; **291:** 1678–80.
11. Okuyama A., Fujisue H., Matsui T., Doi Y., Takeyama M., Nakamuru M., Namiki M., Fujioka H., Matsuda M. Surgical repair of varicocoele effective treatment for subfertile men in a controlled study. *Eur. Urol.* 1988; **14:** 298–300.
12. Robinson L.Q., Grant A., Weston P., Stephenson T.P., Lucas M., Thomas D.G. Experience with the Brindley sacral root stimulator. *Brit. J. Urol.* 1988; **62:** 553–7.
13. Brindley G.S., Personal communication, 1988.
14. Abrahams J.I., Solish G.I., Boorjian P., Waterhouse P.K. The surgical correction of retrograde ejaculation. *J. Urol.* 1975; **114:** 888–90.
15. Pryor J.P. Reconstruction of bladder neck for retrograde ejaculation. In: Gingell C., Abrams P. (eds.): *Controversies and Innovations in Urological Surgery.* London: Springer Verlag, 1988: 433–7.

Further reading

Hargreave T.B. (ed.) *Male Infertility.* Berlin: Springer Verlag, 1983.
Pryor J.P., Lipschultz L.I. (eds.) *Andrology.* London: Butterworths, 1987.
Tanagho E.A., Lue T.F., McLune R.D. *Contemporary Management of Impotence and Infertility.* Baltimore: Williams and Wilkins, 1988.
Wageknecht L.V. *Microsurgery in Urology.* New York: Thieme, 1985.

14

The practice of children's surgery in India

R.K. Gandhi, MS, FRCS (Edin), FACS, FAMS, FCPS

Introduction

The practice of medicine in the tropics differs substantially from that in developed countries, owing to socio-economic factors and the geographical influence.

In a region where more people live below the poverty line than above it, widespread malnutrition, unhygienic living conditions and increased susceptibility to infection are responsible for the prevalence of certain diseases which are specific to the area. The same factors influence the course of so many other universally prevalent diseases, to render them more virulent and vicious. Diseases with pathologic processes having a strong correlation with environmental and climatic conditions (e.g. some parasitic infestations) occur mostly in this region only.

The above considerations apply equally, if not more, to the practice of paediatric surgery. The results of paediatric surgery are vitiated by a high incidence of fœtal immaturity, undernutrition and poor resistance to infection, more frequent and more severe congenital malformations resulting from inadequate antenatal care, ignorance contributing to an inordinate delay in seeking medical advice, and superstitious beliefs and practices denying the benefit of surgery to needy babies.

This chapter is intended to highlight some of the practical problems, knowledge of which would be difficult to acquire in any other setting. It needs to be emphasized that this is assuming increasing importance because of the mixing of people of different ethnic origins, varying cultural backgrounds and differing social habits, resulting from the flow of international traffic. Also, in any affluent country with an unfettered economy, yawning disparities of income are bound to arise, and cities develop pockets inhabited by underprivileged sections of the society. These 'urban slums' then carry health hazards similar to those in a developing country, making a knowledge of these problems relevant and necessary.

With a full realization that it is well nigh impossible to condense one's lifetime experience into a small chapter, an attempt is made here to bring out personal observations and those details that are not commonly known or have not been mentioned in other treatments of the subject.

Staphylococcal pneumonia and its complications

A few decades ago, pneumonia and its resulting complications had a wide and virtually universal prevalence. With improvements in living conditions and the increasing chemotherapeutic control of infections, the incidence rapidly came down in affluent countries and the complications of pneumonia became unusual. Even in developing countries there was a sharp decline, though this was mainly confined to privileged sections of society. Now, however, with the rising incidence of bacterial resistance to antibiotics, there has been a resurgence.

Most of the pneumonias are currently staphylococcal in origin; infections from Pneumococcus, Streptococcus and *H. influenza* are almost eliminated because of the low levels of antibiotic resistance.

The resurgence is seen mostly in deprived sections of society, which are more vulnerable and which cannot readily afford suitable antibiotics. Interestingly, the occasional case of staphylococcal pneumonia occurring in a child from a more affluent section of society is resistant to the common antibiotics.

Pathology

Infants are most commonly affected, one-third of all cases occurring in infants below three months and two-thirds of all cases in infants under one year of age. With a virulent infection, a vulnerable infant may develop fulminant septicaemia and succumb to it. The essential pathology is bronchiolitis involving the terminal minute bronchioles, with necrosis of the wall, intramural micro-abscess formation and peribronchial inflammatory exudation. This gives rise to a partial narrowing of the bronchiolar lumen, which acts as a check valve giving rise to an increased intra-alveolar tension with a breakdown of interalveolar septa to a varying extent and the formation of *pneumatoceles*. Intrapleural rupture of a pneumatocele would result in a spontaneous *pneumothorax* and, if the infection is still active, there may be a *pyopneumothorax* with a bronchopleural fistula. Rupture of a subpleural micro-abscess would, however, give rise to an *empyema*.

Management

The average yearly intake of such cases in the author's hospital practice has been around 70, making an accumulated experience of about 1500 cases in a span of two decades (1967–87). What follows is thus based on experience of the management of a vast spectrum of clinical cases.

Effective chemotherapy based on specific antibiotic sensitivity studies is the main line of treatment. It is advisable, however, not to wait for the sensitivity report, but to start promptly with the antibiotic likely to be most effective, based on one's knowledge of the prevailing disease pattern. It is recommended that for the first 48 hours the antibiotic be administered in heavier dosage and frequently enough to ensure a high sustained blood level of the drug. The chemotherapy should be continued for at least six weeks, or for two weeks after the subsidence of pneumonia as well as its complications, whichever is longer. There is a tendency for the infection to lurk silently and to reappear when the infant is sent back to an unfavourable environment.

Between 1967 and 1977 the antibiotics found to be most effective were chloramphenicol and erythromycin; cephalosporins have since then been the drugs of choice, though in selected cases aminoglycosides have been used parenterally as an initial therapy and oral cephalosporins continued for the remaining period. Supportive measures in the form of small transfusions of fresh blood have been found very effective.

Treatment of complications

Pneumatoceles

The mere presence of one or more pneumatoceles on x-ray does not call for active intervention. With the effective control of infection and subsidence of the primary pathology, and the resulting check valve effect, pneumatoceles are bound to disappear. If, however, any one of them rapidly increases in size and gives rise to increased intrathoracic tension, as indicated by respiratory embarrassment and mediastinal shift, an intercostal catheter should be inserted inside the pneumatocele and connected to the underwater seal until the pneumatocele collapses and the remaining lung expands.

Tension pneumothorax

Tension pneumothorax is indicated clinically by acute respiratory embarrassment, tachypnoea and cyanosis. Radiologically, there is free air in the pleural cavity with a pulmonary collapse accompanied by a mediastinal shift and pleural herniation to the contralateral side. An intercostal drainage will evacuate the air and allow the mediastinum to return to its normal place. The catheter should not be removed for at least 48 hours after the restoration of normalcy.

Empyema

A catheter should be inserted through a proper intercostal space into the pleural cavity for the prompt drainage of pus. The only indication for tapping with a needle is a diagnostic aspiration. The temptation to resort to repeated tappings as a therapeutic measure must be resisted for fear of making the empyema chronic, rendering the pus thick and inducing pleural adhesions with loculations. An intercostal catheter drainage, if resorted to early, permits an effective evacuation of the pus which is quite thin at that time. The largest catheter that the intercostal space can accommodate should be used to ensure that the lumen does not become obliterated quickly by fibrinous deposits, and the catheter should not be removed for at least 48 hours after total evacuation of the pus and full expansion of the lung. In an infant, an intercostal catheter provides an effective and adequate drainage, and it has never been found necessary to resort to rib resection for this purpose.

Often on an x-ray, haziness in the hemithorax persists for some time owing to fibrinous deposits on the pleura. This should not cause any anxiety as the haziness will invariably disappear with time as the deposits start resolving (Figs. 14.1–14.3). At times the deposits are very exuberant, giving rise to a dense radiological opacification. An unwary clinician is likely to mistake this for an extensive pleural thickening, and may even be tempted to undertake an unnecessary thoracotomy and decortication. Given time, such deposits always resolve and the radiological opacification disappears, showing a complete expansion of the lung. In an occasional case where the process of resolution is rather slow, a short course of corticosteroids has been found very helpful in hastening it, with a prompt disappearance of opacification.

Pyopneumothorax

This is the worst and most trying complication, often necessitating patient, painstaking and prolonged management. Effective and continuous intercostal catheter drainage is the prime requirement. At times, if the drainage is unsatisfactory, there should be no hesitation in inserting a second catheter in another intercostal space (double catheter drainage). The essence of the management is complete and continued evacuation of the pus and air so as to allow the lung to fully expand and remain fully expanded until the bronchopleural leak is sealed off and healed (Fig. 14.4). This may at times take weeks. The longest period in my experience has been 14 weeks, at the end of which the leak subsided. Thoracotomy, pleural toilet, decortication and/or pulmonary resection have been required very rarely and should not be undertaken in haste. Only five patients (out of 335 cases) required this. Of these, in two patients the pulmonary destruction was found to be so massive that there was very little lung tissue left that could have expanded and sealed the bronchopleural leak.

Abdominal tuberculosis

Tuberculosis is caused by *Mycobacterium tuberculosis*, mostly of the human type (infection with the bovine type being extremely rare). Lately there has been an increasing incidence of atypical mycobacterial infection, particularly in tuberculous lymphadenitis.[1]

Tuberculosis is prevalent in children from the low socio-economic group because in that social group there is a high incidence of chronic pulmonary tuberculosis in adults who are infective. Overcrowding, poor ventilation and malnutrition facilitate the transmission of infection, and debilitating diseases like whooping cough, measles and gastroenteritis increase the vulnerability to infection and activate the disease in those children with silent infection.

It is hardly surprising that the incidence of tuberculosis in children follows a close parallel to that in adults as the latter are the common source of infection in the children. The interesting observations made by Grzybowski are relevant.[2] He found that chemotherapeutic treatment of 586 cases with smear-positive pulmonary tuberculosis in a developed country like the Netherlands resulted in a cure rate of almost 98 per cent; only 1 per cent of the patients did not respond and continued to be infective. In contrast, a similar management of 474 cases

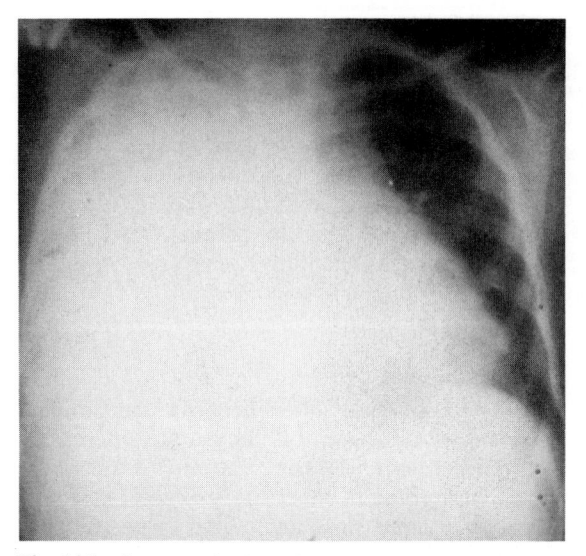

Fig. 14.1 An x-ray of a chest showing a massive empyema on the right side.

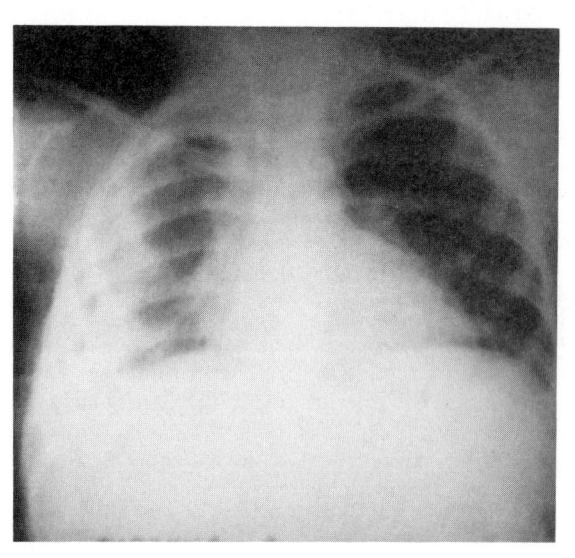

Fig. 14.2 An x-ray of the same chest as in Fig. 14.1 at the end of an effective drainage of the empyema. Note the opacity due to extensive fibrinous deposits in the pleural cavity.

in India yielded a cure rate of only 63 per cent, whereas 10 per cent died and 27 per cent failed to respond and continued to be infective. These observations also emphasize why it is difficult to achieve total control of this disease.

The prevalence of active disease in the Indian population is 15–25 per 100 000,[3] and a quarter of the cases are bacillary. In an estimated population of 750 million, in 1985, there would be about 20 million cases of active tuberculosis with about 5 million bacillary cases.

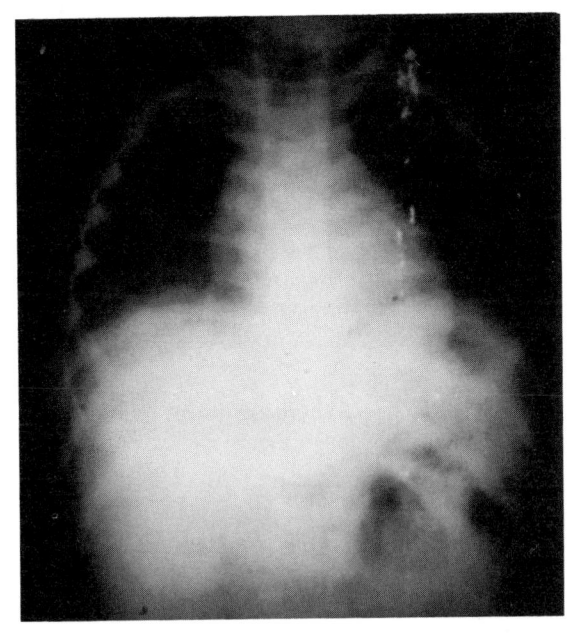

Fig. 14.3 An x-ray of the same chest as in Fig. 14.2 two weeks later, showing complete disappearance of the fibrinous deposits and a fully expanded lung.

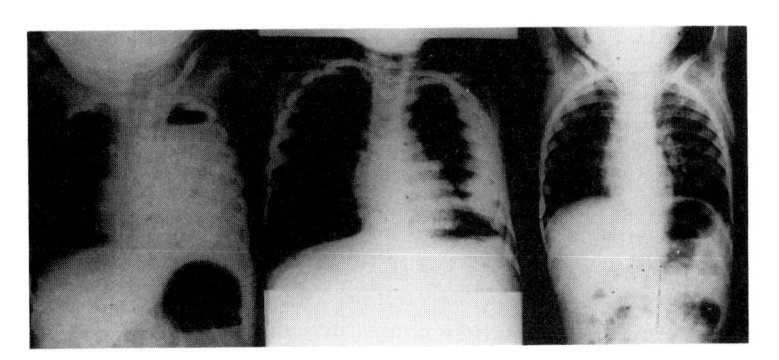

Fig. 14.4 (a) An x-ray of a chest, showing a pyopneumothorax on the left side. (b) At the end of effective drainage. Note the expanded lung and residual opacity. (c) After three weeks. Note the complete disappearance of the opacity and full expansion of the lung.

In spite of the better living conditions in an urban area, the mortality from the disease is still 48 per 100 000 in Delhi,[4] whereas it is as high as 90 per 100 000 in rural areas.

In metropolitan cities like Bombay, 55 per cent of the total population gets tuberculized by the age of 20 years, while in the rural area of Maharashtra State almost 38–40 per cent of the total population gets tuberculized before the age of 15 years.[5] In the population of slums and residents of the one-room tenements in the cities, the rate of acquired primary tuberculosis as detected by tuberculin survey is 40 per cent by the age of 6 years and nearly 80 per cent by the age of 14 years. In most developing countries including India, the present risk of infection is 25 times higher than in developed countries.[6]

Abdominal tuberculosis manifests itself as visceral, peritoneal or lymph glandular. It may appear as a combination of these types.

Visceral abdominal tuberculosis. In this type, any part of the GI tract or a solid abdominal viscus (e.g. liver) may be involved. The two commonly affected areas are the small intestine and the ileocaecal region. The small-intestine involvement usually takes the form of an ulcer which tends to heal with the formation of a stricture, whereas the ileocaecal involvement manifests as a hyperplastic mass which encroaches on the lumen of the terminal ileum and caecum, giving rise to varying degrees of intestinal obstruction.

Peritoneal abdominal tuberculosis. In this variety there is diffuse involvement of visceral as well as parietal peritoneum. The peritoneum becomes studded with minute tubercules which may later coalesce and caseate. The peritoneal involvement is further subdivided into two subtypes:

1. the *adhesive or dry type* (peritonitis sicca), characterized by extensive peritoneal and intra-abdominal adhesions of varying density;
2. the *exudative or ascitic type*, characterized either by free fluid in the peritoneal cavity (generalized ascites), or by a loculated collection of fluid (encysted ascites), if there are pre-existing peritoneal adhesions.

Lymph gland tuberculosis. The commonly affected lymph nodes are those in the mesentery of the terminal ileum, giving rise to a mass in the right iliac fossa or the umbilical region (tabes mesenterica).

The clinical picture

In the absence of complications, the symptoms tend to be vague. Abdominal pain, diminished appetite, loss of weight and mild pyrexia are the common complaints. Infrequently there is diarrhoea and at times steatorrhoea. Diagnosis at this stage can be quite rewarding, though difficult.

Diagnosis is usually made when a child presents with an abdominal mass or masses or with ascites or with an intestinal obstruction. At times the child is brought with a clinical picture of generalized peritonitis, which on exploration is found to result from an intestinal perforation proximal to the stricture. Unusually the presenting feature may be an umbilical fistula with an underlying mass or an intraperitoneal abscess with hectic fever.

One form of abdominal tuberculosis which appears to be specific to children and which has not been commonly mentioned is the peritoneal type. One or more plaque-like, flat, superficial masses are felt in the abdomen. The mass gives the impression of being intra-abdominal as it is deep to abdominal muscles, but can be picked up with the abdominal wall indicating its parietal nature. Underlying the mass there are extensive and dense peritoneal adhesions; these make it very difficult and hazardous to open the peritoneal cavity. It has been found safer to make an incision over the mass, which is exposed after incising the parietal muscles. Without attempting a laparotomy, a biopsy of the mass is taken to confirm the diagnosis. Interestingly this variety responds remarkably and rapidly to the use of steroids in combination with the necessary antituberculous chemotherapy. All the 18 cases treated in our series have done well, the masses disappearing in two to three weeks time, leaving behind no particular sequelae and followed by a virtual cure.

In a 12-year period (1975–87), 223 cases of abdominal tuberculosis were dealt with. Of these, 96 cases were of the peritoneal variety (including the 18 cases just referred to), 61 presented with intestinal stricture, and 45 children were brought with complications like active peritonitis, intraperitoneal abscesses or faecal fistula. Only 21 children were picked out while investigating vague symptoms.

Investigations

Most of the laboratory and radiological investigations (e.g. routine haemogram, erythrocyte sedimentation rate, plain radiograph, barium meal studies) do not provide confirmatory evidence of the disease. The only certain method is a biopsy, which is essential to establish a diagnosis before the patient is submitted to a long-term chemotherapeutic regimen. Laparoscopy, where feasible, is also quite helpful and may obviate the laparotomy. Laparoscopy, however, may be dangerous in the plastic variety or peritoneal type and should be undertaken with extreme caution.

Management

The sheet anchor of management is antituberculous chemotherapy, given in a proper combination and with effective dosage over a sufficiently long period. Surgery is required for those cases that fail to respond to chemotherapy and develop complications.

The recommended chemotherapeutic regimen is as follows:

1. *First three months:*
   Rifampicin 10 mg/kg daily
   Isoniazid 10 mg/kg daily
   Pyrazinamide 30 mg/kg daily
   Streptomycin injections 30 mg/kg daily for 1st month
   alternate day for 2nd month and twice weekly for 3rd month.
2. *Four to six months:*
   Rifampicin
   Isoniazid
   Streptomycin injections twice weekly.
3. *Seven to nine months:*
   Rifampicin
   Isoniazid.
4. *Ten to twelve months:*
   Isoniazid.

Surgical treatment

Cases presenting with complications would need a laparotomy and appropriate surgical correction of the offending pathology, depending on the findings; for example, separation of peritoneal adhesions, stricturoplasty, excision of the affected segment or closure of a perforation.

Surgery should be conservative, confined to correction of the pathology which is most urgent. Residual lesions will be taken care of by the subsequent chemotherapy.

Surgical ascariasis

Helminths and humans have lived together for a very long time, and a number of helminthic parasites still pester mankind, more so in the developing countries. Of all the helminthic infestations, the one with most surgical significance is ascariasis.

Infestation with *Ascaris lumbricoides*, a nematode commonly referred to as roundworm, is widespread. It invades almost every other person in certain rural areas, and every fourth person in cities. Apart from its chronic damaging effect on the nutrition of an individual, this worm is a cause of a number of surgical problems by virtue of its notorious traits. Its protective habit of clumping together results in a mass which can occlude the intestinal lumen; it has a tendency to nibble its way through, giving rise to perforation and peritonitis; and it has a migratory instinct to wander and burrow its way into an orifice, giving rise to biliary or pancreatic obstruction or appendicitis.

Ascarideal intestinal obstruction

This is the most frequent complication of roundworm infestation, accounting for two-thirds of all complications. One or more clumps of roundworms occlude the intestinal lumen. The occlusion is frequently accentuated by spasm of the overlying intestinal wall. There is often congestion and oedema of the mucosa owing to an inflammatory reaction caused by the secretions by the roundworms and by the products of their decomposition. All these factors contribute to making a subacute obstruction into an acute one.

As time passes the intestinal wall undergoes patchy gangrene, with subsequent perforation of the gangrenous area.

Clinical features

The child presents with intermittent colicky pain and vomiting. In the early stages the vomiting will be reflex and will consist of the gastric contents. Later on it will be because of obstruction and will be bilious. A previous history of passing roundworms in the stools or a history of vomiting roundworms may be indicative of roundworm obstruction; but neither of these is confirmatory because a child with roundworm infestation may develop an intestinal obstruction from any other cause and may have the same history.

The diagnostic feature is a palpable roundworm mass. The mass is usually around the umbilicus, it may be irregular in shape, and gentle pressure on the mass may evoke a soft crepitus because of the air trapped between the roundworms or between the mass and the intestinal wall. Serial palpation may reveal a change in the size or position of the mass; this is diagnostic. The mass is non-tender and tends to yield.

Development of tenderness over the mass, or the mass becoming tense and unyielding, are sinister findings indicative of a possible gangrenous change.

Investigations

A plain x-ray of the abdomen reveals multiple fluid levels and a typical mottled appearance due to radiolucent specks interspersed with small areas of opacity (Fig. 14.5). The latter show air-bubbles trapped between the roundworms and are very typical of a roundworm mass. At times there are thin air-streaks or wisp-like radiolucent lines in parallel inside an opaque mass, because of air in the worms' intestinal tracts (Fig. 14.6).

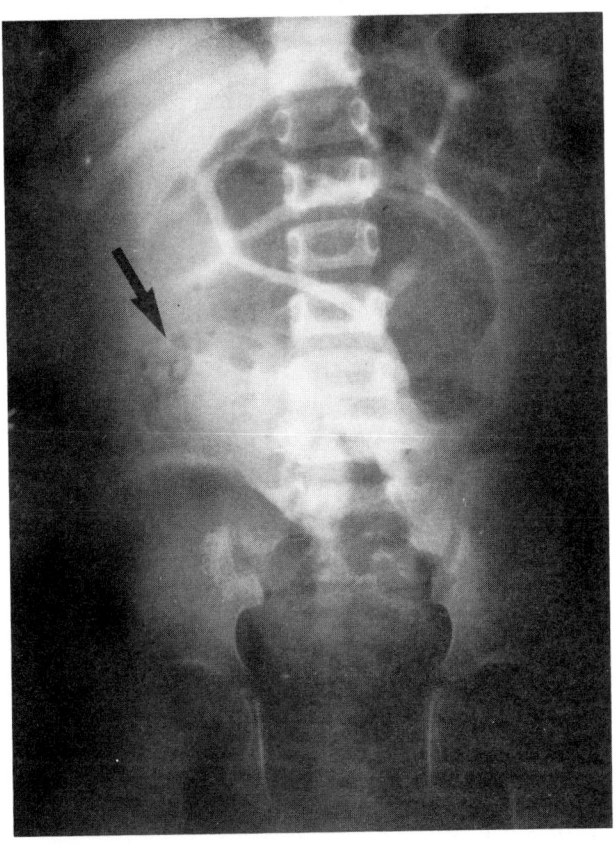

Fig. 14.5 A plain x-ray of an abdomen. An arrow points to a mass of roundworms, showing a typical mottled appearance.

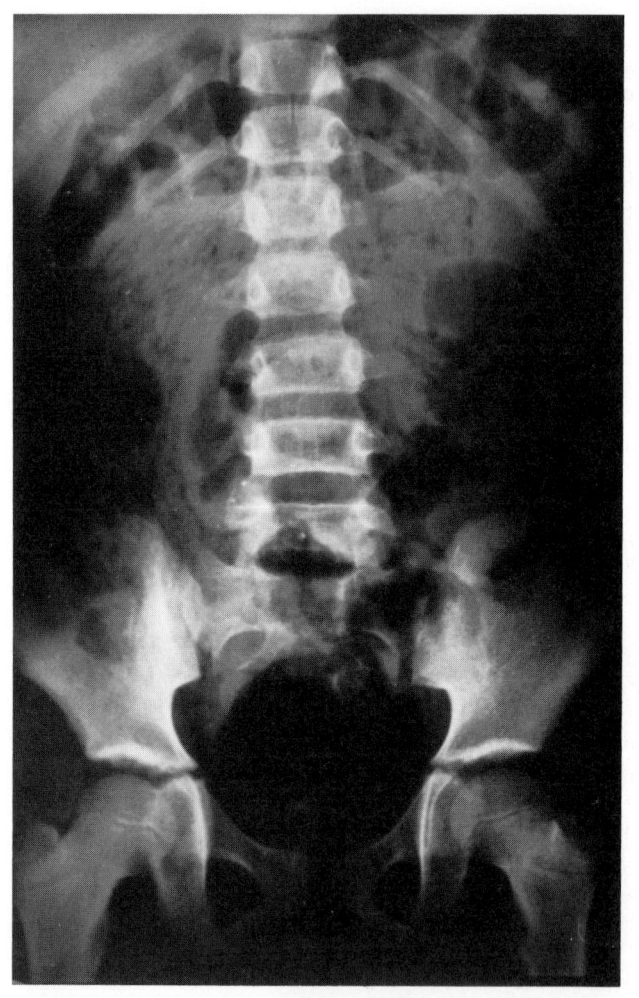

Fig. 14.6 A plain x-ray of an abdomen, showing an opaque roundworm mass in the centre with parallel radiolucent streaks.

Management

Conservative management consists of nasogastric aspiration and parenteral fluids; this may result in relief of the obstruction by the worms disentangling themselves after a period. Use of hypertonic saline enema every 4–6 hours often helps.

Surgical intervention is indicated if the worm mass:

1. becomes tense and tender;
2. becomes fixed in position;
3. does not change in size and shape over a period, with no relief of the obstruction.

Surgical management starts with a laparotomy followed by exteriorization of the intestine together with the mass. The clumped worms are gently kneaded to disentangle them, and subsequently pushed through the ileocaecal valve into the colon from where they are automatically expelled. It is very important that undue pressure over the mass and prolonged squeezing are not employed, for fear of rupturing the already devitalized intestines and/or releasing roundworm toxins, with consequent toxaemia and shock. When it is difficult to dislodge the worms, an enterotomy is carried out proximal to the mass in the healthy intestine and the worms manipulated through the enterotomy and sucked out. It is advisable to use non-absorbable material for closure of the enterotomy as well as the laparotomy wound, because secretions of the roundworms tend to have a proteolytic effect and may absorb catgut very fast.

Roundworm perforation

The child will be brought with acute abdominal pain and vomiting. The patient may have pyrexia and may be very toxic, sometimes restless and delirious. On examination, the abdomen is tender and there is generalized guarding. In ascarideal perforation the guarding is not as severe and boardlike as in a perforation from other causes.

A plain x-ray of the abdomen in the upright position may reveal gas under the diaphragm which, when present, will be confirmatory of the diagnosis.

Management involves an emergency laparotomy after adequate hydration and gastrointestinal decompression. The peritoneal cavity will contain thin seropurulent fluid which should be sucked out. (The absence of thick pus and gummed-up intestines so typical of suppurative peritonitis is because of the proteolytic nature of the roundworm secretions, which tend to make the exudate thin, seropurulent and non-adhesive.) The perforation is located and sutured. In the event of a large ragged perforation involving most of the circumference, a resection of the affected area is indicated.

Unusually, in spite of a diligent search, no perforation is detected even though there are free roundworms in the peritoneal cavity. Presumably the roundworms have burrowed through the different layers of the intestinal wall in a valvular fashion.

The enterotomy, or the intestinal ends after resection, are closed with non-absorbable material for the reason already given above.

Biliary ascariasis

A roundworm lodging itself in the biliary tract is an unusual event. However, when it does occur, it may give rise to obstructive jaundice and in some cases to ascending cholangitis and hepatic abscesses. If the worm dislodges itself or dies and decomposes, the obstruction will be relieved spontaneously. In the event of absence of such a happy outcome, an operative exploration with removal of the roundworms will be required. When facilities are available, an endoscopic visualization and removal of the worms is worth a trial.

Surgical amoebiasis

Entamoeba histolytica essentially affects the colon. The caecum and ascending colon are most commonly involved, the rectum and sigmoid colon being next in frequency. The amoeba lodges itself in mucosal crypts and gives rise to mucosal ulcers with varying degrees of colliquative necrosis of the colonic wall. It may erode into a small venule and enter the portal blood stream, which then carries it to the liver where it will set up an acute inflammatory reaction with or without abscess formation.

The surgical problems resulting from this parasite are gangrenous colitis, colonic perforation and peritonitis, amoeboma, and amoebic abscess of the liver.

Gangrenous colitis

A virulent infection in an undernourished child with low resistance will give rise to fulminating colitis with gangrenous changes in the wall of the colon, which may lead to a colonic perforation. Clinically the child is ill and toxic with abdominal pain and severe dysentery. The abdomen reveals tenderness and guarding over the colon.

Amoebic peritonitis

This results from a perforation of the colon affected with amoebic colitis or a rupture of an amoebic abscess of the liver. The child will have the usual features of peritonitis and there may be gas under the diaphragm on plain x-ray. The child will be very toxic.

The management will involve a laparotomy, evacuation of the pus and closure of the colonic perforation. In a bad case exteriorization of the colon with colostomy may be required. This should be coupled with systemic antiamoebic chemotherapy.

Amoeboma

Normally an amoebic ulcer heals without fibrosis and without a stricture. Unusually, an amoebic ulcer is associated with fibrotic reaction and granulation tissue, giving rise to a firm tender mass, termed amoeboma. The commonest site is the caecum, though it may occur in the sigmoid colon and rarely in the transverse colon. It is extremely unusual in children.

A therapeutic trial with emetine and metronidazole results in a cure and is an important test to differentiate it from other lesions.

Amoebic abscess of the liver

This usually affects the right lobe of the liver. There may be one large multilocular abscess, or the liver may be studded with multiple small abscesses. When it occurs near the superior surface of the liver, it is associated with elevation of the right dome of the diaphragm and sometimes with basal pleuritis.

When it affects the anterior and inferior surfaces, it gives rise to an enlarged and tender liver palpable below the costal margin.

A clinical triad of pain in the right hypochondrium, pyrexia and hepatomegaly should raise the suspicion of an amoebic abscess of the liver, more so when there is a history of a recent attack of amoebic dysentery.

A plain x-ray may reveal an elevation of the right dome of the diaphragm and pleural reaction. The white blood cell count reveals marked polymorphonuclear leucocytosis. A radio-isotope hepatogram will show a cold area in the liver.

Repeated aspiration of the hepatic abscess with a wide-bored needle coupled with the systemic use of antiamoebic drugs—emetine and metronidazole—results in a cure. It is very rarely necessary to carry out open drainage of the abscess.

Acknowledgements

My sincere thanks are due to my colleagues Professor (Mrs) S.S. Deshmukh, Dr V.S. Wainganker and Dr V.M. Rege, and to the administrators of K.E.M. Hospital and Sir H.N. Hospital, for their helpful roles in the preparation of this chapter.

References

1. Gandhi R.K., Deshmukh S.S. Incidence of atypical mycobacterial infection in tuberculous cervical lymphadenitis in children: a preliminary report. *Ind. J. Surg.* 1978; **40:** 101.
2. Grzybowski. Impact of chemotherapy on the epidemiology of pulmonary tuberculosis. *Ind. J. Tuber.* 1988; **35:** 50–8.
3. Pamra S.P. Problems of tuberculosis in developing countries. *Clin. Notes Chest Med.* 1980; **1:** 266–71.
4. Goyal S.S., Mathur G.P., Pamra S.P. Tuberculous trends in an urban community. *Ind. J. Tuber.* 1978; **25:** 77.
5. Shah P.M., Udani P.M. Medical examination of rural school children in Palghar taluka. *Ind. Pediat.* 1968; **5:** 343.
6. Bleiker M.A., Styblo K. The animal tuberculosis infection rate and its trends in developing countries. *IUAT.* 1978; **53:** 295–8.

15

Benign diseases of the breast

John Hadfield, CBE, TD, MS, FRCS

Since my chapter appeared in Volume 1 of this series in 1976 there has been much interest in this field and much work on the subject has been forthcoming. In most studies the results have been of value and have advanced knowledge. In a few, the patients treated have been small in numbers, the time of follow-up too short for meaningful deductions and the conclusions drawn have shown ignorance of the published work on the subject and of the basic pathology of the underlying lesions. The surgeon who is asked to give a second opinion when the previous treatment has failed and the disease has recurred may find that his treatment needs to be prolonged and the patient is inconvenienced.

In this chapter I make no effort to cover the whole large subject of benign breast disease, but have taken up areas of progress, controversy, misconception and the common problems of patients seen in my clinic over the last 30 years and treated primarily by me or referred to me for a second opinion.

Breast cysts

Breast cysts present as single or multiple lumps of varying size. In a previous study of 300 patients followed for a 15-year period,[1] the majority of patients were around the age of 40 years and presented with a painless, discrete, spherical lump in the breast substance or periareolar region. About one-quarter of the patients had pain as a first symptom. The duration of the history was from weeks to months, depending on the symptoms and the patients' disposition. Many patients reported a change in the size of the lump with their periods; others described lumps which had disappeared spontaneously.

Cysts in this series were located equally in left and right sides, the majority occurring in the upper and outer quadrant. At first examination, about 10 per cent of the patients had more than one cyst in the same breast. In patients previously treated for a cyst, over one-third had developed another cyst at a different site in the breast on follow-up. The diameter of the cysts varied from a few millimetres up to 3–4 cm.

Treatment and management is based on the following simple classification:

1. *simple cyst:* a single cyst in a clinically normal, nodular or granular breast;
2. *cystic carcinoma* (Fig. 15.1);
3. *a carcinoma*, coincidental with, but separate from a breast cyst;

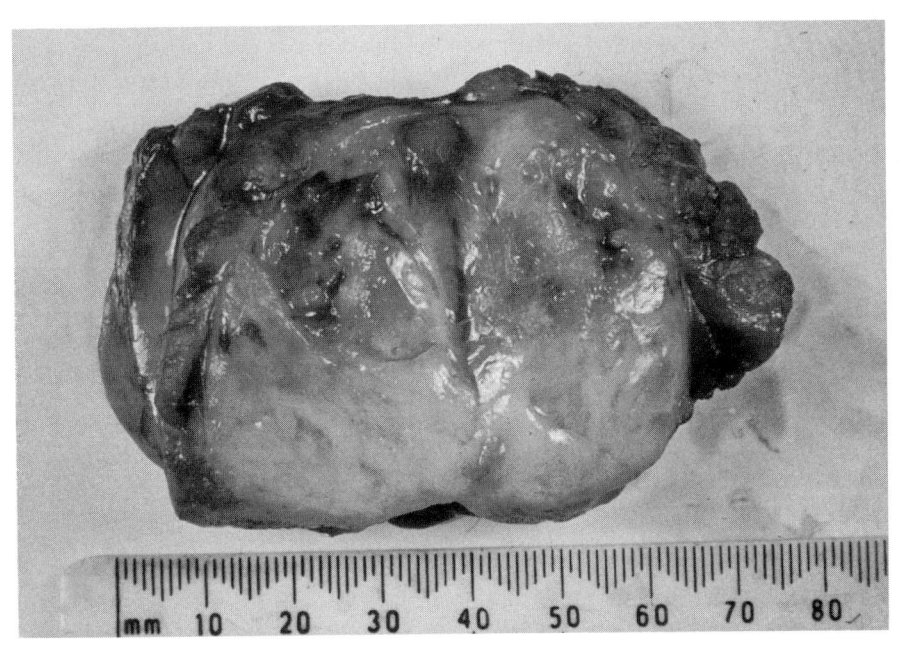

Fig. 15.1 A breast cyst opened to show carcinoma inferiorly. The blood-stained aspirate was cytologically positive.

4. *multiple cysts:* blue-domed cysts occurring in a nodular or granular breast;
5. *cysts associated with the duct system.*

The routine on demonstrating a discrete mobile mass clinically is to attempt to diagnose and treat the patient at the first visit. This is made possible by the diagnostic radiologist and the surgeon running simultaneous sessions.

My preferred form of management is to see and examine the patient as the first step. At that stage a needle exploration of the lump is carried out. If the lump is cystic, it is aspirated to dryness and the patient sent on for mammography and for ultrasound examination at the radiologist's discretion. Prior attempted aspiration of a breast lesion before imaging does not increase the risk of the imaging technique failing to reveal a cancer. If the lesion was cystic, the fact that aspiration completely emptied the lump must be checked by simple palpation, but the evidence of the imaging is superior to simple palpation alone.

Some surgeons prefer to have ultrasound and/or mammography carried out on receipt of the doctor's referral letter, the patient attending the clinic later to see the surgeon with these results. Others order ultrasound and/or mammography after clinical examination and bring the patients back later at that session or on another occasion for aspiration if indicated.

Aspiration remains the mainstay in the treatment of breast cysts. Some clinicians order a cytological examination of all cyst aspirates. In the majority of cases this is either negative or unhelpful, but it is always indicated if the aspirate is blood-stained or a lump remains after aspiration—though surgical removal of that zone of the breast is always in any case mandatory. If the cyst has recurred on follow-up and the previous mammogram was negative, a further aspiration and review are carried out. Large cysts often need more than one aspiration. Before discharge from the clinic all patients should be advised and taught to check the breasts regularly for lumps and report back if one is found, as there is an increased tendency for further cysts in patients who have previously had one.

The last problem is the cyst which recurs after repeated aspiration. An attractive approach here is to inject a sclerosant after aspiration. This has been tried in breast cysts and for a longer time with hydroceles. A recent report[2] suggests encouraging results using the antigonadotrophin Danazol. It appears to have fewer side reactions than other agents, which often produce for a varying period of time a tender, red breast.

The necessity for surgical excision is uncommon. At Stoke Mandeville Hospital we use it for a recurrent single cyst which does not resolve by other means. We prefer an incision over the lump rather than the cosmetic circumareolar incision. The latter involves burrowing through the breast substance to reach the cyst and can be complicated by an embarrassing haematoma, especially in a large, soft breast.

Even after surgery, there can be further trouble with breast cysts since the condition is multifocal. In the rare case of multiple recurrent cysts destroying the breast substance and untreatable by other means, we would consider a subcutaneous mastectomy and prosthesis, especially as these patients are often in the older age group.

Microcysts demonstrated by imaging techniques are usually treated by aspiration by the radiologist at the time of examination. They will be discussed later.

Excision of the major duct system of the breast

The technique of this operation remains virtually the same since it was first designed by Adair and described by Hadfield[3,4] and Urban.[5] This is confirmed by a recent account by Preece,[6] where he describes the method used by Professor Hughes's group in Cardiff. From time to time reports have been published or patients referred with postoperative problems. The majority of these are caused by technical mistakes, incomplete or inadequate surgery. The most common, in my experience, are as follows.

Partial necrosis of the nipple, or necrosis at the edge of the circumareolar incision. When the nipple flap is reflected it is not uncommon to find thin-walled veins which bleed easily and run across the flap. They can be controlled by pressure between the surgeon's thumb and finger and diathermy or catgut ligature where they emerge from the breast on the opposite side to the incision. Diathermy on the flap or at the incision will cause necrosis. Also, the flap should be the full thickness of the areolar skin.

Necrosis of the skin edge, or thick scars. Both of these sequelae can be avoided by careful haemostasis away from the edge and by retracting the skin flap manually with gauze or wound hooks. Tension on the skin edge is avoided by fixing the under-surface of the areola to the surface of the reconstructed dead space left by the removal of the major duct system, using fine catgut sutures. The commonest causes of skin necrosis are too many tight, or subcuticular Dexilon sutures. We use a few fine mono-filament Prolene 40 sutures. The Cardiff group recommend the Douati dermal suture.[6]

Postoperative nipple discharge. This is caused by incomplete removal of the major ducts either as they enter the nipple (A), by dividing them flush with the nipple base or missing some as they enter the nipple laterally or on the opposite side (B), (Fig. 15.2).

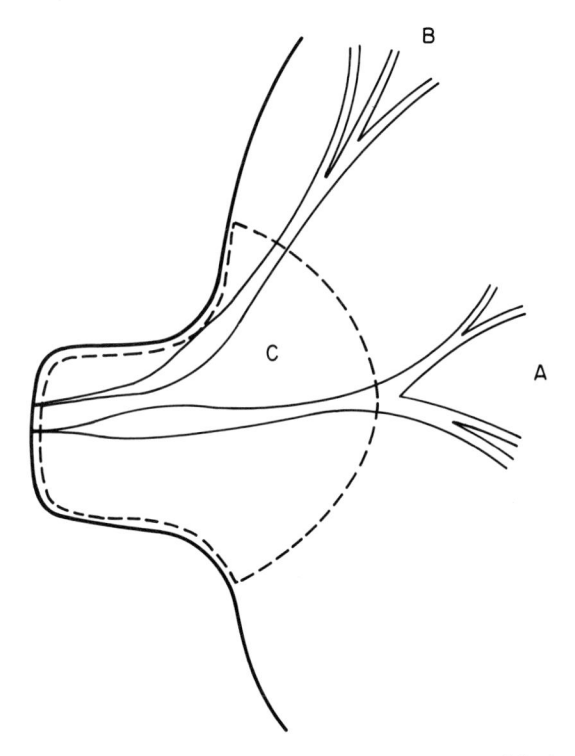

Fig. 15.2 The anatomy of the major duct system of the breast (diagrammatic), showing the arrangement of the major ducts (A), the area for excision (C) and how they may be missed at operation (B).

Poor cosmetic results. These are the consequence of three mistakes. First, there may be inadequate or incomplete eversion of the nipple. Many of those patients have a thick fibrous core and inversion of the nipple from periductal mastitis. This can be avoided by excising the fibrous core and placing an everting catgut purse-string suture around the base of the nipple.

Another cause of poor cosmesis is inadequate obliteration of the dead space of the major ducts and failure to build it up to be slightly convex.

Infection after this operation has been reported in a few small series. Much of this can be avoided by good haemostasis and adequate wound drainage. We do not use antibiotics for all cases, but reserve this mainly for fistula and abscess patients.

Mammillary fistula

This condition has three aetiologies, namely:

1. a fistulous track opening in the para-areolar region lined by granulation tissue and communicating with a single abnormal squamous-lined breast duct[7] (in discussing the aetiology the authors favoured a congenital rather than an infective lesion);

2. a fistula in association with the duct ectasia complex of periductal mastitis or para-areolar abbcess;

3. postoperatively following inadequate or incomplete treatment for the conditions described in (2) above (Fig. 15.3).

In all these circumstances we advise excision of the major duct system which, if done correctly, will render the patient symptom-free with a good result.

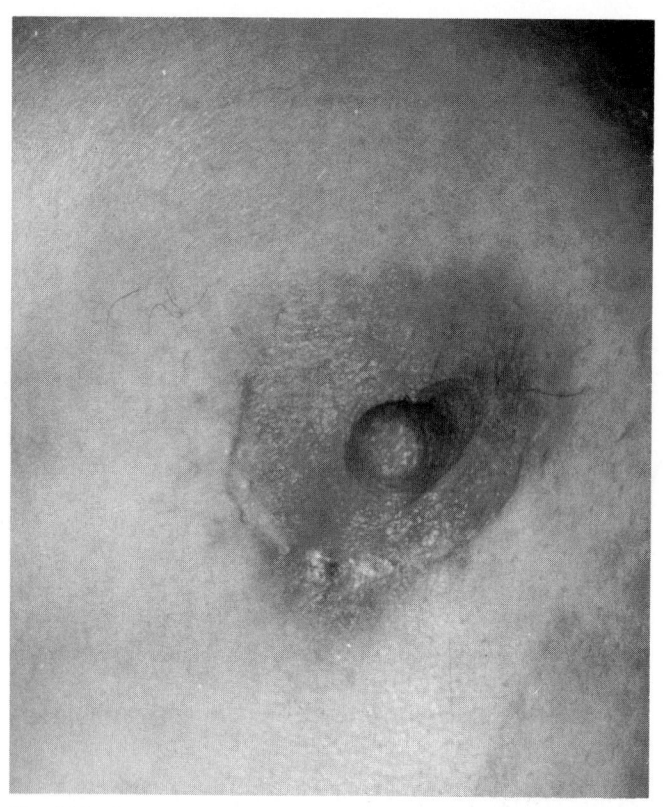

Fig. 15.3 Postoperative mammillary fistula following incomplete treatment for a para-areolar abscess.

Duct ectasia

Antibiotics are used in the presence of demonstrable sepsis. Some surgeons advise laying open the fistula and allowing it to heal by granulation.[8] It is conceivable that this technique might be used for aetiology (1) above, but it is entirely inapplicable for the others as it does not remove the underlying disease and primary cause.

Duct ectasia

Duct ectasia or a generalized dilatation of the major duct system of the breast is a common benign breast condition.[9] It is bilateral, asymmetrical and has a similar incidence to breast cancer (Fig. 15.4). It is a common cause of nipple discharges, which vary from blood-stained to colourless, white, green or brown and may be serous or viscid.[10] In duct ectasia the discharge appears at several duct orifices, whereas in duct papilloma or carcinoma only one duct is involved. Duct ectasia may alternatively present as a para-areolar abscess due to secondary infection of the dilated major ducts with anaerobic secondary invading organisms and associated periductal mastitis.

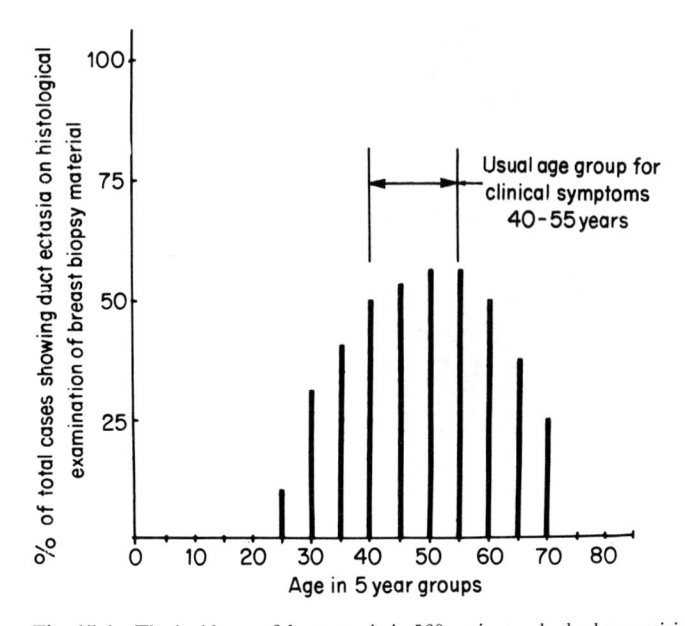

Fig. 15.4 The incidence of duct ectasia in 560 patients who had an excisional biopsy for an undiagnosed breast lump without a clinical nipple discharge.

Periductal mastitis may also present as a hard, red, hot solid lump in the breast which may be mistaken for a cancer, acute abscess or 'mastitis'.[11,12,17]

Lastly, duct ectasia may be demonstrated on mammography as a coarse granular calcification which may be localized or widespread (Fig. 15.5). This may be the healed stage of the dead or damaged tissues and the thickened fibrous walls of the ducts.

214 *Benign diseases of the breast*

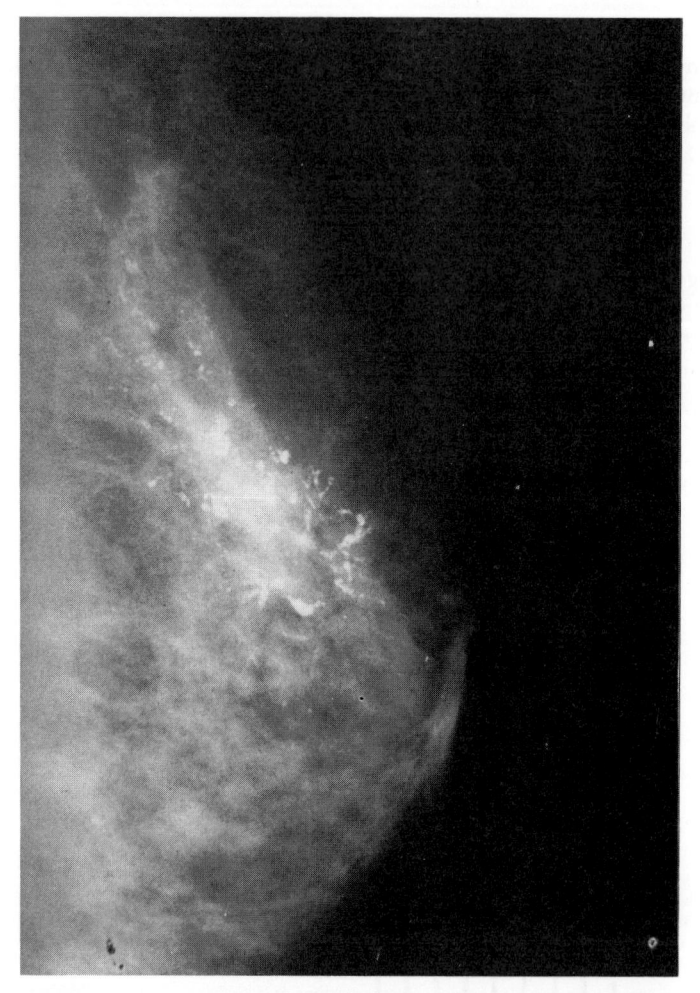

Fig. 15.5 Periductal mastitis — the final lesion. A mammogram showing coarse granular calcification related to the duct system.

The micro-photographs in Fig. 15.6 show the ductal lesions, while the accompanying diagram shows the mechanism by which the thin-walled, dilated ducts laden with lipoid-filled macrophages break down to become the fluid of the nipple discharge. This also passes through the thin and damaged dilated duct wall to become the initial lesion of plasma cell[16] or periductual mastitis.[11] The influence of infection in the development of this lesion is discussed in references 12, 13 and 14.

A discussion of the detailed pathology of duct ectasia has been made elsewhere.[11,16]

Para- and sub-areolar abscess

The incidence of acute breast abscess, often associated with pregnancy and lactation, is now uncommon, but can vary with geographic pathology. Para- and sub-areolar abscesses remain, however, and can cause problems (Fig. 15.6). Aetiologically, they are related to the duct ectasis/periductal mastitis/mammillary fistula complex.[18] Clinical presentation starts as a para- or sub-areolar abscess which bursts, forming a fistula which apparently heals over only to recur.

Secondly, they may persist following incomplete or inadequate surgery, or antibiotic therapy only. When associated with duct ectasia, which is often the case, the abscess may be multifocal below the nipple, often undermining it and causing loss of viability of the overlying skin.

Where there is an established abscess we advise culture of the pus and determinations of antibiotic sensitivity, with adequate incision and drainage under antibiotic cover. The cavity is left open and allowed to obliterate itself from below, otherwise recurrence is inevitable. At a later stage excision of the major duct system is required, using the standard technique, to remove the underlying pathological lesion.

In other patients where there is an established fistula we advise culture of the fistulous tract followed by excision of the major duct system *en-bloc* with the associated fistula. Some surgeons carry this out under antibiotic cover for all patients. We tend to use antibiotics when there is proven infection.

The patient with a longstanding recurrent para-areolar abscess treated by recurrent incision and drainage with courses of antibiotics and with a recurrent fistula is a complex problem (see Fig. 15.3). We treat first by establishing the microbiology of the organisms and the use of antibiotics with adequate open drainage. Often healing will not be complete owing to a thick-walled para- or sub-areolar cavity with the damaged areolar skin forming the roof. This can only be cured by removing the underlying pathology with the major ducts. This can be done through the incision for laying the abscess open. When final healing has occurred the healed area of incision has much the same colour and texture as the areola.

Benign microlesions

Mammography has demonstrated a large number of microlesions, many of which are benign. Although mammography and ultrasound examination, needle biopsy and cytological or histological examination, or cyst aspiration may be diagnostic, in some cases a wire- or dye-marked biopsy will be needed to make a final differentiation from malignancy. The standard procedure is carried out with postoperative radiological checking on the material removed. It is of paramount importance that the microlesion has both been found and examined fully from the clinical and medico-legal point of view. This problem has been discussed by Eidken.[19]

216   *Benign diseases of the breast*

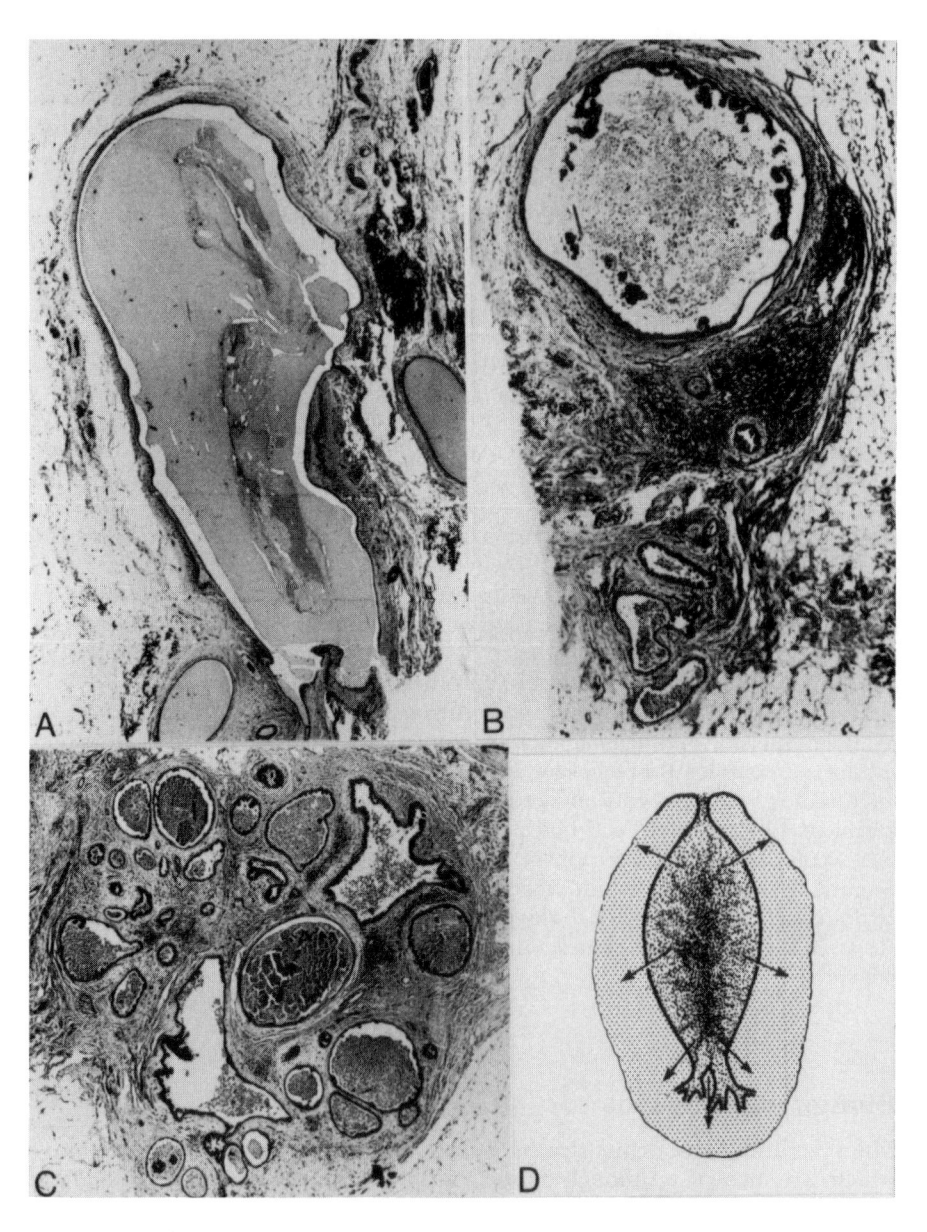

Fig. 15.6   Duct ectasia: a compound picture of the three grades of duct, from the same specimen and affected by this disease. Patches of periductal mastitis can also be seen. (a) Major duct (× 10), showing dilatation of the lumen in which secretion is present and atrophy of the lining epithelium. (b) Intermediate duct (× 20) which is dilated and filled with secretion. (c) Minor ducts (× 20), showing varying degrees of dilatation, periductal mastitis and distension of their lumens with secretion. (d) Periductal mastitis formation (diagrammatic). The lipoid-rich secretion in the duct is passing through the damaged duct wall to initiate the periductal mastitic reaction. (Reproduced from reference 11 with the kind permission of the Royal College of Surgeons of England)

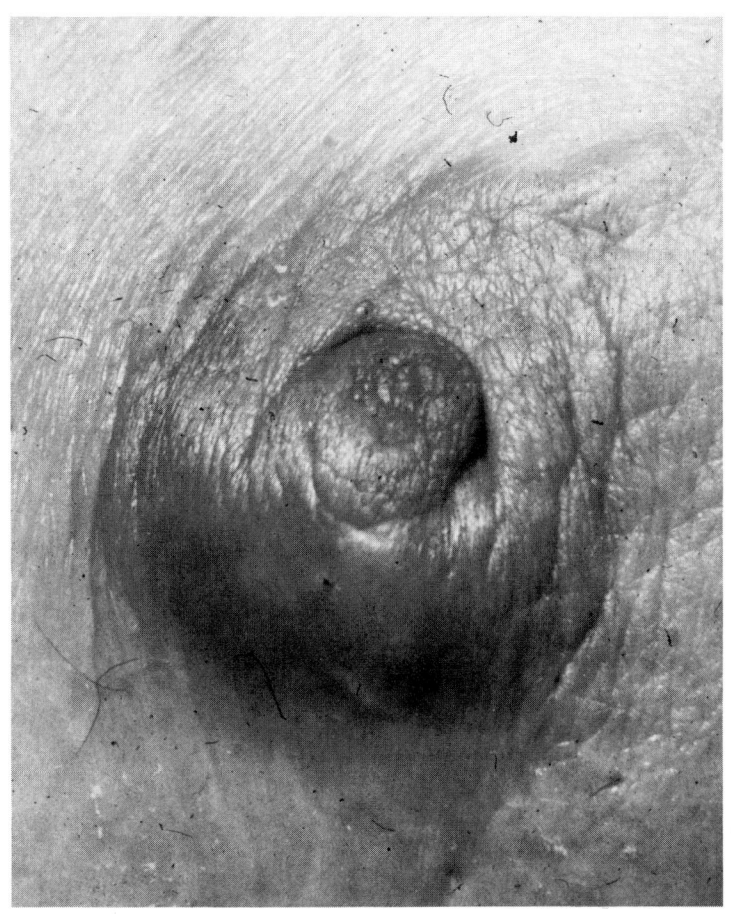

Fig. 15.7 A para-areolar abscess in the breast of a woman aged 45 years. No previous history of breast disease was given.

References

1. Hadfield G.J. Benign diseases of the breast. In: Hadfield G.J., Hobsley M. (eds.): *Current Surgical Practice*. London: Edward Arnold, 1976: 250–61.
2. Hinton C.P., Williams M.R., Roebuck E.J., Blamey R.W. Danazol in the treatment of multiple breast cysts. *Breastnews*. 1986; **2:** 11–12.
3. Hadfield G.J. Excision of the major duct system for benign disease of the breast. *Brit. J. Surg.* 1960; **47:** 472–7.
4. Hadfield G.J. Further experience of the operation for excision of the major duct system of the breast. *Brit. J. Surg.* 1968; **55:** 530–5.
5. Urban J.A. Excision of the major duct system of the breast. *Cancer*. 1963; **16:** 516–20.
6. Preece P. How I do a subareolar duct excision. *Breastnews*. 1987/1988; **2:** 9–12.
7. Patey D.H., Thackray A.C. Pathology and treatment of mammary duct fistula. *Lancet*. 1958; **2:** 871–3.
8. Atkins H.J.B. Mammillary fistula. *Brit. Med. J.* 1955; **2:** 1473–4.

9. Bundred N.J., Dixon J.M., Chetty U., Forrest A.P.M. Mammillary fistula. *Brit. J. Surg.* 1987; **74:** 466–8.
10. Birkett J. *The Diseases of the Breast and their Treatment.* London: Longman, 1850.
11. Hadfield G.J. The pathological lesions underlying discharges from the nipple in women. *Ann. R. Coll. Surg. Eng.* 1969; **44:** 323–33.
12. Walker J.C., Sandison A.T. Mammary duct ectasia. *Brit. J. Surg.* 1964; **50:** 57–64.
13. Zuska J.J., Crile G., Ayres W.W. Fistulas in lactiferous ducts. *Amer. J. Surg.* 1951; **81:** 312–17.
14. Pearson H.E. Bacteroides in areolar breast abscesses. *Surg. Gyn. Obst.* 1967; **125:** 800–2.
15. Leach R.D., Eykin S., Philips I., Corrin B. Anaerobic subareolar breast abscesses. *Lancet.* 1979; **1:** 35–7.
16. Hadfield G.J., Levine A. The breast. In: Hadfield G.J., Hobsley M., Morson B.C. *Pathology in Surgical Practice.* London: Edward Arnold, 1985: 7–21.
17. Adair F.E. Plasma cell mastitis: a lesion simulating mammary carcinoma. *Arch. Surg.* 1933; **26:** 735–49.
18. Scholefield J.H., Duncan J.L., Rogers K. Review of a hospital experience of breast abscesses. *Brit. J. Surg.* 1987; **74:** 469–70.
19. Edeiken S. Mammography and palpable cancer of the breast. *Cancer.* 1988; **61:** 263–5.

IATROGENIC SURGICAL DISEASE

Introduction

John Hadfield, Michael Hobsley and Tom Treasure

The term iatrogenic, by dictionary definition, means conditions produced by the medical practitioner. It therefore involves every branch of treatment and management by drugs, medicines, anaesthetic agents, surgical operations, radiological examinations, especially those using contrast media or invasive methods and radiotherapy.

The examples presented in this section of the book are not given in order to suggest that the problem can be solved by banning a form of treatment, but rather in an effort to clarify how surgeons can strive to make the treatment safe or at least safer.

Nothing stands still: new concepts, new techniques, new endeavours in all spheres of management are not just desirable, but essential for progress and better results. Both our patients and medical science would be the eventual losers if problems were solved only by using defensive medical practices. The results would be tragedy for everyone.

Either during an operation or following surgery there may be damage to the tissue being operated upon or injury to anatomically related structures. The injury may be unavoidable if the pre-existing disease has altered the anatomical relations. This risk is particularly serious if there have been pre-existing inflammatory changes. The risk of surgical injury is related to the degree of experience of the surgeon performing the operation and his anatomical knowledge of the region. On the other hand, it should be accepted that a junior and less experienced surgeon can only be expected to perform to the best of his ability. He will not be expected to have the expertise and experience of his senior colleague. Yet he must at least know his limitations, because matters go from bad to worse when an inexperienced surgeon faced with damage that he recognizes does not know how to deal with the situation. Equally, even when the greatest care is exercised damage may occur.

It is also important to appreciate that, though the damage may be done during the operation, the effects may not become manifest until later. An example of this is injury to the middle colic artery: the sloughing of the transverse colon may not occur for several days.

In our present state of knowledge, some complications appear to be inevitable despite all reasonable precautions. This statement applies, for example, to postoperative thromboembolism, the occurrence of which cannot be ascribed to any fault of the surgeon provided that he has taken the reasonable precautions.

Informed consent by the patient and counselling by the surgeon means, in effect, that the risks, problems, results and complications of the operation must be discussed. This is conducted with absolute straightforwardness, attempting to inform the patient and the relatives fully and kindly without generating fear or suspicion. In any operation, no plans can be definite until the operating field is exposed and final decisions can be made.

Few surgeons have a large personal experience of the problems of iatrogenic surgical disease, and even for those who have any experience this is usually confined within their speciality. In the planned situation the operating surgeon can arrange, if necessary, for a colleague to be present to deal with the problems at the time when they arise.

In the unforeseen situation, a senior colleague is called at once and he may deal with it himself or call in a specialist colleague to help. This is preferable, as long as the patient can stand prolonged surgery and anaesthesia, rather than closing up and re-opening later when the operation area may have dense vascular adhesions and the function of the damaged organ may become disarranged. In either of these circumstances, the patient and his relatives must be fully informed. Full and detailed notes of the whole situation must be made and kept at the time of operation and during follow-up. The patient's general practitioner and the surgeon's defence union should be fully informed both at the time of the incident and at follow-up. It cannot be too fully stressed that good follow-up by the surgeon in charge of the patient, or at least by his staff under his close and continued supervision, is obligatory.

When the diagnosis is made preoperatively, as with the initially planned procedure, the surgeon in charge may, if he has sufficient experience, take it on himself or he may seek the help of a colleague who has special knowledge or experience of the situation.

Patients always, and rightly, fear the immediate consequences and those that can occur later. For instance, a patient needing an axillary or a groin dissection for a neoplastic lesion of the upper or lower limb will be told of the possibility and consequences of the ensuing lymphoedema. The degree of disability depends on the patient and his work. However, if at the time of treatment care of the lymphoedema is instituted early in a regular clinic and the progress monitored, the patient will not only accept the condition, but will become involved in treating it and obtaining a good result. This could equally apply to speech therapy following damage to the recurrent laryngeal nerve. Patient groups like the Ileostomy Association are an example of this doctor–patient support.

The groups of circumstances which our expert contributors discuss in this section embrace a wide field, but the topics have been chosen for the fact that they do occur regrettably more often than one might think or certainly wish. The thrust is not only what to do given the acute or delayed problem, but also how to prepare for the unforeseen and try to prevent trouble.

The contribution and place of the medical defence unions and the medico-legal implications and future developments in this respect are of interest to everyone involved in the management and treatment of sick patients. The Royal College and all bodies involved in the training of doctors are deeply conscious that this must be an important part in any trainee doctor's professional training course.

For all these reasons, this section is addressed not only to the trainee, but to the trainer as well.

16

The philosophy of medical defence: a 'bridge over troubled waters'

J.W. Brooke Barnett, MB, BS

Background

It is difficult for any doctor now to envisage what practising medicine was like before medical defence had been invented. The advantages of medical defence are now taken for granted: the disadvantages of not having such a system are no longer remembered. It is a salutary experience to look back a century to see what the medical profession endured in those days.

In 1884, Dr David Bradley of Whittington Moor near Chesterfield was charged by the police with criminal assault on a female patient who had had an epileptic fit in his surgery.[1] Throughout his trial he maintained his innocence, but in spite of this, and the fact that there was no corroborative evidence, the prosecution secured a verdict of guilty and Dr Bradley was sentenced to a two-year prison sentence with hard labour. He did not have the means to brief a lawyer with experience in such cases. It was, in fact, Mr Lawson Tait who, when not in dispute with the Council of the Royal College of Surgeons, found time to rescue him. He wrote to the *British Medical Journal*[2] stating that at a recent meeting of the Birmingham and Midland Counties branch of the British Medical Association the following resolution was passed: 'that this meeting, having heard a statement of the case of Dr Bradley, recently convicted of a felonious assault at the Leicester Assizes, desires to express its opinion that this case is eminently one in which a reconsideration of the verdict of the jury is demanded'.

Pressure from the medical profession, led by Mr Lawson Tait, caused the Home Secretary to review the evidence given at the trial and to conclude that it was not sufficient to support a conviction. Dr Bradley was granted a free pardon, but only after he had been in gaol for eight months.

A series of criminal and civil actions against doctors who had no adequate means of defending themselves led to the foundation of the first medical defence organization—the Medical Defence Union (MDU) — and appropriately Lawson Tait became its first president. Before that, appeals for money to pay doctors' legal expenses after a trial were commonplace. Sir William Jenner, president of the Royal College of Physicians, took a prominent part in appealing for funds. However, it was not a rational solution to the problem. The obvious solution was to collect money in advance and retain medical and legal experts.

And so, on 23 October 1885, the Medical Defence Union was registered under the Companies Act 1862. Dr Francis Bond of Gloucester wrote to the *British Medical Journal*:[3]

'*Sir*,—I have just received a circular inviting me to join an association which has been formed under the above name for the purposes of defending, or assisting in defending, its members in cases where actions involving questions of principle to the profession, or cruel and groundless charges, are brought against them; of suppressing unauthorized practitioners; and of offering its assistance, as far as may be deemed judicious, in promotion or modification of any Bill or movement initiated for the benefit of the medical profession. These objects appear to be excellent, and the former two of them, at any rate, fulfil entirely the condition which alone justifies them being made the excuse for establishing a new association, namely, that they are, at the present time, a decided "want" . . . [These matters touch] most nearly the interests of every member of the profession, for they affect the question of his self-preservation, which, in medicine, as in other cases, is Nature's first law.'

It was the intention that local committees would be formed and that these would unite. The Medical Defence Union was founded at the same time as two other famous unions—the Rugby Union and the Mothers' Union—with perhaps not dissimilar charitable objects! As a result of this unique idea two other organizations were founded in the following years:

1892: the London and Counties Medical Protection Society, later to be known as the Medical Protection Society (MPS)
1902: the Medical and Dental Defence Union of Scotland (MDDUS).

Adverse conditions facing the medical profession in other countries led to the Medical Defence Union and the Medical Protection Society becoming worldwide organizations.

These defence societies have truly kept the balance between the power of the state, the interests of patients and the professional reputations of doctors. A former president of the MDU, Dr Seymour Cochrane Shanks, consultant radiologist at University College Hospital, described the union as having two functions (both equally important): to protect the doctor and to compensate the patient when compensation was due.

It is also salutary to examine how the defence societies have kept this balance between the interests of the patient, the doctor and the state.

The state

Criminal courts

The state in this context is represented in criminal proceedings against doctors. The most celebrated criminal trial concerning a doctor, *Regina* v. *Bodkin Adams*,[4] took place in 1956. Dr Bodkin Adams was accused of murdering a patient. The death sentence was then the penalty for those found guilty of murder. Dr Bodkin Adams was represented by the MDU. Owing to the experience and skill of the union's solicitors and counsel, it was possible to dispel the rumours and gossip which were the basis for the prosecution's case. Finally the case turned on the contemporary evidence in some long-forgotten nurses' notebooks which contradicted the faulty recollections the nurses were giving on behalf of the prosecution. Dr Bodkin Adams was acquitted and eventually returned to his general practice in Eastbourne—a fair trial and a fair judgement, with the MDU holding the balance between life and death.

The defence of a doctor in a criminal court not only protects his reputation but sometimes also establishes a principle in law for the whole profession. This was the outcome of a criminal charge against an eminent gynaecologist, Mr Aleck Bourne,[5] in 1938, which ended not only in his acquittal but also set the interpretation of the law on abortion for the next three decades, until the Abortion Act 1967 and the regulations in 1968 came into operation. Mr Bourne was represented by the Medical Protection Society.

Coroners' courts

It has been a long-established service provided by the defence societies that they represent members at coroners' courts. Happily in the UK there have been few instances in the last 20 years in which coroners have overstepped their remit and impugned a doctor's reputation. However, the defence societies, by representing members, have played a valuable part in seeing that the interests of the state, the relatives and the doctor are fairly balanced.

Administrative tribunals

In all countries in the world there has been a proliferation of administrative tribunals to which doctors are subject. In the UK there are, for example, the following tribunals:

1. the Preliminary Proceedings Committee and the Professional Conduct Committee of the General Medical Council (GMC);
2. the Health Committee of the GMC;
3. the Clinical Complaints Procedure in hospitals in the National Health Service, in which two independent consultants adjudicate on a clinical complaint;[6]
4. the committees in the NHS Hospital Service set up to investigate 'untoward incidents';[7]
5. the 'three wise men' procedure;[8]
6. disciplinary committees[9] to investigate an NHS hospital doctor's competence and conduct;
7. the investigation of administrative complaints in the NHS Hospital Service by the Health Service Ombudsman;
8. the Medical Service Committees of the Family Practitioner Committees which, for NHS general practitioners, investigate complaints in relation to their terms of service (on appeal to the Secretary of State legal representation is permitted).

It has been said that a doctor in the UK is subjected not only to double jeopardy but to quadruple jeopardy. The defence societies have indeed kept the balance between the legitimate right of a patient to have a complaint investigated and the right of a respondent doctor to have his account of what he did heard fairly and judged objectively.

Litigation

Most surgeons look to their defence organization when they receive a letter from a solicitor alleging negligence. Many take it for granted that this service, which has been built up over a hundred years, is readily available and provides skilled and experienced doctors and expert lawyers and counsel. Indeed, some patients' organizations have complained that the defence societies do more than hold the balance between patients and doctors: that they have a positive advantage, particularly with access to expert medical witnesses. There have been several notable actions in recent years in which the doctor has been accused of negligence.

Consent

Failure to obtain 'informed consent' as a basis for litigation against doctors was not a prominent part of the defence societies' work until the 1980s, when plaintiffs who might not have a good case for negligence against a doctor tended to add as a makeweight to a Statement of Claim: 'Had I known that the outcome of the operation would not have been 100 per cent successful, I would never have undergone it.' It is, of course, easy with hindsight to make such allegations, and very difficult for the surgeon to remember many years after the event what he had said to the patient.

(a) *Hatcher* v. *Black*

The first celebrated action concerning consent, *Hatcher* v. *Black*,[10] took place in 1954. The patient sued the surgeon for failing to warn her that her voice might be affected after a thyroidectomy. The surgeon took the view that this was a rare occurrence and that it would only increase the patient's anxiety to name this as one of the possible complications. In the event, the left recurrent laryngeal nerve was damaged and the patient's voice was affected. Lord Denning in his summing-up said:

> 'But in a hospital, when a person goes in who is ill and is going to be treated, no matter what care you use there is always some risk. Every surgical operation involves risks. It would be wrong, and indeed bad law, to say that simply because a misadventure or mishap occurred, thereby the hospital and the doctors are liable. Indeed it would be disastrous to the community if it were so. It would mean that a doctor examining a patient, or a surgeon operating at a table, instead of getting on with his work, would forever be looking over his shoulder to see if someone were coming up with a dagger. For an action for negligence against a doctor is for him like unto a dagger. His professional reputation is as dear to him as his body, perhaps more so, and an action for negligence can wound his reputation as severely as a dagger can his body. You must not therefore find him negligent simply because something happens to go wrong, as for instance if one of the risks inherent in an operation duly takes place or because some complications ensue which lessen or take away the benefits that were hoped for or because, in a matter of opinion he makes an error of judgement. You should only find him guilty

of negligence when he falls short of the standard of a reasonably skilful man. In short, when he is deserving of censure—for negligence in a medical man is deserving of censure.'

This fair judgement was given in favour of the surgeon supported by the Medical Defence Union.

(b) *The Sidaway case*

Another action which has determined the law on consent concerned a Mrs Sidaway[11] who had undergone a successful cervical (C5–6) laminectomy under a well-known neurosurgeon. The patient returned to the same surgeon some years later when she was suffering severe symptoms relating to a disc lesion at C4–5. A further laminectomy was carried out but unfortunately she became partly paralysed. She claimed that had she known this was the outcome of the operation then she would not have agreed to it.

American and Canadian judgements in favour of informing a patient of 'all material risks' were quoted by her counsel. Such a procedure may protect the doctor but is not necessarily in the best interests of the patient. The Law Lords rejected these propositions and dismissed her appeal. It was held that a surgeon was under a duty to disclose to a patient any substantial risk involving grave adverse consequences inherent in the surgery. Even if a surgeon took a different view, although supported by a responsible body of surgeons, it would be open to the courts to conclude that no reasonably prudent medical man would have withheld information about a risk that was so obviously necessary for the patient to know before the patient could make an informed decision. The Medical Protection Society represented the neurosurgeon. The defence was hampered by the fact that there was no record as to what the neurosurgeon had said to the patient, and by the time the action came to trial the neurosurgeon had died.

Negligence

(a) *The Bolam case*

In 1957 the Medical Defence Union represented a member who had followed an accepted form of treatment at that time—ECT without relaxants. The patient, Mr Bolam,[12] suffered fractures of both hips. It was contended many years later, after the procedure had been modified, that the doctor was negligent in not giving relaxants. Judgement was eventually given in favour of the doctor. The judge said:

> 'I must explain what in law we mean by "negligence". In the ordinary case which does not involve any special skill, negligence in law means this: some failure to do some act which a reasonable man in the circumstances would do, or doing some act which a reasonable man in the circumstances would not do: and if that failure or doing of that act results in injury, then there is a cause of action. How do you test whether this act or failure is negligent? . . . In one case it has been said you judge it by the conduct of the man on the top of a Clapham omnibus . . . But where you get a situation which involves the

use of some special skill or competence, then the test as to whether there has been negligence or not is not the test of the man on the top of the Clapham omnibus, because he has not got this special skill. The test is the standard of the ordinary skilled man exercising and professing to have that special skill . . . it is well-established law that it is sufficient if he exercises the ordinary skill of an ordinary competent man exercising that particular art . . . in the case of a medical man, *negligence means failure to act in accordance with the standards of reasonably competent medical men at the time* . . . as long as it is remembered that there may be one or more perfectly proper standards: and if he conforms with one of those proper standards, then he is not negligent . . . the real question you have to make up your mind on . . . is whether the defendants, in acting in the way they did, were acting in accordance with a practice of competent respected professional opinion . . . if you are satisfied that they were acting in accordance with a practice of a competent body of professional opinion, then it would be wrong for you to hold that negligence was established . . . Finally bear this in mind, that you are now considering whether it was negligent for certain action to be taken in August 1954, not in February 1957; . . . you must not look with 1957 spectacles at what happened in 1954.'

Hence this has become known as the Bolam test.

(b) *The Whitehouse case*

Perhaps the most celebrated case in recent years was that of *Whitehouse* v. *Jordan*,[13] in which it was alleged that Mr Jordan, an experienced gynaecologist, had in attempting a forceps delivery pulled too hard and too long before doing a Caesarean section, which resulted in a brain-damaged child. The Medical Defence Union represented Mr Jordan. The case was finally heard in the House of Lords in 1981 when Mr Jordan was exonerated of all negligence.

Several features of the case are noteworthy. First, the long process of law took from 1970 when the delivery occurred to 1981 when judgement was given in favour of the obstetrician in the House of Lords. Secondly, the standard of care expected of a doctor was reaffirmed by Lord Denning in the Court of Appeal. He said: 'We must say, and say firmly, that in a professional man, an error of judgement is not negligent.' The House of Lords corrected this to read '. . . is not necessarily negligent'. Thirdly, many obstetricians predicted that patients would be subjected to unnecessary Caesarean sections had the judgement been given against the obstetrician. Lord Justice Lawton in his judgement said:

'In my judgement negligence was not proved against [the doctor]. I have come to this conclusion with sorrow, knowing as I do what anguish the parents have suffered and the grave disabilities which the infant plaintiff will have to bear until death. As long as liability in this type of case rests on proof of fault, judges will have to go on making decisions which they would prefer not to make. The victims of medical mishaps of this kind should, in my opinion, be cared for by the community, not by the hazards of litigation.'

No-fault compensation

Not only Lord Justice Lawton but many others have expressed their support for a system of compensating patients without them having to go through the long and often dispiriting process of the law which is no less harrowing for the doctor, even though he has the backing of his defence society. In 1973 the Pearson Commission[14] recommended that the experience of the schemes in New Zealand and Sweden be studied before any recommendations be made in relation to the UK. The British Medical Association has twice expressed its support for a no-fault compensation fund which is provided and run by the government. Since then attention has been focused on the Swedish system which was the subject of a special study by the Medical Defence Union and by the medico-legal correspondent of the *Lancet*.[15] There has also been a study on medical negligence by the Centre for Socio-Legal Studies in Oxford, funded by the King's Fund, which sets out the disadvantages of the present tort system and evaluates alternative systems such as no-fault compensation.[16] Also in 1988, the Bar Conference debated the 'pros' and 'cons' of no-fault compensation. The Medical Defence Union was represented, and the views of the union that the advantages of no-fault compensation outweigh the disadvantages were clearly expressed.[17]

Conclusions

As these examples demonstrate, the defence societies have for more than a hundred years kept a balance between the interests of patients, doctors and society. It has been and still is an altruistic interest based on all members of the medical profession supporting each other in adhering to these ideals. There are signs now of such ideals being eroded by the possibility of some members of the profession seeking a commercial alternative to medical defence which might give a short-term financial advantage at the expense of long-term problems as seen in the USA. In looking at the philosophy of medical defence, the profession as a whole would be wise to look back and see the advantages of the balance which the defence societies have maintained between the interests of patients, doctors and society. This has meant that the societies have had to interpret medicine to the legal profession and law to the medical profession. In doing so, and in looking to the future of increasing litigation against the medical profession, one can truthfully say the defence societies do provide *a bridge over troubled waters*.

References

1. Forbes R. *Sixty Years of Medical Defence*. London: Medical Defence Union, 1948.
2. Tait L. The case of Dr Bradley (letter). *Brit. Med. J.* 1885; **I:** 403.
3. Bond F.J. The Medical Defence Union (letter). *Brit. Med. J.* 1885; Nov. 7: 895–6.
4. *Regina* v. *Bodkin Adams*. *Brit. Med. J.* 1957; **I:** 712–13, 771–2, 828–34, 889–94 and 954–5.
5. *Rex* v. *Bourne* (1938). *All England Law Reports* **1938:** 3.615–21.
6. Department of Health and Social Security. *Complaints Relating to the Exercise of Clinical Judgement by Hospital Medical and Dental Staff*. London: HMSO, HC(81)5, 1981.
7. Ministry of Health. *Reporting of Accidents in Hospitals*. London: HMSO, HM(55)66, 1955.

8. Department of Health and Social Security. *Prevention of Harm to Patients Resulting from Physical or Mental Disability of Hospital or Community Medical or Dental Staff.* London: HMSO, HC(82) 13 1982.
9. *NHS (Service Committees and Tribunals) Regulations.* London: HMSO, SI 74/455 as amended in 1978 by SI 87/455. 1974.
10. *Hatcher* v. *Black* (1954). *The Times,* 2 July. Medical Defence Union (1955) Annual Report (1954–5), 33–4, London.
11. *Sidaway* v. *Board of Governors of the Bethlem Royal Hospital and the Maudsley Hospital and Others.* Times Law Report, 24 Feb. 1984.
12. *Bolam* v. *Friern Hospital Management Committee* (1957). *All England Law Reports* **1957:** 2.118.
13. *Whitehouse* v. *Jordan* (1980). *All England Law Reports* **1981:** 1.267–88. Medical Defence Union (1981) Annual Report, 10–13.
14. *Report of Royal Commission on Civil Liability and Compensation for Personal Injury.* London: HMSO, Cmnd 7054, 1978.
15. Brahams D. The Swedish medical insurance schemes. *Lancet.* 1988; **I:** 43–7.
16. Ham C., Dingwall R., Fenn P., Harris D. *Medical Negligence — Compensation and Accountability.* London: King's Fund Institute, 1988.
17. Brahams D. Medicine and the law—barristers debate medicolegal issues. *Lancet.* 1988; **II:** 858.

17

Facial palsy

R.A. Williams, MA, FRCS, FRCS(Ed),
M. Hobsley, TD, DSc, PhD, MChir, FRCS

Intracranial damage

Acoustic neuromas or cerebello-pontine angle meningiomas stretch the facial nerve and may flatten it, so that it looks as if its function must be in peril. However carefully it is dissected off a large tumour, a postoperative palsy may well occur. The operating microscope, the argon laser and the ultrasonic aspirator have been used to make this procedure as atraumatic as possible.[1]

Anatomical and functional preservation of the facial nerve can be achieved in all small tumours,[2] but only in 20 per cent of large ones; there is an average figure of 80 per cent for medium-sized tumours.[3]

In 1968, House[4] reported 72 per cent with no weakness after a year and 5 per cent with total loss of VII nerve function; but by 1978 his figure for preservation by translabyrinthine route went up to 96.6 per cent in a series of 500 acoustic neuromas.[5]

Within the petrous temporal bone, iatrogenic facial palsy may occur after surgery to the middle ear or mastoid. Removal or cauterization of infected polyps, tympanoplasty or (rarely) stapedectomy can damage the nerve. This is sometimes just a result of the local anaesthetic and vasoconstrictor used and wears off within hours. However, the commonest pathology associated with postoperative facial palsy is cholesteatoma. This can distort the anatomy and expose the nerve. Other procedures such as ultrasonic or cryosurgical labyrinthectomy put the facial nerve at risk.

The paralysis may be immediate and complete, incomplete or delayed. It is most important to note the onset, as management of these groups differs radically.

If the patient has an *immediate complete* palsy, there is general agreement that the nerve should be explored as soon as possible. This may involve decompressing an oedematous nerve, removing a spicule of bone, performing a primary repair or a nerve grafting. The results of these procedures are generally good, and the earlier they are carried out the better. However, these are difficult operations and should only be performed by those with experience and training of nerve suture techniques. So referral to another centre involving delay is justified, as results remain good with decompression up to four weeks.[6]

If the palsy is *incomplete*, and especially if it is known that the nerve is intact anatomically, any packing or dressing should be removed from the operation cavity. Most surgeons also give a short course of steroids in the hope of reducing oedema.

If the palsy is *delayed*, the management is not so generally agreed or obvious. It is important to note if the facial nerve is functioning immediately after the operation. Just noting closure of the eye is not good enough as this can be achieved by the III nerve to some extent. However, if the VII nerve is functional then it must be anatomically intact. The first and agreed action is as for an incomplete palsy: to remove the pack and to monitor nerve function by electromyography. For a few days, before degeneration, nerve stimulation peripheral to the lesion will still be noted without any volitional motor unit action potentials.

Ninety per cent degeneration within six days and fibrillation within 3–8 weeks both indicate total damage.[7] Polyphasic action potentials are a sign of regeneration.[6]

Many authorities recommend decompressing the facial nerve surgically at 4–6 weeks if degeneration appears to be complete. Recovery often follows, but there is no way of knowing if this would have occurred anyway. Decompression can cause further damage.[8] However, if a segment of nerve is found to be damaged by a spicule of bone, or fibrotic, presumably from a period of compression, then it is reasonable to assume that decompression, repair or grafting would have been worthwhile. Four to six weeks has been found to be the best time, as results worsen as the period between the damage and the decompression extends beyond this.[9] At about four months, spontaneous recovery from regeneration may be about to become apparent so surgery at that stage is debatable.[6]

Most authorities accept now that a delayed palsy which has become complete within 2–3 weeks should be referred to an expert in this particular field, with a view to decompression before six weeks.

Extracranial damage

The common group of operations associated with surgical damage to the extracranial facial nerve are those on the parotid gland.

There are three possible situations. Either the surgeon knows that he has to destroy the nerve in advance of starting the operation; or he knows that there is no reason for destroying the nerve so that if there is, in the event, some damage then it has been caused unnecessarily by him; or finally he may have to start the operation not knowing whether he will be able to conserve the nerve or whether in the best interest of his patient he may have to destroy part or even the whole of the nerve. The last of these three is the commonest situation and requires that the surgeon undertakes the fullest possible discussion with the patient before the operation.

Likelihood of damage unknown

The usual circumstance is that the surgeon is operating to remove a lump in the parotid region. The points he must make when he has reached his decision to operate must include the following:

1. The lump is in the parotid region and most such lumps turn out to be parotid tumours.[10]

2. Most parotid tumours are benign.[11] However, they ought usually to be removed because (a) even if they are benign they tend to grow, become more unsightly, produce symptoms such as pain and become technically more difficult to remove, and (b) they may be malignant.

3. Even when benign, parotid tumours have the unpleasant property that fragments broken off the main tumour mass and lying in the wound can produce implantation recurrence.[12] Any attempt at preliminary biopsy to ascertain the nature of the lump carries an appreciable risk of implantation recurrence. Therefore, the form of biopsy to be used must be excision-biopsy, removing the lump with a wide margin of normal tissue.

4. As part of its normal anatomy the parotid gland has the facial nerve and its terminal branches running through it. The nerve is at risk during the removal of the lump, particularly because of the necessity to maintain a wide margin around the lump. To safeguard the integrity of the nerve, the surgeon first finds the nerve at the fixed point at which it emerges from the skull. He follows the branches through the gland, keeping as close as possible to the nerves because the better he can see them the less likely is he to cut them by accident. At the conclusion of the operation the nerve and its branches have been completely exposed and the lump has been removed with the widest possible margin.

5. *Provided that the anatomical integrity of the nerve and all its named branches has been preserved, there is never any permanent residual weakness of the muscles of facial expression. Temporary weakness immediately after the operation is so common as to be considered normal*: it ranges from only just detectable to being complete. However, the median duration for complete recovery is two months, although the occasional patient may have a paresis that lasts much longer than this, even up to two years.[13]

6. Occasionally it becomes apparent during the operation that the lump, instead of pushing aside the facial nerve, is invading the nerve, which appears to be growing straight into the tumour. In these circumstances it is clear that the lump is malignant. It is even more important than with other lumps that a wide margin be maintained around the lesion, and it is thus necessary to sacrifice whichever element or elements of the facial nerve system are involved. In these circumstances total recovery of the facial nerve muscles can no longer be confidently expected, although the division of a single branch, or two neighbouring named branches, usually produces no permanent incapacity. The surgeon would undertake immediate treatment to repair the nerve where that is possible, but the results of such repairs cannot be guaranteed.

7. In the event that a primary repair is impossible or fails, secondary manoeuvres are still possible in the future.

8. Finally, it should be emphasized that if the patient refuses permission to destroy the nerve in the event that that proves necessary, avoidance of the operation will not save the function of the facial muscles since continued growth of the tumour will itself eventually destroy the nerve.

The author has met with refusal of permission to destroy the nerve if necessary in only two out of a large number of cases.

No permanent facial nerve damage expected.

The preoperative discussion is modified when the surgeon proposes to remove the superficial parotid because of a parotid duct calculus,[14] or the whole parotid because of Sjogren's syndrome[15] or other more obscure causes of chronic or recurrent parotitis, in each case with preservation of the facial nerve. It is important that in this situation the decision to operate is patient-driven, and that the patient's symptoms are sufficiently severe as to cause him to demand relief, even at the expense of a temporary facial nerve paresis. The information about the danger to the nerve and about the surgical technique used to avoid cutting the nerve is the same as in the group with a lump, and so is the information about the duration and variable severity of the subsequent paresis.

Permanent facial palsy expected

If the surgeon proposes an operation that will inevitably destroy the whole facial nerve—for example a radical parotidectomy[16] — the preoperative discussion must concentrate on the effects of a complete paralysis of the facial muscles on one side and on methods of alleviating the associated sypmtoms. Watering of the affected eye owing to the lack of blinking and the resultant tendency to conjunctivitis is controlled by the frequent use of artificial tear eyedrops, together with lateral tarsorrhaphy or other minor operations to correct ectropion. Food tends to collect between jaw and cheek. Speech may be interfered with by difficulty in controlling the lips.

Prevention of iatrogenic damage to the facial nerve

Any of the established techniques for finding and protecting the facial nerve can be followed. The author describes[17] establishing a space in the neck in front of the anterior borders of three muscles, the sternomastoid, the posterior belly of the digastric and the stylohyoid; another space in the face between the cartilage of the external auditory meatus posteriorly and the gland itself anteriorly; and then a combination of blunt and sharp dissection to whittle away the bridge of superficial tissues between these two spaces until the trunk and primary bifurcation of the nerve are identified. The nerve and its branches are then followed forwards by a similar technique; a pair of artery forceps is passed along the superficial aspect of the nerve to create a tunnel in the tissues overlying the nerve for a few millimetres beyond what can be seen of it, the points of the forceps are elevated to break through the superficial tissues and the band of tissues thereby isolated is divided with scissors. During this manoeuvre, the blades of the artery forceps have themselves protected the nerve from damage.

Methods of repair

A damaged facial nerve may be sutured or grafted. There are also static procedures to provide some symmetry to the face.

Within the internal auditory meatus, Dott[9] and Samii[18] described free grafting from the intracranial part of the nerve to the extratemporal end. Only a few cases were reported.

Direct anastomosis was not successful until House[4] described a method of rerouting the nerve to shorten its course.[5] Even so a graft was often required.[4]

Within the petrous temporal bone direct anastomosis may be possible. Rerouting is not as good as free grafting, which is the method of choice if there is a gap, and the great auricular nerve is often used.

Outside the skull the distal end of the facial nerve can be anastomosed to part of the hypoglossal nerve to provide some tone and movement. This is referred to as a '7–12 hook up' by some authors.[6] Results are good at rest but not so natural on smiling when there may be some mass movement. House considers that there is approximately 50 per cent restoration of facial function with a good anastomosis.[4]

Within the parotid, direct primary end-to-end repair may be possible. In the authors' experience the fewer sutures the better, perhaps even one or two. Other experts describe more complicated techniques. If the gap is too large an interposed nerve graft is used, and the great auricular nerve is most suitable. The nerve is found at the anterior border of the sternomastoid at the start of the parotidectomy and has to be divided anyway to achieve adequate access so, making a virtue out of necessity, a segment about 5 cm can usually be excised.

Cross-facial anastomosis[19] involves exploring branches of the facial nerve at the upper, anterior and lower borders of the parotid on the non-paralysed side. These are joined to branches on the paralysed side using sural nerve, a long length of which can be excised from the calf through a series of small incisions tunnelling between them. The routes of the cross-connections can be the forehead, upper lip and chin. Results are, however, rather disappointing, but various combinations of grafts and repairs have been described by Stennert.

Microvascular muscle transfers

The ipsilateral gracilis muscle is normally used. It is detached with its neurovascular pedicle and transferred to the face where its proximal end is attached to the temporalis. The vessels are then joined to the superficial temporal or facial, whichever are most appropriate, and the previous sural nerve grafts identified and joined to the nerve to gracilis. The muscle is divided distally into smaller bundles and attached to the various territories of the face. One group has described a series of 40 patients with a complete facial nerve palsy of whom 35 were improved by the combination of these two modern techniques.[20]

Static procedures

A variety of static procedures can be used to improve the balance and symmetry of the face at rest. These include the weighting of the upper eyelid with a gold pellet, correction of ectropion and the raising of the angle of the mouth by a suspensory band of autogenous material, fasica lata or non-absorbable foreign material such as nylon.

However, static procedures do not re-animate the face and endeavour is now concentrated on producing re-innervation, preferably of the patient's intrinsic facial musculature, by a combination of nerve grafts.[19]

References

1. Giannotta S.L., Pulec J.L., Goodkin R. Translabyrinthine removal of cerebellopontine angle meningiomas. *Amer. J. Neurosurg.* 1985; **17:** 620–25.
2. King T.T., Morrison A.W. Translabyrinthine and transtentorial removal of acoustic nerve tumours. *J. Neurosurg.* 1980; **52:** 210–16.
3. Glasscock M.E., Kveton J.F., Jackson C.G., Levine S.C., McKennan K.X. A systematic approach to the surgical management of acoustic neuroma. *Laryngoscope.* 1986; **96:** 1088–94.
4. House W.F., Hitselberger W.E. Preservation of the facial nerve in acoustic tumour surgery. *Arch. Otolaryngol.* 1968; **88:** 107–10.
5. House W.F., Luetji, C.M. *Acoustic Neuroma: Diagnosis and Management.* Baltimore: University Park Press, 1978.
6. May, M. Trauma to the facial nerve. *Otolaryngol. Clinics Amer.* 1983; **16:** 661–70, 1983.
7. Coker N.J., Kendall K.A., Jenkins H.A., Alford B.R. Traumatic intratemporal facial nerve injury: management rationale for preservation of function. *Otolaryngol. Head Neck Surg.* 1987; **96:** 262–9.
8. May M., Klein S. Facial nerve decompression complications. *Laryngoscope*, 1983; **93:** 299–305.
9. Dott N.M. Facial paralysis: restitution by extra-petrous nerve graft. *Proc. R. Soc. Med.* 1958; **51:** 900.
10. Patey D.H., Hand B.H. Diagnosis of mixed parotid tumours. *Lancet.* 1952; **ii:** 310–11.
11. Hobsley M. Salivary tumours. *Brit. J. Hosp. Med.* 1973; **10:** 553–62.
12. Patey D.H., Thackray A.C. The treatment of parotid tumours in the light of a pathological study of parotidectomy material. *Brit. J. Surg.* 1957; **45:** 477–87.
13. Stevens K.L., Hobsley M. The treatment of pleomorphic adenomas by formal parotidectomy. *Brit. J. Surg.* 1982; **69:** 1–3.
14. Suleiman S.I., Thomson J.P.S., Hobsley, M. Recurrent unilateral swelling of the parotid gland. *Gut.* 1979; **20:** 1102–8.
15. Watkin G.T., Hobsley M. Natural history of patients with recurrent parotitis and punctate sialectasis. *Brit. J. Surg.* 1986; **73:** 745–8.
16. Corcoran M.O., Cook H.P., Hobsley M. Radical surgery following radiotherapy for advanced parotid carcinoma. *Brit. J. Surg.* 1983; **70:** 261–3.
17. Hobsley M. Head and neck. In: Kirk R.M., Williamson R.C.N. (eds.): *General Surgical Operations.* London: Churchill Livingstone, 1980: 350–75.
18. Sammi M. Intra-cranial reconstruction of facial nerve after lateral basal fracture. In: Sammi, Brihaye (eds.): *Traumatology of the Skull Base.* Berlin: Springer, 1979.
19. Stennert E. Indications for facial nerve surgery. *Adv. Oto-Rhino-Laryngol.* 1984; **34:** 214–26.
20. O'Brien B.McC, Morrison W. *Reconstructive Microsurgery.* London: Churchill Livingstone, 1987: 478–80.

18

The laryngeal nerves

Malcolm H. Wheeler, MD, FRCS, and
Stephen H. Richards, FRCS

The recurrent laryngeal nerves were probably first described by Galen[1] as early as the second century, but their relevance to the operation of thyroidectomy remained hidden until Kocher's remarkable contributions rendered this procedure both safe and acceptable.[2] Other great surgical pioneers such as Wolfler and Billroth[3,4] recognized the risk of injury to these nerves, and, even today, damage to the recurrent laryngeal nerves remains a potential hazard of thyroid surgery, the reported incidence ranging from zero to 13 per cent.[5-8]

Although most attention has been paid to the recurrent laryngeal nerve, in recent years considerable emphasis has also been rightly placed on the need to avoid damage to the superior laryngeal nerve at thyroidectomy.[9,10] An understanding of the anatomy and function of the laryngeal nerves is an essential prerequisite for a meaningful consideration of the causes of nerve damage, the methods of protecting the nerves at surgery and subsequent management of any injury which might occur.

Anatomy

The recurrent laryngeal nerve (RLN)

This nerve arises from the vagus nerve and loops around the aortic arch on the left side and the subclavian artery on the right, passing posterior to the carotid artery to ascend towards the tracheo-oesophageal groove on each side. The nerve then ascends parallel and closely related to the trachea, possessing an extremely variable relationship to the inferior thyroid artery and its branches, usually dividing itself into two or more branches, before coursing backwards to enter the larynx behind the inferior cornu of the thyroid cartilage (Fig. 18.1). It is this variability of course, propensity for branching and the relationship to the thyroid gland, inferior thyroid artery and adjacent fascial layers which render the nerve liable to damage at surgery.[11] These various factors will each be considered in detail later.

The superior laryngeal nerve (SLN)

This nerve arises from the nodose ganglion of the vagus nerve near its exit from the jugular foramen of the skull. The nerve divides high in the neck into an internal branch which enters the larynx through the thyrohyoid membrane and an external branch which descends in close relationship to the inferior pharangeal constrictor muscle before entering the cricothyroid muscle.

This external branch of the superior laryngeal nerve is particularly vulnerable at thyroidectomy because of its proximity and variable relationship to the superior thyroid artery and the superior pole of the thyroid gland.

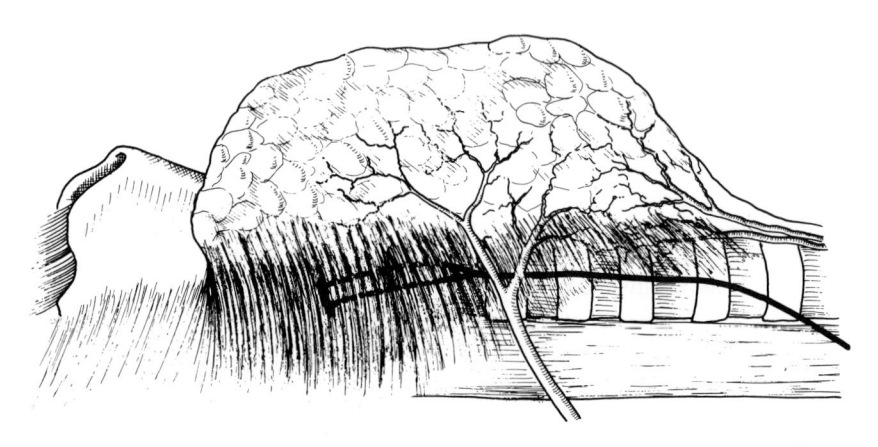

Fig. 18.1 Commonly occurring anatomy of the recurrent laryngeal nerve which is ascending anterior to the tracheo-oesophageal groove, passing deep to the main branches of the inferior thyroid artery and dividing into two branches before passing deep to the ligament of Berry and entering the larynx beneath the inferior cornu of the thyroid cartilage.

Physiology and function

The recurrent laryngeal nerve is motor to the intrinsic laryngeal muscles supplying the abductors and adductors. The external branch of the superior laryngeal nerve is motor to the cricothyroid muscle, whilst its internal branch is primarily sensory to the mucous membrane of the larynx.[12]

Damage to the laryngeal nerves may be complete or incomplete, unilateral or bilateral. It had been suggested that the abductor fibres of the recurrent nerve are more susceptible to injury than the adductor fibres,[13,14] but this view is no longer tenable. Complete unilateral paralysis of a recurrent nerve causes the vocal cord to be immobile in a position between the inspiratory and phonation positions, the so-called paramedian position.[15] The opposite cord is able to swing across the midline to compensate during phonation and, therefore, the voice although initially hoarse may soon appear to recover apart from susceptibility to fatigue and difficulties when singing. Unilateral palsy rarely causes any breathing difficulties under normal circumstances, but during extreme physical activity the aperture between the cords may not be able to provide adequate compensatory enlargement and audible stridor can result. In some patients contracture and cord fibrosis may occur at a later stage and then airway problems can supervene.[16]

If both the recurrent and superior laryngeal nerves (external branch) are damaged, the affected vocal cord will be held in an abducted inspiratory position because under these circumstances the tensor muscle of the cords, the cricothyroid, is also paralysed.[15] Although the airway is satisfactory the voice is initially husky because the opposite normal cord is unable to move sufficiently far across the midline to reach the paralysed cord. Hoarseness later improves after a period of weeks or months as fibrosis draws the paralysed cord closer to the midline and compensatory movement across the midline occurs in the unaffected cord.

Isolated injury to the external branch of the superior laryngeal nerve does not interfere with cord abduction and may therefore be easily overlooked at postoperative indirect laryngoscopy.[10] Cord tension, however, is impaired, with the affected cord on laryngoscopy being either normal or showing slight bowing at its centre.[17] The resulting disability is likely to be subtle, the voice tiring easily and disturbances occurring in the speaking range and upper singing register. Naturally these changes are disastrous to a professional person such as an opera singer who is dependent upon the absolute quality of the voice.

When the internal branch of the superior laryngeal nerve is damaged, usually in association with injury to the other laryngeal nerves, the combination of sensory loss[18] and muscle paralysis causes an unpleasant proneness to aspiration and spillage of liquids into the larynx (*vide infra*).

Bilateral recurrent nerve damage is a clinical catastrophe which should be absolutely avoidable. It results in total inability to abduct or adduct vocal cords which are fixed in the paramedian position.[19] There may be no initial obvious airway embarrassment, unless there is associated laryngeal oedema;[20] but after a few months there will be atrophy fibrosis of the cords, and, as fibrosis and fixation progress, the cords move closer together. The voice continues to improve, but now there is increasing difficulty in breathing, with stridor and marked limitation on physical exertion. A tracheostomy is frequently necessary.

Causes of nerve damage

Damage to the recurrent laryngeal nerve

The RLN is vulnerable to damage at thyroidectomy because of its variable position, course and relationship to key anatomical structures in the neck.[5,11] If damage is to be avoided an accurate knowledge of the normal anatomy and these variations is of paramount importance. Vulnerability is somewhat greater on the right than the left, because of the obliquity of the nerve's course in the lower third and its distance from the trachea compared with the course of the left nerve. Only rarely does the RLN lie precisely in the tracheo-oesophageal groove. In the lower part of the neck the nerve may occasionally be displaced anteriorly in relation to the trachea for no apparent reason, and then its course and proximity to the inferior thyroid veins are such that the nerve may be damaged when these vessels are ligated and divided (Fig. 18.2).[21]

It has long been recognized that the RLN and inferior thyroid artery have a complex and extremely variable relationship which is a potent source of nerve vulnerability. Not surprisingly a large number of workers have studied this nerve/artery relationship and many confusing results have been reported.[18,21–23] However, certain clear general principles emerge, and it seems that at least eight important relationships can be identified, with the nerve most frequently lying deep to the artery or its branches, but identical relationships on each side only being seen in approximately 30 per cent of cases.[5] The nerve may pass between the main arterial divisions or intermingle with the smaller, more distal glandular branches. These associations often cause fixation of the nerve in an arterial fork, bringing the structure out of its usual position into one of great danger (Fig. 18.3).

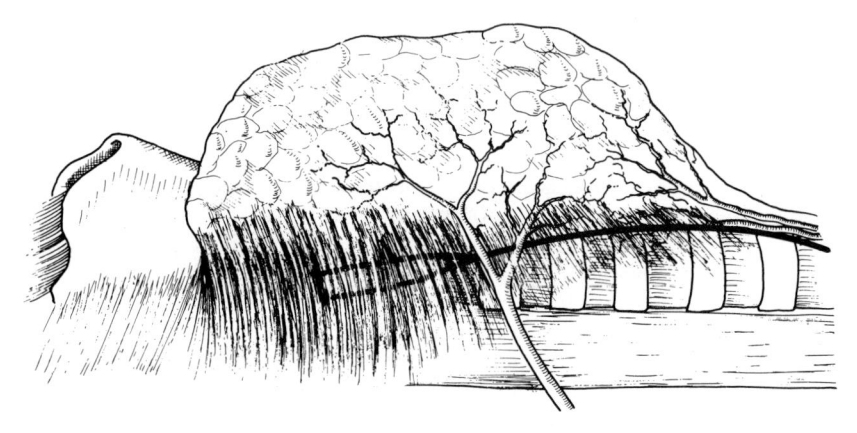

Fig. 18.2 Recurrent laryngeal nerve displaced anteriorly into a vulnerable position where it may be ligated and divided with the inferior thyroid veins.

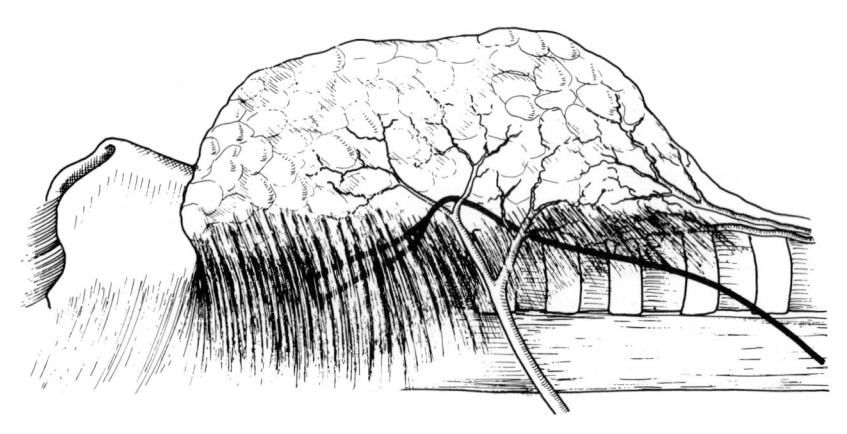

Fig. 18.3 The recurrent laryngeal nerve is rendered vulnerable by anterior fixation to the thyroid in a fork formed by the glandular branches of the inferior thyroid artery.

The fascial layers of the neck and their relationship to the RLN are important factors contributing to the risk hazard. In the lower third of its course the nerve is covered by fairly thin fascia and areolar tissue which constitutes no particular problem. The RLN in its middle and upper third has crucial relations to the fascial layer[24,25] attaching the thyroid to the cricoid and upper tracheal rings, the so-called suspensory ligament of Berry. Almost invariably the nerve in its upper third passes deep to this fascial structure and is vulnerable because of fixation and difficulties in its identification as it frequently adopts a curving looping course before entering the larynx (Fig. 18.4). In its middle third, the RLN may lie deep to Berry's ligament, within its layers or even superficial to the ligament, being intimately related under these circumstances to the posteromedial aspect of the thyroid lobe.

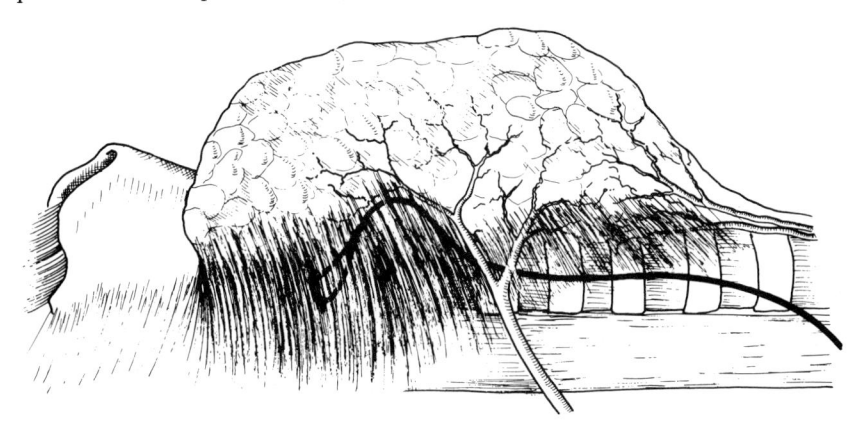

Fig. 18.4 Fascial fixation by the ligament of Berry has caused anterior displacement of the recurrent laryngeal nerve before entry into the larynx. This looping curve renders the nerve vulnerable during ligation of the small branches of the inferior thyroid artery.

The intimate relationship of the nerve to the thyroid gland must be appreciated if damage is to be avoided. The nerve never pierces the actual thyroid capsule or the gland itself, but it is not uncommon for tunnelling to occur[21] owing to the irregular growth of thyroid nodules (Fig. 18.5), particularly if the nerve is already fixed to the gland by an arterial division or fascial band. Similar tunnelling and fixation is often seen in malignancy as a result of enlarged metastatic nodes. The recurrent nerve may of course be directly involved in the primary tumour mass.

A large goitre may render the nerve vulnerable, particularly in the middle and lower thirds of its course, because of the potential for displacement of the nerve from its most usual course. Damage is also possible in these circumstances as a result of the traction and force which may be all too readily applied to mobilize and deliver the large gland. This is particularly true with a gland which has extended into a retrosternal position.[5]

It is usual for the RLN to divide into at least two branches before entering the larynx, and up to six such divisions have been described.[26–28] Each of the branches has both adductor and abductor fibres, and so division of a single branch is not an adequate explanation for the various cord positions which may be seen after nerve damage. Subtotal thyroidectomy for the vascular diffuse goitre of Graves' disease, often accompanied by troublesome bleeding which can obscure normal anatomy, places the nerve at greater risk than the relatively

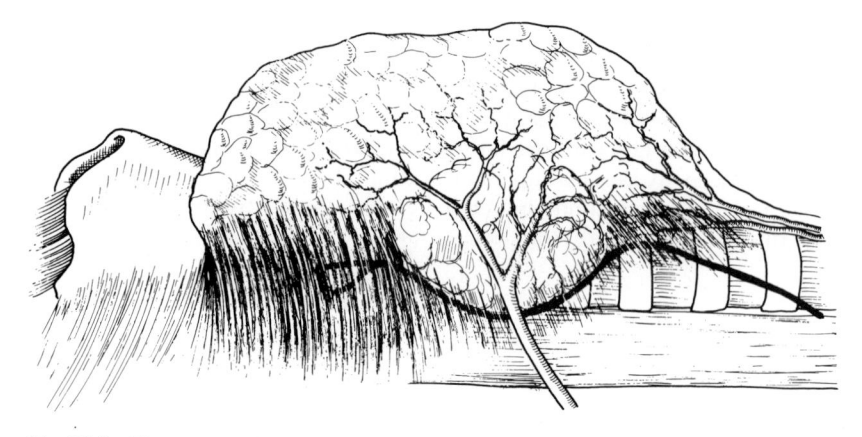

Fig. 18.5 The recurrent laryngeal nerve has been distorted and displaced from its most usual course by a posteriorly situated thyroid nodule. Occasionally tunnelling of the nerve may occur between the nodule and the adjacent thyroid lobe.

straightforward lobectomy procedure for a benign colloid nodule. Second and third thyroid explorations for recurrent disease, benign or malignant, are technically challenging, and there is little doubt that the recurrent laryngeal nerve is in more danger of being damaged than in an initial thyroidectomy.[29]

The anomalous recurrent laryngeal nerve has been of great interest to the thyroid surgeon, but the vulnerability of such a nerve has probably been exaggerated. The most usual anomaly consists of a right recurrent laryngeal nerve arising directly from the vagus at the level of the cricoid and passing behind the common carotid artery to enter the larynx behind the inferior cornu.[30] This unusual course is due to failure of development of the fourth aortic arch on the right and is associated with an origin of the right subclavian artery from the aorta distal to the left subclavian vessel, passing posterior to the oesophagus. As the nerve in its upper third has a similar course to normal it should not be at particular risk, and in the lower part of the neck it is absent and therefore at no risk. The hazard is due to failure to recognize the high origin of the nerve and its sweeping course medially, so that a ligature could be placed around the inferior thyroid artery and include the nerve (Fig. 18.6). Although this anomaly is extremely rare on the left, it has been described in association with situs inversus.[31]

It is relevant to examine the precise mode of nerve injury which may occur during thyroidectomy. Experimental studies have indicated that nerve division by sharp instrument or compression in a ligature are inevitably followed by permanent palsy. Crushing in a haemostat and stretching, perhaps during delivery of a retrosternal goitre, are likely to give rise to a temporary palsy which will recover after a period of weeks or months.[32]

Prevention of damage

The essential prerequisites for a safe thyroidectomy procedure, free of any significant risk of permanent damage to the recurrent laryngeal nerve, are

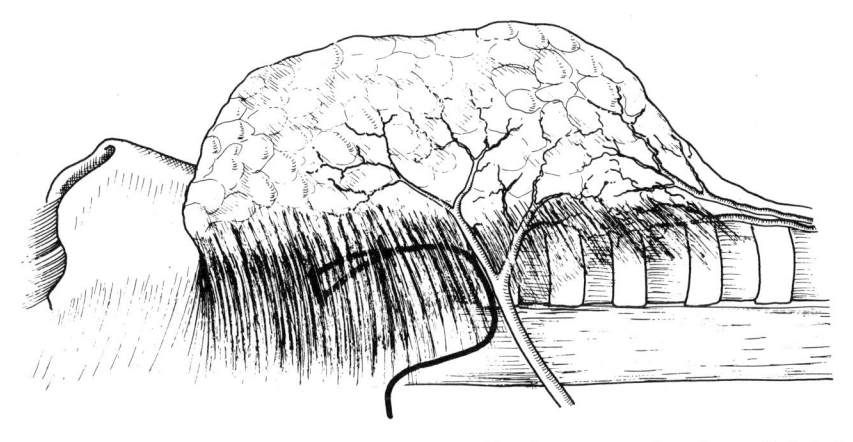

Fig. 18.6 Aberrant right recurrent laryngeal nerve arising from vagus and passing medially before turning to enter the larynx. This nerve may be at risk when a ligature is placed around the inferior thyroid artery.

a complete awareness by the surgeon of the normal nerve anatomy and its many possible variations and a discipline of identifying the nerve throughout its course in the neck, particularly at the upper third of its course where it is most vulnerable. Many thyroid procedures are performed for a unilateral solitary nodule, and the basic procedure of a choice is total lobectomy and isthmusectomy. If nerve preservation is to be ensured identification is mandatory.

It has not always been accepted that identification of the recurrent laryngeal nerve at operation is either necessary or desirable. Prioleau[33] considered it to be a dangerous practice to expose the nerve, and said 'it is an axiom in thyroid surgery that a recurrent laryngeal nerve seen is injured'. Crile[34] thought that the RLN was more sensitive to exposure than a normal peripheral nerve and might even be damaged by wound exudate and subsequent fibrosis. These views were certainly not supported by the experimental studies of Judd and colleagues[32] and the subsequent clinical experience of Lahey,[6] who in 1938 advocated routine exposure of the RLN at operation in order to avoid nerve injury, later quoting an incidence of nerve damage of less than 0.3 per cent in many thousands of cases managed by this method.[16] Riddell,[7] introducing the concept of 'nerves at risk', showed that identification of the RLN reduced the injury rate, but thought that once the surgeon had totally familiarized himself with the various aspects of the anatomy in a series of operative dissections, he might then discontinue deliberate dissection of the nerve.

On the basis that it is a fundamental surgical principle to identify a structure, for example the common bile duct, at cholecystectomy in order to avoid damage to that structure, it would seem reasonable to apply the same rules to the RLN. Wade clearly demonstrated that this technique reduced the damage, quoting no injuries in 100 consecutive patients, and thought that dissection also facilitated haemostasis, adequate resection of the thyroid and identification and prevention of damage to the parathyroid glands.[5] If the RLN is injured when identified it is likely to be a transient palsy and recovery will follow.

Initial identification of the RLN in its lower third is frequently possible by palpating the nerve as a cord like structure which can be rolled against the trachea. Palpation alone is insufficient, and so direct visualization can be achieved by gently opening the fascial layers over the nerve with a haemostat, the jaws being opened along the line of the nerve. Visualization in the region of the inferior thyroid artery with precise definition of the nerve/artery relationship and any fixation by the arterial branches to the thyroid is then achieved. A potential pitfall for the unwary exists when the RLN appears to pulsate if it passes superficial to the inferior thyroid artery and may therefore be mistaken for a vessel and ligated. In the operation of unilateral lobectomy the small arterial branches must all be individually clipped and tied close to the thyroid gland staying on the thyroid capsule. To identify the nerve as it passes further towards the larynx through the area of Berry's ligament where it is at greatest risk, this suspensory fascia must be divided. This manoeuvre is most safely accomplished by staying close to the thyroid and picking up superficial layers one at a time with fine haemostats, being absolutely certain at each stage that only fascia and small arterial branches are included. The recurrent nerve is soon seen at a deeper level glistening with its fine accompanying arterial blood vessel aiding identification. Careful scalpel dissection along the thyroid capsule rather than the use of scissors is most effective. The parathyroid glands are teased laterally with their blood supply intact and mobilization of the lateral lobe of the thyroid continued. It will be noted that the main inferior thyroid artery trunk is not ligated.

The inferior cornu of the thyroid cartilage is a most dependable landmark for the point of entry of the RLN into the larynx.[35] The cornu can be palpated easily and aids identification of the remainder of the nerve's course in its upper one third, although the nerve may often loop forward under the fascia before curving back towards the inferior cornu.

Wade drew attention to the possibility of nerve injury during ligation of the superior thyroid pedicle when the goitre lies unusually low in the neck, and under these circumstances a precise identification of the nerve is mandatory.[5]

If the operation is for the vascular goitre of Graves' disease, a small remnant (3–4 grams) will be left posteriorly, and it is essential that the nerve is identified before the thyroid gland is incised and that any haemostats placed along the edge of these remnants do not encroach upon or include the nerve. Similarly, sutures placed in the remnant for haemostasis must be meticulously inserted to avoid the nerve, and if the technique of suturing the remnant to the larynx is employed, traction on the thyroid tissue and nerve must be avoided.

Not all surgeons use suction drains after thyroid surgery, particularly when the procedure has been a simple unilateral lobectomy; but if these drains are used it is important to avoid placing them in close proximity to an exposed nerve for fear of inducing suction damage.

Preoperative indirect laryngoscopy should always be performed by an independent otorhinolaryngologist, as the occasional patient will already have a laryngeal nerve palsy, unsuspected owing to some unrelated cause such as a viral infection.[36] A large nodular goitre, particularly if retrosternal, may also paralyse a recurrent laryngeal nerve, and if pressure has been longstanding recovery may not take place even when the offending goitre is resected. A malignant goitre may, of course, produce nerve damage by a combination of pressure and direct invasion. Such preoperative information is vitally important and will often influence the precise surgical procedure performed, it being necessary for the surgeon to take even more than the usual care to avoid damaging the opposite nerve and thus inducing a catastrophic bilateral nerve palsy.

Postoperative assessment by indirect laryngoscopy usually on the fourth or fifth day should be performed, as assessment on the basis of audible phonation is likely to be unreliable. A hoarse voice is very common immediately after any surgical procedure involving endotracheal intubation and is no guide to identification of the patient with a nerve palsy. Observation of the cords by the anaesthetist at extubation may be helpful, but is less reliable than indirect laryngoscopy.[37] It must be remembered that endotracheal intubation for any procedure, even an inguinal hernia, is associated with a small incidence of recurrent laryngeal nerve damage, presumably as a direct effect of pressure damage from the cuff of the endotracheal tube.[38]

If the recurrent nerve is identified at surgery, but still damaged, the majority of such palsies will be transient and recovery occurs in weeks or months.

Damage to the external branch of the superior laryngeal nerve (ESLN)

This nerve lies close to the superior thyroid artery and its branches (Fig. 18.7) and is highly vulnerable during ligation of the superior pole vessels, as in up to

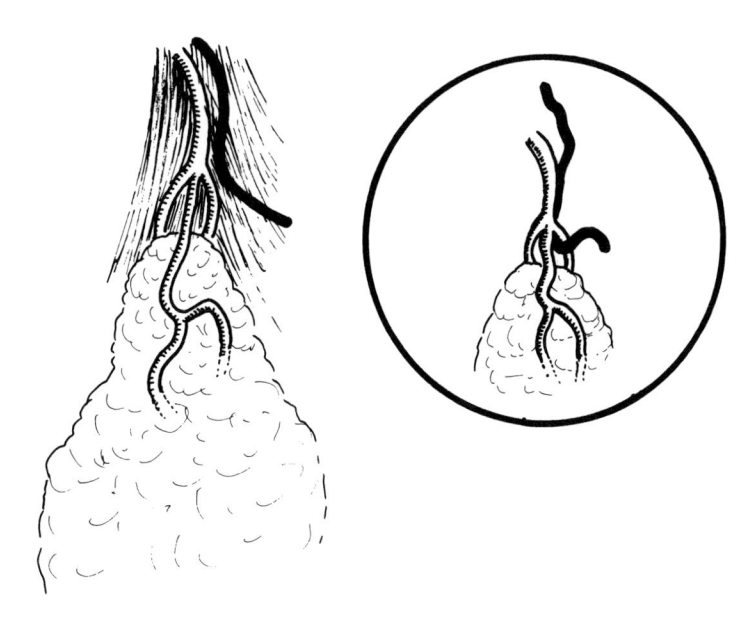

Fig. 18.7 The external superior laryngeal nerve (ESLN) descending medial to the superior thyroid artery before entering the cricothyroid muscle. The inset shows the vulnerable ESLN passing between branches of superior thyroid artery.

18 per cent of patients the nerve may course laterally and even be found passing between the branches of the superior thyroid artery.[10] In the majority of cases (80 per cent), however, the nerve lies medial to the upper pole vessels and surrounding fascia, and in 20 per cent of cases runs its distal course through the pharyngeal constrictor muscle, precluding any identification at surgery without muscle dissection. Such a dissection is unnecessary as the nerve is at no risk in these latter circumstances. The exterior laryngeal nerves can be identified by opening up the cricothyroid space, initially with forceps and then with a small pledget swab. The superior thyroid vessels are retracted laterally and the caudal part of the pharyngeal constrictor muscle inspected. The ESLN is usually readily identified on this muscle. Mass ligation of the superior pole vessels is inadvisable, and the individual branches should be skeletonized and tied close to the superior pole to avoid damaging the ESLN.

Damage to this nerve, and indeed to the recurrent laryngeal nerve, may occur as a result of indiscriminate use of diathermy, either directly or by heat conduction from a vessel coagulated some distance away from the nerves. It is an excellent discipline to avoid the use of diathermy whenever possible once the thyroid gland has been exposed and the dissection of the nerves and parathyroid glands initiated.

Treatment

Management of vocal cord paralysis following thyroid surgery varies considerably according to whether the palsy is unilateral or bilateral, and whether the superior laryngeal nerve is involved.

Unilateral paralysis of the recurrent laryngeal nerve

Most cases of vocal cord palsy following thyroid surgery are unilateral and transitory. Spontaneous improvement usually occurs within six weeks owing to recovery of nerve function, or because the mobile cord moves across the midline to make contact with the paralysed one. In order to reduce oedema of the nerve, and thereby help to forestall degeneration, steroid therapy should be given. Prednisolone 15 mg t.d.s. for 10 days is administered orally and the dose then gradually reduced to zero over the subsequent 10 days. This treatment should commence within seven days of operation, and this factor underlines the importance of early routine indirect laryngoscopy after thyroidectomy.

If recovery does not take place within six weeks then degeneration of the nerve has probably occurred and recovery will be delayed for six to twelve months whilst the nerve regenerates. During this period speech therapy plays an important part in preserving function in the non-paralysed muscles of the larynx, and in maintaining the patient's morale.

Should the paralysed vocal cord remain immobile for 18 months or more, then failure of nerve regeneration is diagnosed and subsequent recovery cannot be expected. If the paralysed cord is near the midline, and has good tone, then phonation is good, and further treatment unnecessary. However, when the cord is more laterally placed, or is severely lacking in tone, the patient often has a degree of hoarseness which interferes with his employment, especially in such occupations as school teaching, broadcasting or lecturing. In such cases good lasting improvement is obtained by injecting a suspension of Teflon into the larynx on the paralysed side and this brings the fixed cord nearer the midline.[39] This procedure is carried out by direct microlaryngoscopy under general anaesthesia.

Bilateral recurrent nerve palsy

The problems of patients with bilateral RLN palsy differ markedly according to the position of the vocal cords, and treatment has to be varied accordingly. When the vocal cords are fixed in adduction (i.e. in or near the midline) then the main symptoms will be those of airway obstruction. If, on the other hand, the cords are fixed in abduction the problems will be those of poor phonation and sputum retention.

Bilateral paralysis in adduction

When the immobile cords are nearly in apposition there is always some degree of airway obstruction, and if this is causing respiratory embarrassment then emergency tracheostomy is indicated. The need for such a procedure is usually clear in that the patient has a loud inspiratory stridor and the accessory muscles of respiration are brought into action. A rising pulse rate denotes that the heart is having to make increasing effort to maintain oxygenation; this, together with deteriorating Po_2 and Pco_2 readings, are valuable signs indicating that operation should not be delayed. Certainly one should not await the development of cyanosis before taking the patient to the operating theatre. A postponed decision may result in an emergency procedure having to be carried out under adverse circumstances with the patient in bed. The operation can be carried out under local infiltration analgesia, but if there is time, and if the services of an experienced anaesthetist are available, then it can be performed in a more leisurely manner under general anaesthesia with a cuffed laryngeal tube in position.

Whether they have had an emergency tracheostomy or not, most of these patients recover partially or completely within a few weeks. The few who still have an inadequate airway after 18 months can be offered the operation of arytenoidectomy where one vocal cord is permanently fixed in a lateral position.[40] This procedure improves the airway, allowing the tracheostomy to be closed, but often results in a serious worsening of the voice. A number of patients therefore choose to retain their tracheostomy as the lesser of two evils.

Bilateral paralysis in abduction

In the early stages, the treatment of this rare condition is directed towards prevention and treatment of any pulmonary complications caused by inability to cough effectively. Physiotherapy directed towards coughing and breathing exercises, and postural drainage, should be commenced as soon as possible. Humidification helps to render the sputum less tenacious, but the degree to which it is used should be carefully controlled by monitoring the viscosity of the patient's sputum. Antibiotics are given to forestall and treat pulmonary infection.

Should these measures prove inadequate then tracheostomy is indicated in order to remove the bronchial secretions by suction and to enable the patient to cough more effectively. This may need to be supplemented with repeated bronchoscopy if there is evidence of segmental pulmonary collapse. The tracheostomy tube should be cuffed so as to prevent any tendency to aspirate food or saliva into the trachea.

Fortunately the above are temporary emergency measures only and usually are soon rendered unnecessary by spontaneous recovery of function in one or both cords. If one cord does not recover then the voice can be improved by Teflon injection. Permanent tracheostomy for bilateral vocal cord palsy in abduction is sometimes unavoidable in patients who have brain-stem pathology, but is extremely rare following thyroid surgery.

Superior laryngeal nerve palsy

Damage to the external motor branch of the superior laryngeal nerve, as described above, causes only subtle voice changes[41] which can improve spontaneously or may require a course of speech therapy. The main clinical problem resulting from damage to the internal branch of the superior laryngeal nerve is aspiration of food and liquids into the respiratory passages owing to loss of sensation in the supraglottic area of the larynx.

In unilateral cases the aspiration is usually slight and improves rapidly. The patient should be reassured and encouraged to swallow slowly and carefully whilst inclining the head and trunk towards the sound side, thereby encouraging the bolus to gravitate to the pyriform fossa of the normal side. In more severe cases a gastro-oesophageal tube is passed and the patient advised to spit out rather than to swallow his saliva. At the same time regular physiotherapy is given to forestall pulmonary complications. If the latter are seriously threatening then a temporary tracheostomy is required with insertion of a cuffed tube into the trachea to protect the lower airways. Even if there is no recovery of nerve function most patients are able to learn to swallow satisfactorily and permanent tracheostomy is hardly ever required.

Repair of the divided recurrent laryngeal nerve

There is no evidence that repair of the transected recurrent laryngeal nerve will result in useful recovery of vocal cord function even if this is undertaken immediately after sectioning. Reports of success from this procedure during the early years of this century were probably due to failure to appreciate that adduction of the cords can be produced by a functioning superior laryngeal nerve.[42] A section of the RLN followed by immediate resuturing in dogs produces regeneration of the nerve and electromyographic responses but no useful return of function.[43] Anastomosis of the divided phrenic nerve to the RLN has met with rather more success as reported by Colledge[44] and Ormerod.[45] Again the main improvement was in adduction for which persisting function in the SLN was probably responsible.

There appears, therefore, to be no place for exploration of the recurrent laryngeal nerve in cases of post-thyroidectomy vocal cord palsy. Such a procedure would not help the crushed nerve which usually regenerates spontaneously.[46] Furthermore, exploration of this nature could seriously endanger the nerve that is only slightly traumatized. However, in the unusual event of the surgeon accidentally dividing the nerve and recognizing this at the time of operation, it would be reasonable to proceed immediately to undertake a suture anastomosis of the divided ends using the same microsurgical technique as has been used in the facial nerve with good results.

References

1. Galen C. *On Anatomical Procedures: the Later Books* (translated by Duckworth W.L.H.). Cambridge: Cambridge University Press, 1962.
2. Kocher T. Uber Kropfextirpation und irhe Folgen. *Arch. Klin. Chir.* 1883; **29:** 254.
3. Wolfler A. Uber die Entwickelung und den Bau des Kropfes. *Arch. Klin. Chir.* 1887; **29:** 1.
4. Wolfler A. Die Kropfextirpation an Hoft Billroth's Klinik von 1877 bis 1881. *Wien. Med. Wochenschr.* 1882; **32:** 6.
5. Wade J.S.H. Vulnerability of the recurrent laryngeal nerves at thyroidectomy. *Brit. J. Surg.* 1955; **43:** 164–80.
6. Lahey F.H., Hoover W.B. Injuries to the recurrent laryngeal nerve in thyroid operations. *Ann. Surg.* 1938; **108:** 545–62.
7. Riddell V.H. Injury to recurrent laryngeal nerves during thyroidectomy. *Lancet.* 1956; **ii:** 638–41.
8. Roy A.D., Gardiner R.H., Niblock W.M. Thyroidectomy and the recurrent laryngeal nerves. *Lancet.* 1956; **i:** 988–90.
9. Moosman D.A., De Weese M.S. The external laryngeal nerve as related to thyroidectomy. *Surg. Gynaecol. Obstet.* 1968; **127:** 1011–16.
10. Lennquist S., Cahlin C., Smeds S. The superior laryngeal nerve in thyroid surgery. *Surgery.* 1987; **102:** 999–1008.
11. Bowden R.E.M. The surgical anatomy of the recurrent laryngeal nerve. *Brit. J. Surg.* 1955; **43:** 153–63.
12. Williams A.F. Nerve supply of laryngeal muscles. *J. Laryngol. Otol.* 1951; **65:** 343–8.
13. Semon F. On the proclivity of abductor fibres of the recurrent laryngeal nerve to become affected sooner than the adductor fibres. *Arch. Laryngol.* 1881; **2:** 197–222.
14. Kratz R.C. The identification and protection of the laryngeal motor nerves during thyroid and laryngeal surgery: a new microsurgical technique. *The Laryngoscope.* 1972; **82:** 59–78.
15. Gisselsson L. Laryngeal paralysis following thyroidectomy. *Acta Chir. Scand.* 1949; **99:** 154–62.
16. Lahey F. Exposure of the recurrent laryngeal nerves in thyroid operations. *Surg. Gynaecol. Obstet.* 1944; **78:** 239–44.
17. Dedo H. The paralysed larynx: an electromyographic study in dogs and humans. *The Laryngoscope.* 1970; **80:** 1455–519.
18. Nordland M. The larynx as related to surgery of the thyroid based on an anatomical study. *Surg. Gynaecol. Obstet.* 1930; **51:** 449–59.
19. Holinger L.D., Holinger P.C., Holinger P.H. Etiology of bilateral abductor vocal cord paralysis: a review of 389 cases. *Ann. Otol.* 1976; **85:** 428–36.
20. Wade J.S.H. Respiratory obstruction in thyroid surgery. *Ann. R. Coll. Surg. Engl.* 1980; **62:** 15–24.
21. Fowler C.H., Hanson W.H. Surgical anatomy of the thyroid gland with special reference to the relations of the recurrent laryngeal nerve. *Surg. Gynaecol. Obstet.* 1929; **49:** 59–65.
22. Reed A.F. The relations of the inferior laryngeal nerve to the inferior thyroid artery. *Anat. Rec.* 1943; **85:** 17–23.
23. Ziegelman E.F. Laryngeal nerves: surgical importance in relation to the inferior thyroid arteries, thyroid gland and larynx. *Ann. Otolaryngol.* 1933; **18:** 793–808.

24. Berlin D.D. The recurrent laryngeal nerves in total ablation of the normal thyroid gland. *Surg. Gynaecol. Obstet.* 1935; **60:** 19–26.
25. Berry J. Suspensory ligaments of the thyroid gland. *Proc. Anat. Soc. Gr. Brit Ir.* 1877; (*J. Anat. Physiol.* 1877–78; **22:** IV–V).
26. Armstrong W.G., Hinton J.W. Multiple divisions of the recurrent laryngeal nerve. *Arch. Surg.* 1951; **62:** 532–9.
27. Morrison L.F. Recurrent laryngeal nerve paralysis: a revised conception based on the dissection of one hundred cadavers. *Ann. Otol. Rhinol. Laryngol.* 1952; **61:** 567–92.
28. Thompson N.W., Olsen W.R., Hoffman G.L. The continuing development of the technique of thyroidectomy. *Surgery.* 1973; **73:** 913–27.
29. Beahrs O.H., Vandertoll D.J. Complications of secondary thyroidectomy. *Surg. Gynaecol. Obstet.* 1963; **117:** 535–9.
30. Pemberton J. de J., Miller J.M. Anomaly of the right inferior laryngeal nerve. *Arch. Surg.* 1941; **42:** 712–18.
31. Henry J.F., Audiffret J., Denizot A., Plan M. The non-recurrent inferior laryngeal nerve: review of 33 cases including 2 on the left side. *Communication to Ninth Annual Meeting, American Association of Endocrine Surgeons,* Boston, 1988.
32. Judd E.S., New G.B., Mann F.C. The effect of trauma upon the laryngeal nerves. *Ann. Surg.* 1918; **67:** 257–62.
33. Prioleau W.H. Injury of laryngeal branches of vagus nerve in thyroid surgery. *South Surg.* 1933; **1:** 287–92.
34. Crile G.W. The prevention of abductor paralysis in thyroidectomy. *Surg. Gynaecol. Obstet.* 1929; **49:** 538–9.
35. Wang E.A. The use of the inferior cornu of the thyroid cartilage in identifying the recurrent laryngeal nerve. *Surg. Gynaecol. Obstet.* 1975; **140:** 91–4.
36. Faaborg-Andersen K. Recurrent laryngeal nerve paralysis of unknown aetiology. *Acta Otolaryngol.* 1954; **118** (Suppl.): 68–75.
37. Blackburn G., Salmon L.F.W. Cord movements after thyroidectomy. *Brit. J. Surg.* 1961; **48:** 371–3.
38. Holley H.S., Gildea J.E. Vocal cord paralysis after tracheal intubation. *JAMA.* 1971; **215:** 281–4.
39. Dedo H., Urrea R.D., Lawson L. Intra-cordal injection of Teflon in treatment of 135 patients with dysphonia. *Ann. Otol. Rhinol. Laryngol.* 1973; **82:** 661–7.
40. Woodman D.G. A modification of the extra-laryngeal approach in arytenoidectomy for bilateral abductor paralysis. *Arch. Otolaryngol.* 1946; **48:** 63–5.
41. Kark A.E., Kissin M.W., Auerbach R., Meikle M. Voice changes after thyroidectomy: role of the external laryngeal nerve. *Brit. Med. J.* 1984; **289:** 1412–15.
42. Rice D. Laryngeal reinnervation. *Laryngoscope.* 1982; **92:** 1049–59.
43. Dedo H.H. Electromyographic and visual evaluation of recurrent laryngeal nerve anastomosis in dogs. *Ann. Otol. Rhinol. Laryngol.* 1972; **80:** 664–8.
44. Coledge L. On the possibility of restoring movement of paralysed vocal cord by nerve anastomosis: an experimental inquiry. *Brit. Med. J.* 1925; **1:** 547–8.
45. Ormerod F.C. The repair of recurrent nerve paralysis. *J. Laryngol. Otol.* 1941; **56:** 151–8.
46. Boles R., Fritzell B. Injury and repair of the recurrent laryngeal nerves in dogs. *Laryngoscope.* 1969; **79:** 1405–18.

19

Bile duct injuries

Maurice Mercadier, MD, FRCS

Iatrogenic injuries to the bile duct are still all too frequent, their incidence varying between 0.3 and 0.5 per cent. They are serious complications in terms of mortality, morbidity and costs. Quite often, after the initial repair, they are associated with the possible necessity of repeated operations of increasing complexity, handicapping the lives of the patients who are in their most active and productive stages of life. This is indeed important, because these injuries concern mainly young adults, and especially women, the sex ratio being 3 : 1, in accordance with the high incidence of cholelithiasis in women.

Aetiology

Almost all iatrogenic injuries to the bile ducts occur during biliary surgery, and more rarely during difficult operations such as gastrectomy, excision of a duodenal diverticulum, liver resection or pancreatic surgery, or even endoscopic sphincterotomy.

Biliary surgery

Cholecystectomy and choledocholithotomy, often considered as routine operations, can occasionally become very difficult when the gall bladder and the hepatoduodenal ligament are inflamed or fibrotic. In any case, even when apparently easy, these procedures require expertise based on perfect knowledge of bile duct anatomy, the arterial supply, and their variations (Fig. 19.1).[1,2]

In fact, the most important predisposing factor is poor surgical technique (i.e. a subcostal incision made too short or too oblique, a paramedian incision made too low or too short, insufficient exposure of the hepatoduodenal ligament and specially of the cystic duct).[3-7]

The common duct may be mistaken for the cystic duct during introduction of the cannula necessary to perform peroperative cholangiography. The result is a partial or total division of the common duct below the level of the junction of the cystic duct and the common duct.

Bile duct injury often occurs when the cystic duct is closely adherent to the common bile duct as they course together within a common sheath. The common duct is mistaken for the cystic duct, and ligated and divided.

252 *Bile duct injuries*

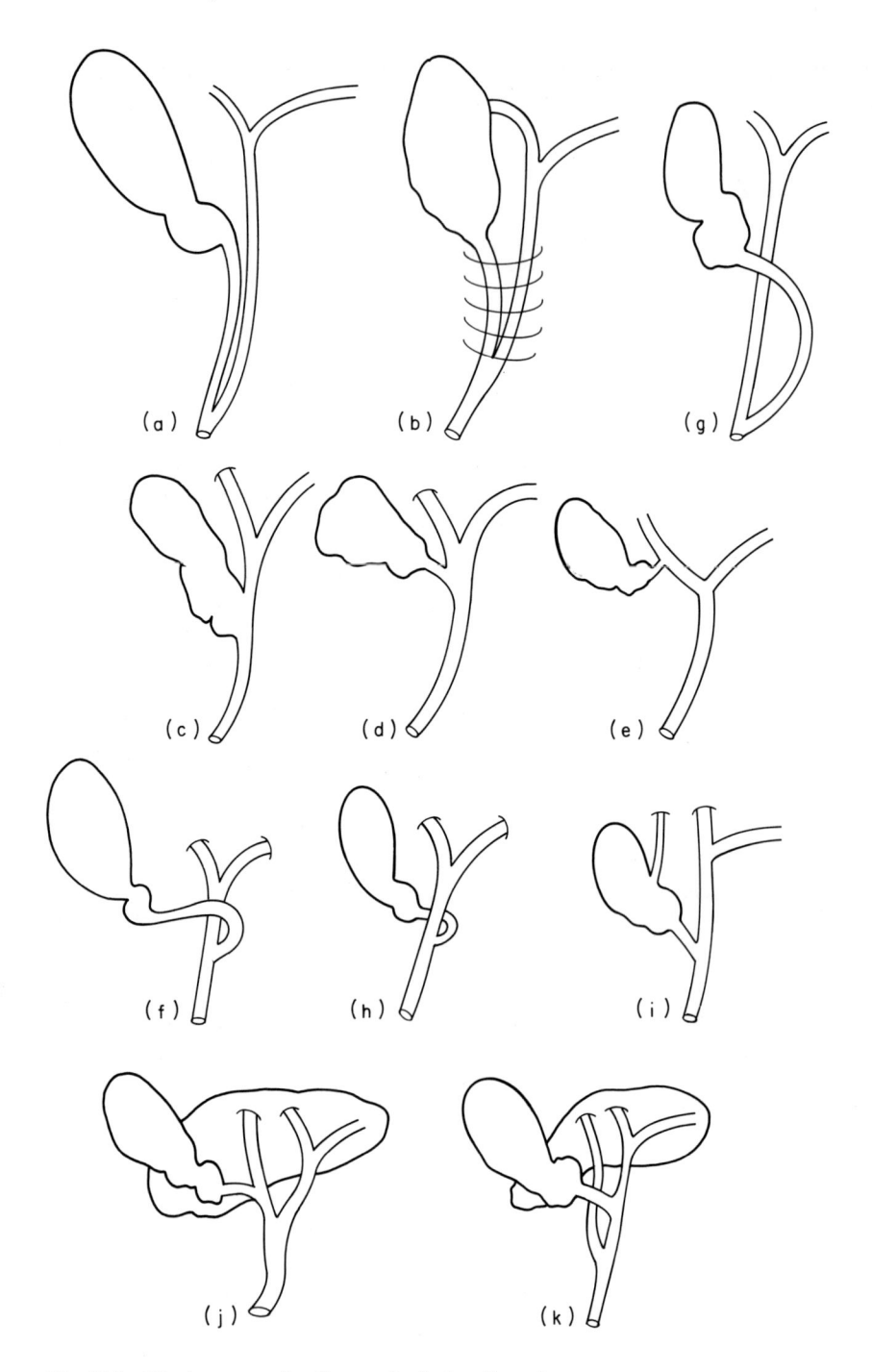

Fig. 19.1 Bile duct anomalies. See text for further discussion.

Frequently, the cause of injury is the implantation of an anterior or posterior spiral cystic duct in the common duct or the common hepatic duct, or the high implantation of the cystic duct in the common hepatic duct or the right hepatic duct. In such instances, the main bile duct is confused with the cystic duct and divided. Another cause of bile duct injury is the presence of an abnormal anterior or posterior right hepatic duct which traverses the triangle of Calot to join the fundus or the body of the gall bladder.[1] Injury occasionally results from the cystic duct being too short or absent.

Extensive traction on the gall bladder during fundus-down choleystectomy leads to extreme bending of the junction of the common hepatic duct and the common bile duct and creates a situation likely to result in ligature and excision of a segment of the common hepatic and bile ducts.

Avulsion of a friable cystic duct by excessive traction is quite rare but possible, the result being a lateral wound of the common bile duct.

Quite often, the main cause of bile duct injury is a difficult cholecystectomy, when dense and extensive fibrosis obscures the triangle of Calot so that the gall bladder lies against the common hepatic duct. In such instances, dissection within the triangle may cause a lateral breach, complete division, or segmental resection of the hepatic duct.

The bile duct injury is occasionally the result of a spontaneous postinflammatory biliary fistula between the fundus, whether or not it contains any stones, and the common hepatic or common bile ducts. In such instances, the bile duct is largely compromised, but its continuity may not be entirely broken.[4]

In rare cases, attempts to control haemorrhage arising from a divided, inflamed, friable or tortuous cystic or right hepatic artery during cholecystectomy for acute cholecystitis may damage the common hepatic duct or one of the hepatic ducts, especially when clamps are applied blindly. In such cases, the artery and the duct are either ligated or divided simultaneously, leading to destruction of the bile duct confluence and blood supply.

On the other hand, rough handling of a metal probe, bougie, or forceps in the exploration of the common bile duct may create a hole in the posterior aspect of the duct, or provoke the passage of the instrument into pancreatic tissue and eventually cause pancreatitis.

Difficult extraction of stones located in the bile duct via the cystic stump, or a duct incision too short, may also cause avulsion of a segment of the duct wall.

Other procedures

Biliary injury may also occur during liver resection for tumours or cysts, especially if the lesions involve the hilum where the biliary tree is likely to suffer damage during dissection.

Injury to the common duct can occur during a difficult gastrectomy when the pyloric region is adherent to the common bile duct.

Several cases of low common bile duct injuries have been reported after excision of a duodenal diverticulum, and recently, retroperforations of the lower portion of the common duct during endoscopic sphincterotomy have been described.

Prevention

Almost all operative injuries to the bile (Fig. 19.2) ducts can be prevented by adequate exposure of the bile ducts and careful management of accidental haemorrhage.[8]

Cholecystectomy complications

During cholecystectomy, no structure should be clamped, ligated or divided before the entire and complete triangle of Calot, bounded by the right borders of the common hepatic duct and the right hepatic duct, the upper surface of the gall bladder and the cystic duct, have been identified. During dissection, excessive traction on the fundus should be avoided to prevent avulsion of the cystic artery or bending of the main bile duct. Once the triangle of Calot has been exposed, the initial manoeuvre should be the identification, dissection and ligation of the cystic artery, close to the gall bladder to avoid damage to the common or right hepatic duct, as well as to the hepatic or the right hepatic artery; secondly, the precise point of junction of the cystic duct with the common duct must be clearly demonstrated; thirdly, a catheter must be introduced into the cystic duct to perform an operative cholangiography demonstrating the anatomy of the main bile ducts and allowing the detection of any variations.

If substantial accidental bleeding occurs, for instance when a friable artery is torn, a pack should be applied to the bleeding site for haemostasis, the blood removed by gentle suction, the bleeding point located and suture-ligated with thin silk. Torrential haemorrhage can be controlled by Pringle's manoeuvre.

When extensive fibrosis or inflammatory oedema makes dissection of Calot's triangle difficult, the common bile duct should be opened distally and a probe inserted proximally to allow safe dissection of the common hepatic duct and the fundus. But if adhesions are firm, or if an abscess is present, it may be safer to postpone cholecystectomy, removing the stones in the gall bladder and leaving the patient with a temporary cholecystostomy.

Choledocholithotomy complications

To avoid any injury during choledocholithotomy, the exploration should be performed with soft probes, and the stones extracted with appropriate biliary forceps or Dormia's basket via a long incision, avoiding any harmful manoeuvres. When the common duct is thin and the stones are small, operative exploration is difficult and extraction may be dangerous. In such instances, it is wise to abandon the surgical procedure, as the small stones may pass asymptomatically or can ultimately be extracted by endoscopic sphincterotomy.

Other operations

To avoid injury during difficult gastric procedures, or the resection of a localized pancreatic lesion or duodenal diverticulum, it is wise to perform a supraduodenal choledochotomy and to gently insert a probe into the distal common duct, which helps greatly in identifying the duct during dissection.

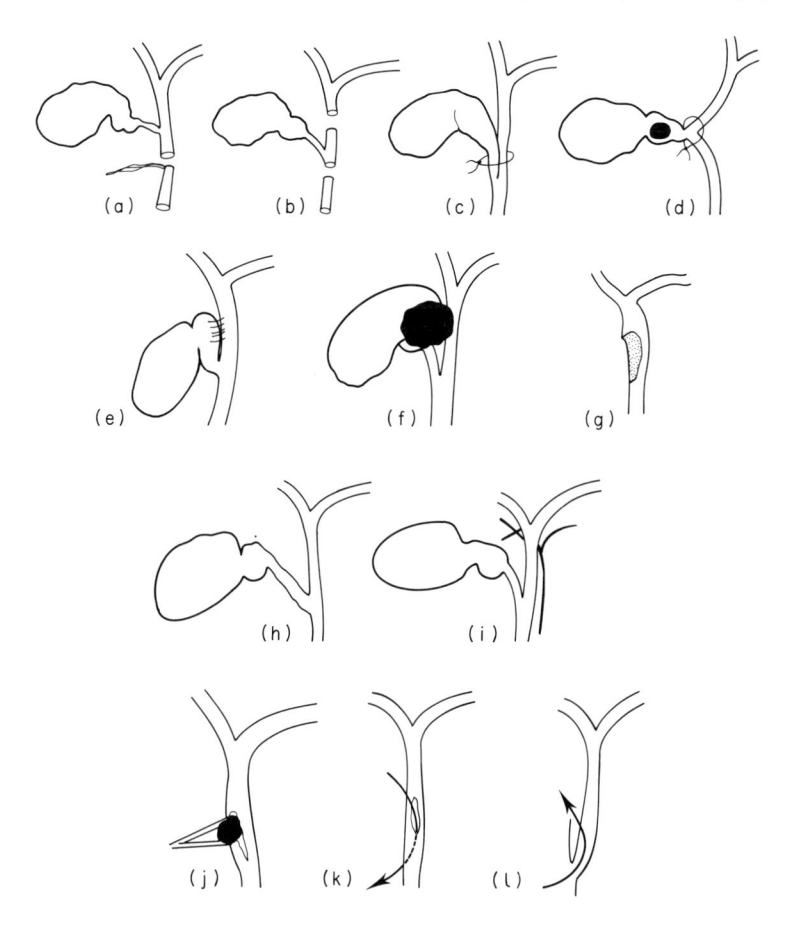

Fig. 19.2 Technical errors.

Injuries recognized during operation

By means of precise control of the operative field and routine cholangiography during operations involving the biliary tract, about 15 per cent of iatrogenic bile duct injuries are discovered at the time of operation. The wound is frequently revealed by the unexpected presence of bile in the operative field, under the liver surface or near the hepatoduodenal ligament. Occasionally, the operative cholangiography shows the dye emerging from a leak at the level of the biliary tract. In rare cases, the injury is discovered indirectly when two ducts joined side-by-side are discovered by routine pathological examination of the specimen.

Repair

If the surgeon is well trained in biliary surgery, he can undertake immediate biliary repair, but he quite often faces an arduous task, as the bile ducts are of a narrow calibre and a precise mucosa-to-mucosa apposition is difficult to obtain. Healing without fibrosis and stricture is difficult to achieve in such conditions. In any event, the first objective is to ascertain precisely the extent of the injury. This is achieved by careful dissection of the bile duct, gentle instrumental exploration of the biliary tree, and above all operative cholangiography demonstrating precisely the location and size of the biliary injury.

To repair the bile duct injury, the following principles must be observed: minimal dissection and mobilization of both extremities of the injured duct so as to maintain a good blood supply; accurate mucosa-to-mucosa apposition of the two ends of the bile duct; avoidance of any tension at the level of the anastomosis; use of very thin monofilament suture material; stitches tied on the outside; use of a thin rubber splint brought out through the bile duct at a site distant from the anastomotic line. [9,10]

The surgeon is faced with quite different situations according to the site of the injury, the size of the duct damaged and the nature of the injury. Minimal injuries, such as a small side hole resulting from the perforation of the bile duct by the cannula in the course of operative cholangiography or by a false passage created by a probe or forceps, require a simple transverse suture of the defect. The bile duct is then drained for at least two weeks with a thin T-tube.

Injury to an accessory duct is quite often impossible to repair by end-to-end anastomosis. The best way to avoid a biliary fistula is to ligate the duct firmly with a through-and-through non-absorbable suture.

Injuries to the posterior, anterior or right hepatic ducts are not uncommon, and they are quite difficult to manage. End-to-end anastomosis over a drain produces the best results. Nevertheless, the incidence of postoperative biliary fistula or stricture reaches the vicinity of 25 per cent in such cases.

Incomplete section of the main bile duct may be managed by the insertion of the short limb of a T-tube between the two edges of the wound.

Complete section without loss of length is quite rare. In this case, end-to-end anastomosis is mandatory, the thin T-tube being brought out of the bile duct at a site distant from the anastomotic line.

Complete section with loss of length generally involves the distal part of the hepatic duct and the proximal part of the common duct, where the main bile duct was mistaken for the cystic duct. If loss of length is not very substantial, and the calibre of the duct is not too small (greater than 5 mm), end-to-end anastomosis may be considered after full mobilization of the duodenum and head of the pancreas to avoid any tension. If the two ends cannot be apposed without tension, an immediate biliary–intestinal anastomosis is necessary. In the past, the hepaticoduodenostomy was considered to be the best operation, but complications such as a major fistula with considerable loss of bile and duodenal fluids or secondary severe stenosis of the anastomosis have been reported quite frequently. In such cases, an end-to-side Roux-en-Y hepaticojejunostomy with a 60–70 cm long jejunum limb is preferable, as this operation avoids not only chymal reflux into the bile ducts but also reduces the severity of a possible leak. Stricture at the hepaticojejunal anastomosis is caused by a granulating area at the anastomosis as a result of distraction resulting from the weight of the loop. The best technique for avoiding this complication is to pass a balloon catheter through the liver to lie within and beyond the anastomosis: tension on the catheter as it traverses the abdominal wall prevents distraction of the suture line until healing is complete. While the catheter is *in situ* bile drains into the loop through holes above and below the balloon.[11]

When the injury is not circumferential and the defect large, it is impossible to suture the irregular wound transversely. As the use of a vein patch or a piece of omentum have been shown to be unsuccessful, it is better to excise the retained part of the duct wall and perform a large end-to-side hepaticojejunostomy.

Injuries to the confluence of the hepatic ducts are quite rare, as the right and left hepatic ducts are separated. To restore the continuity between the two bile ducts and to perform a hepaticojejunostomy is a difficult task, especially if small vessels are bleeding. In this instance, the haemorrhage must be controlled first. A stent is inserted into each duct and then brought out through the liver and the abdominal wall. A safer secondary repair, when the patient is in better condition, is then possible.

When the bile duct is very thin (less than 5 mm) and the wall sclerotic, the same procedure may be chosen.

Follow-up

After bile repair, the most important factor is estimation of the patency of the duct. A rise in the alkaline phosphatase levels means that stricture should be suspected and proper imaging studies of the biliary tree must be performed, using real-time echography and HIDA scanning. These simple investigations provide details which help select the appropriate therapy if a new stenosis is recognized.

Results

It is difficult to determine the exact number of bile duct injuries recognized immediately, and more difficult to appreciate the rate of failure of these operations, as only good results are published.

Injuries recognized in the early postoperative period

In 85 per cent of cases, the bile duct injury is discovered after the operation.[12,13]

Bile peritonitis

Extravasation of bile in the peritoneal cavity, seen in 11 per cent of cases, is a very serious postoperative complication and is usually secondary to absent or ineffective drainage of the operative field. When bile is infected, the patient's condition is often serious. Shock, fever, abdominal pain and paralytic ileus are the main symptoms and signs of bile peritonitis. If the bile is sterile, large volumes of fluid may accumulate within the peritoneal cavity, and the diagnosis of bile peritonitis is often delayed until the abdomen becomes distended and the collection recognized by echography/or paracentesis.

Immediate and definitive repair of the biliary wound is usually impossible, as the bile ducts are collapsed and friable. Treatment consists of life-saving measures, including evacuation of bile and lavage of the abdominal cavity, and insertion of a tube into the proximal end of the duct to divert the bile outside the abdomen. The result is the formation of an external biliary fistula, which can be repaired two months later.

Biliary fistula

External extravasation of bile, as seen in 36 per cent of cases, is a postoperative manifestation of an unrecognized operative injury. It usually appears on the very day of the operation, with the bile staining the dressing.

Many authors refuse to reoperate immediately. I do not share their feelings. In two cases, I have successfully repaired the bile duct on the first postoperative day. In the first case, it was possible to perform an anastomosis between a right anterior hepatic duct and a Roux-en-Y jejunal loop. In the second case, an end-to-end anastomosis was performed between the common hepatic and the common ducts divided at their junction. A thin transanastomotic stent, exteriorized below the anastomosis, was left in place for two weeks in each case.

When the biliary fistula is not reoperated within a few hours after the bile duct injury, repair is quite impossible. The bile ducts may be small and the exposure of the healthy bile duct mucosa necessary for adequate anastomosis can be very demanding. In such instances, treatment is limited to maintenance of adequate nutrition and control of infection with suitable antibiotics if the bile is infected. The volume of bile gradually diminishes; the drain can then be pulled out gradually day by day until there is spontaneous closure of the fistula. Occasionally, a subhepatic abscess can occur, requiring drainage of pus by a further incision and insertion of a large latex drain.

When, after several weeks, the fistula dries up, the bile ducts are usually enlarged and biliary stricture is present. Operation can be planned as soon as infection is controlled by specific antibiotics and the general status of the patient has been restored.

Biliary obstruction

In 38 per cent of cases, jaundice is the first symptom of an iatrogenic ligature of the bile ducts. Nevertheless, other causes of icterus must be ruled out, such as (1) intrahepatic cholestasis following a long and difficult operation associated with the administration of large amounts of blood; (2) toxic jaundice secondary to the use of halothane; and (3) infectious jaundice.

Biliary obstruction appearing as soon as the second or third postoperative day is usually accompanied by rapid increase of jaundice followed by pruritus. There is no pain and no fever. The level of the bilirubin reaches 100–150 mg/l at the end of the first week. Alkaline phosphatase and transaminases, especially SGPT, rise quickly. The diagnosis of biliary obstruction is quite obvious by the end of the second week.

In such cases, I prefer to delay the biliary repair until the fourth week when a biliary stricture with enlargement of the proximal bile ducts is established. The nutritional state of the patient is maintained or improved by hyperalimentation. In the presence of cholangitis, administration of broad-spectrum antibiotics is a valuable adjunct. If the patient is anaemic, he may require a blood transfusion.

Conclusions

The best treatment for an iatrogenic wound of the biliary tract is prevention by adequate education of surgeons in the performance of a safe technique of cholecystectomy. Great care must be exercised during other biliary tract operations, difficult gastrectomies, pancreatic operations, endoscopic biliary tract investigations and operations in order to preserve the bile ducts. It is very important for every surgeon to be aware of the variants of biliary duct anatomy. This is the reason why I use routine peroperative cholangiography in association with careful dissection of the blood supply to avoid any unexpected bleeding.

Injuries recognized during the operation must be repaired immediately by a specific technique suited to the specific wound. On the other hand, injuries recognized in the early postoperative period do not require immediate repair except in the case of bile peritonitis.

In either case, the morbidity rate is quite high, and yet the precise number of fatalities is difficult to assess accurately.

Consequent on technical surgical improvement, iatrogenic wounds of the biliary tract should progressively disappear.

References

1. Netter F.H. Normal anatomy of the liver, biliary tract and pancreas. In: Oppenheimer E.(ed.): *The Ciba Collection of Medical Illustrations*, Vol. 3, *The Digestive System*, Pt. III. New York: CIBA, 1967: 2–25.
2. Northover J.M., Terblanche J. A new look at the arterial supply of the bile duct in man and its surgical implication. *Brit. J. Surg.* 1979; **66:** 379–84.
3. Negri A. *Accidents Opératoires au Cours des Interventions sur les Voies Biliaires*. Rapport au 21è Congrès Argentin de Chirurgie, Buenos Aires, 1950.
4. Hepp J., Grimoud J., Mercadier M. *Les Fistules Biliaires*. Rapport du 54è Congrès Français de Chirurgie, Paris. Masson, 1952.
5. Vilkaris S. Operative injuries to the bile ducts. *Acta Chir. Scand.* 1960; **199:** 83–92.
6. Rosenquist H., Myrin S.O. Operative injury to the bile ducts. *Acta Chir. Scand.* 1960; **119:** 92–107.
7. Mouchet A., Marquand J., Garcin J.P., Guivarc'h M. A propos des plaies opératoires de la voie biliare principale et de leur reparation. *Mem. Acad. Chir.* 1968; **94:** 173–82.
8. Blumgart L.H., Thompson J.N. The management of benign strictures of the bile ducts. *Curr. Prob. Surg.* 1987: 13–17.
9. Braillon G., Guillemin G. Réparation immédiate des plaies opératoires de la voie biliaire principale. *Lyon Chirurgical*. 1970; **66:** 58–9.
10. Hepp J. Le chirurgien devant une section fraiche accidentelle de la voie biliaire principale. *Med. Chir. Dig.* 1981; **10:** 214–15.
11. Smith R. Hepaticojejunostomy for very high strictures of the hepatic ducts with transhepatic intubation: a technique. *Brit. J. Surg.* 1980; **51:** 186–94.
12. Longmire W.P. Early management of injury to extrahepatic biliary tract. *JAMA*. 1966; **119:** 92–107.
13. Bismuth H., Lazorthes F. *Les traumatismes opératoires de la voie biliaire principale*. Paris: Monographies de l'Association Française de Chirurgie, 1981: 7–45.

20

Spinal cord damage associated with surgery of the descending aorta

G. Keen, MS, FRCS

One of the greatest tragedies that can befall an active child is the development of severe and disabling neurological damage after an apparently straightforward operative procedure to resect a coarctation. The consequent deprivation and anguish to the patient, family and surgeon, to say nothing of probable litigation, makes this a subject worthy of serious consideration.

Operations on the descending thoracic aorta are also performed for acute traumatic rupture, dissection and aneurysm. All these operations involve cross-clamping the aorta above and below the abnormality and steps must be taken to protect the kidneys and spinal cord from the effects of ischaemia. If aortic occlusion is maintained for longer than about 20 minutes at normal temperatures, the risk of paraplegia becomes very great.[1] In addition, steps must be taken to avoid left ventricular strain. In experiments, animal aortic cross-clamping at this level without bypass results in a marked rise in left ventricular, left atrial and pulmonary artery pressure.

The potential for damage to the spinal cord arises on account of its variable, and sometimes precarious, blood supply. The spinal cord is at risk not only during operations on the thoracic aorta but also in orthopaedic and neurological operations on the thoracic spine, particularly those for the mechanical correction of scoliosis. Although the risk of paraplegia in operations for traumatic rupture of the aorta and of acute dissection is high (indeed, in these conditions the patient may present with paraplegia), the incidence after operations for coarctation of the aorta is fortunately low. Nevertheless, since many operations for these conditions are undertaken worldwide, there is a group of patients suffering paraplegia as a consequence and, because of the understandable reluctance of surgeons to publish these tragedies, this number is probably considerably underestimated.

Anatomy

The traditional concept of the blood supply to the spinal cord is that the anterior spinal artery forms a single continuous channel which flows uninterrupted from the cervical to the lumbar region. There are, however, many variations. The first accurate description of the circulation of the spinal cord was in 1881 by Adamkiewicz.[2] He showed that the anterior spinal artery is not always a

Anatomy 261

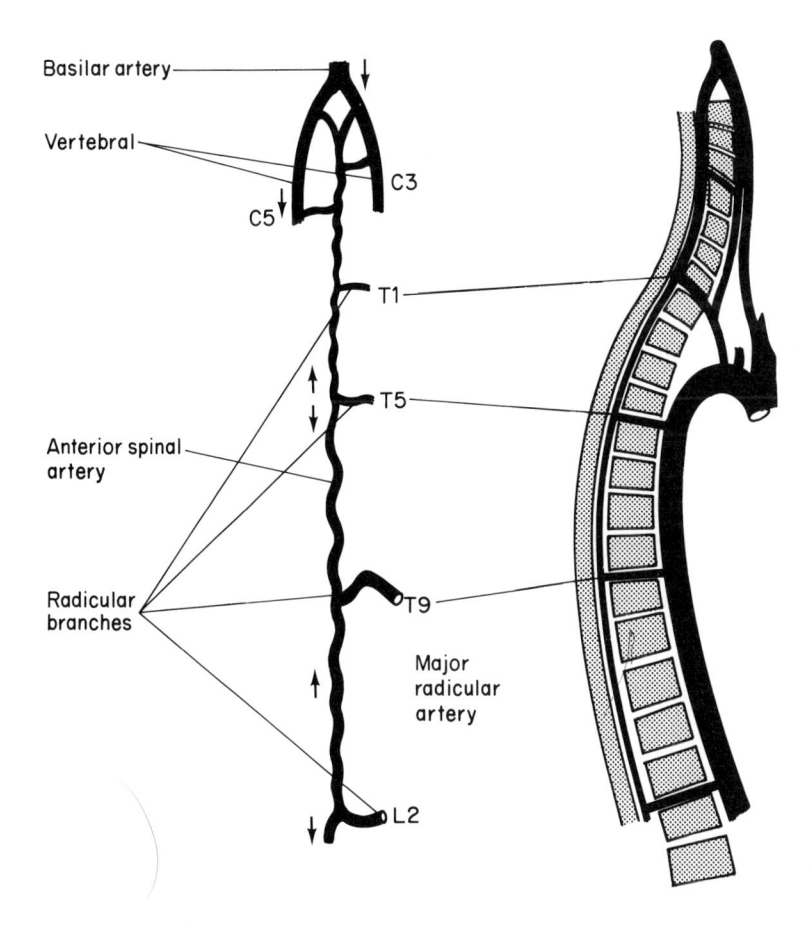

Fig. 20.1 Segmental blood supply of the anterior spinal arteries via the radicular branches of the intercostal and other aortic vessels together with a supply from the vertebral arteries. The anterior spinal artery is shown as a continuous vessel, but common variations make the continuity of the anterior spinal artery precarious and undependable.

continuous vessel and that not every intercostal vessel in the thoracic region will have a radicular branch to supply the anterior spinal artery (Fig. 20.1).

The anterior spinal artery is interrupted at one or more levels, creating a functional division in the blood supply to the cord. The upper division, which is the upper cervical and thoracic regions, is supplied by branches of the vertebral arteries which form the anterior spinal artery and by a number of spinal arteries which vary in location, the most constant branch accompanying a radicular branch of C4, which receives its blood supply from the superior intercostal vessels. The middle division, from the middle of the lower thoracic region of the cord, has the poorest segmental blood supply and is usually dependent on one radicular artery which commonly arises from T7, T8 or T9. The lower or lumbar division is supplied almost exclusively by the unpaired great radicular artery of Adamkiewicz, and this artery shows considerable variation. When it arises from a lower thoracic intercostal vessel the branch to the middle division may be absent, and when the great radicular artery arises in the lumbar region the blood supply to the lower thoracic cord is poor in the absence of T7–T9 radicular branches. Under normal circumstances, there is little exchange between the territories of the various radicular arteries, and variations in number and origin of important radicular arteries result in potential areas of ischaemia. In effect, occlusion of intercostal vessels may be harmless in one patient and unpredictably dangerous in another (Fig. 20.2).

Clinical significance

If a long section of aorta must be replaced there is a risk of permanently interrupting the blood supply of the spinal cord as intercostal arteries are ligated. Even when temporary occlusion of the aorta is required, as with coarctation and traumatic rupture, there is a risk that ischaemia will result. The variable anatomy and unpredictable consequences apply in both cases.

In the case of coarctation the surgeon has the opportunity to determine whether the collateral circulation which is part of this condition is adequate to the distal aorta after cross-clamping. The only safe measure is to record intra-aortic pressures below the distal clamp during surgery. Although the majority of patients with coarctation of the aorta will maintain a high distal pressure after cross-clamping (i.e. above 50 mmHg mean), patients undergoing surgery for acquired conditions, and who have no collateral circulation, will produce no distal aortic pressure following cross-clamping. In my view those patients with coarctation of the aorta who after cross-clamping produce little or no distal pressure, and all patients having surgery for acquired diseases, should have some form of shunt if unacceptable risks are to be avoided.

Somatosensory evoked potentials

A most attractive method of assessing spinal cord function during these operations is by the continuous monitoring of somatosensory evoked potentials. The stimulation of various sensory systems will produce a signal identifiable by an electroencephalogram on the relevant part of the surface of the brain provided that the transmitting nerve is intact. This has been understood for many years in ophthalmic surgery where the flashing of a light before the eye is picked up as a signal at the occipital cortex, provided that the optic nerve and other tracts are intact. Similarly, stimulation of the peroneal or tibial nerves will produce a continuous signal on the cerebral cortex provided that the spinal cord is intact. This simple concept is, unfortunately, much more difficult to transfer to clinical practice than superficial consideration might suggest. The equipment used is specialized and interpretation of the signals produced are best supervised by neurophysiologists and trained technicians in the operating theatre. Experience has shown that once the technique has been learned a trained member of the team, usually the anaesthetist, will be able to interpret normal and abnormal cerebral responses to peripheral stimulation during surgery (Fig. 20.3).

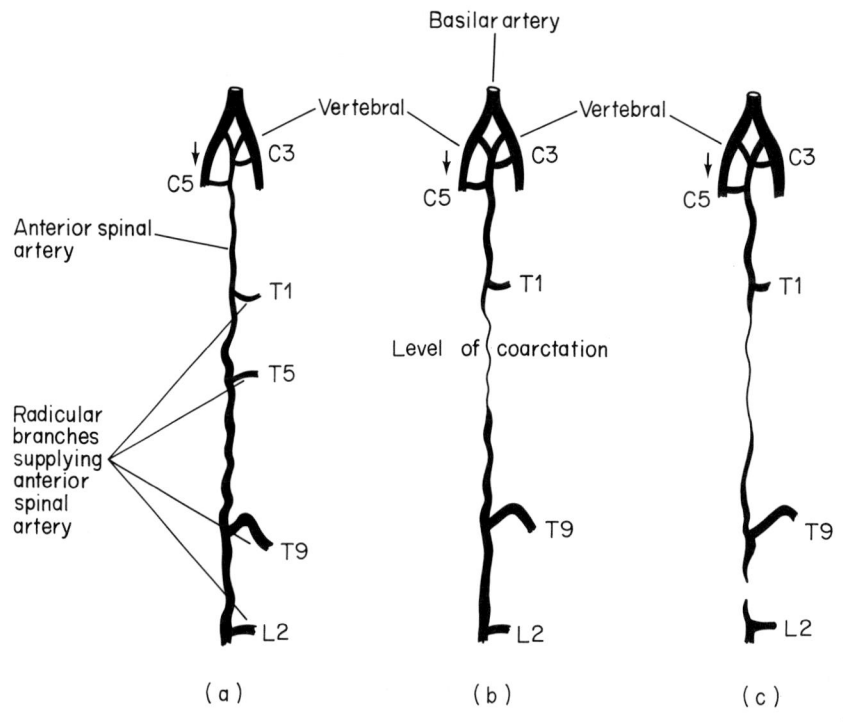

Fig. 20.2 Variations in the supply to the anterior spinal artery. In (a) the spinal artery is supplied by many good radicular vessels, but in (b) there is clearly limitation of anterior spinal artery flow between T1 and T9. In (c), owing to the poor radicular supply from the intercostal vessels, there is discontinuity in the anterior spinal artery between T1 and T9 and again between T9 and L2, and it is in such cases that the spinal cord is endangered during operations on the descending thoracic aorta. The large radicular artery at the level of about T9 (the artery of Adamkiewicz) is a very constant and reliably large branch to the lumbar cord.

Spinal cord monitoring

Laschinger and his colleagues undertook an investigation of the experimental and clinical assessment of the adequacy of partial bypass in the maintenance of spinal cord blood flow during operations on the thoracic aorta using spinal cord impulse conduction (somatosensory evoked potentials).[3,4] They concluded that maintenance of a distal aortic pressure greater than 60–80 mmHg will uniformly preserve spinal blood flow in the absence of critical intercostal exclusion. Should distal aortic pressure be inadequate, early reversible changes in the somatosensory evoked potentials will alert the surgeon; and failure to institute measures to reverse these changes may result in paraplegia.

With the availability of these methods many centres (commonly in the United States and two or three in the United Kingdom) are modifying their techniques and are using somatosensory evoked potentials. Inquiry at these centres shows that a prolonged learning process is required before the interpretation of data is of sufficient accuracy for this to become a clinically reliable technique, and consequently it must be regarded as an experimental technique in the hands of learner groups. Although this appears to be a formidable problem, it is clear that we have a duty to develop these techniques and to transmit them to the operating theatre—for surgery of the thoracic aorta and for scoliosis.

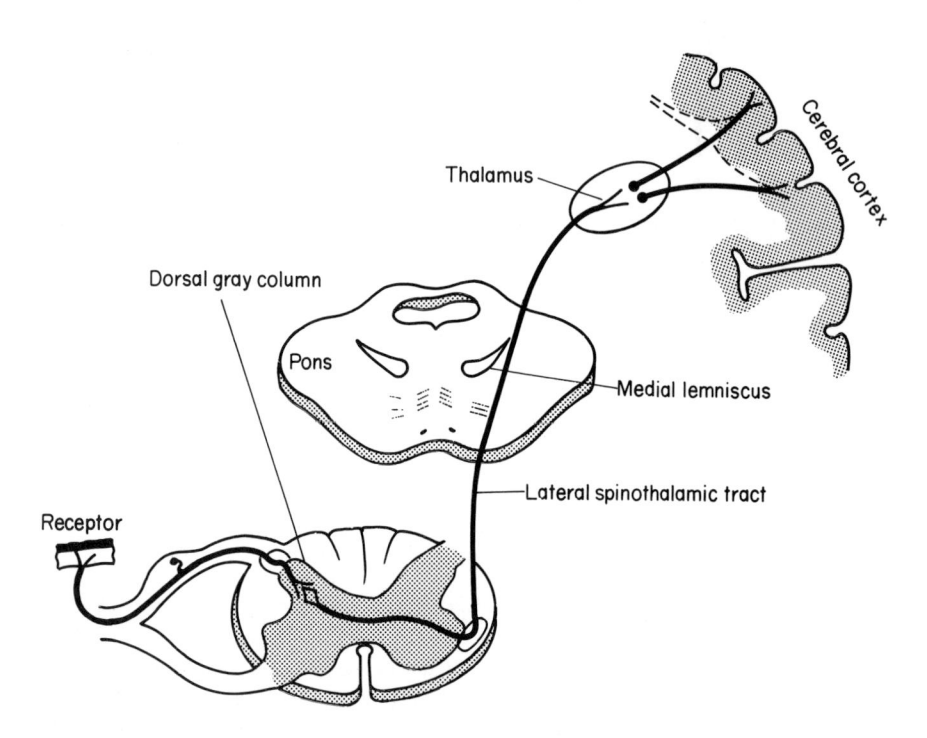

Fig. 20.3 Somatosensory evoked potentials: stimulation of a peripheral receptor will produce a signal at the cerebral cortex provided the pathways are intact.

The initial and revenue costs of such a system are high, and so is the cost of training appropriate personnel; but the equipment and personnel in any one city could be made available to help those surgeons or neurologists who might from time to time need this assistance. It has, of course, yet to be proved that in the present state of our knowledge the use of somatosensory evoked potentials offers greater reliability than the monitoring of distal aortic pressure. Pollock and his colleagues in Glasgow, who are evaluating somatosensory evoked potential monitoring, believe that their initial experience is promising and that its intraoperative use can identify quickly the patient at risk of ischaemic cord damage and allow alternative repair methods, avoiding cross-clamping, to be used.[5] Although they believe that the technique holds great promise, they are of the opinion that much work remains to be done before an appropriate degree of refinement is obtained. A complicating factor is that cortical somatosensory evoked potentials are subject to attenuation by anaesthesia and by hypotension. This increases the difficulty of obtaining good-quality recordings in the operating theatre, which is never an ideal electrophysiological environment.

Although somatosensory evoked potentials are used to measure the function of the entire spinal cord, and some contribution to the potentials may be transmitted by the anterior part of the spinal cord, the main pathway is via the dorsal columns. So far, in acute conditions — for example, in trauma, spinal operations or vascular insults — the somatosensory evoked potential does seem to be a sensitive indicator for global spinal cord function. This is not necessarily the case in chronic paraplegia.

Clearly, we do not yet have sufficient information to know whether in man paraplegia, or at least paraparesis, may occasionally result when somatosensory evoked potentials have not been abolished. This will be difficult to discover with the given incidence of neurological sequelae. The exact relationship of intraoperative somatosensory evoked potential changes to the occurrence and severity of postoperative neurological sequelae has so far not been established.

Paraplegia after abdominal aortic surgery

This may be encountered in up to 6 per cent of descending thoracic aortic aneurysm operations but is rare after abdominal aortic aneurysm surgery, few cases being reported in the literature.[6] The accepted explanation involves the existence of a large infrarenal 'arteria radicularis' which could be injured or occluded in the course of aneurysm repair. Because such a collateral exists in almost half the population despite the rarity of this complication, some other factor must be involved. Interdependence of the anterior and posterior spinal arteries distal to the mid-thoracic spine plays some role.

At least half of the reported cases followed emergency aneurysmectomy, and only one-third either were not hypotensive or did not experience a prolonged period of occlusion above the renal arteries. Those cases not attributable to prolonged or proximal aortic occlusion may be explained on the basis of atheroembolism, or thrombosis of this artery, or a major lumbar supply to the distal cord. Half the patients with this complication died and, whereas almost half recovered some neurological function, only two recovered fully.

Techniques of aortic bypass and spinal cord protection[7]

Left atriofemoral bypass

Left atriofemoral bypass is employed in many cases in which surgery of the descending thoracic aorta is undertaken (Fig. 20.4(a)). This technique allows satisfactory operating conditions preventing proximal hypertension and left ventricular strain during aortic cross-clamping, and also ensures adequate distal perfusion. Heparinization and its reversal by protamine pose no undue problems, but should intra-abdominal or intracerebral bleeding be taking place (as in traumatic rupture of aorta) heparinization might aggravate this.

The patient is positioned on the operating table in the right lateral position—that is, with the left chest uppermost—with the pelvis rotated 45° backwards and the left hip joint fully extended, the chest being thus exposed for full thoracotomy and access provided to the femoral vessels. The left femoral artery is first prepared for cannulation and the left chest is opened widely through the 4th intercostal space. Before mobilization of the aorta the pericardium is opened posteriorly to the phrenic nerve and the left atrial appendage snared by a purse-string. These precautions allow for immediate left atriofemoral bypass should haemorrhage occur during dissection. A large-bore cannula is introduced into the left atrium, whence blood is drained by gravity into a reservoir and thence returned via a roller pump to the femoral artery. Specific steps must be taken to ensure that no air enters the left atrium during this procedure. Heparinization is required in a dosage of 3 mg (300 U)/kg body weight and is subsequently reversed with protamine. A distal flow rate of 40 ml/kg body weight per minute ensures adequate decompression of the proximal aorta with adequate perfusion of the kidneys and, it is hoped, the spinal cord. During perfusion the radial arterial pressure should be maintained at 80 mmHg and urine should be passed.

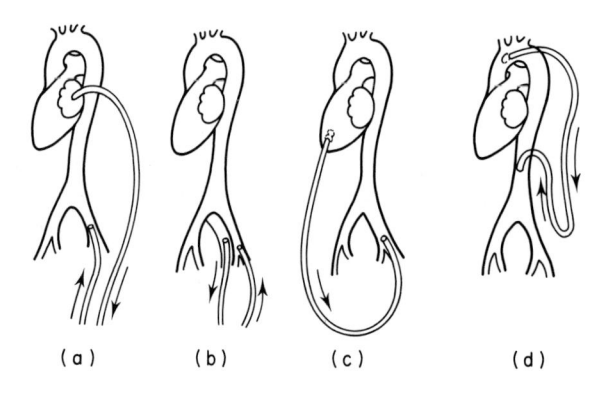

Fig. 20.4 Methods of supporting the circulation below a descending aortic cross-clamp (as described in the text). (a) Left atrial to femoral arterial bypass, requires pump but no oxygenator. (b) Femoro-femoral bypass requires oxygenator and pump. (c) and (d) Left ventriculo-aorto and aorto-aortic bypass with a heparin-bonded shunt require neither oxygenator nor pump.

Femoral venous-to-arterial oxygenation

This technique was described in 1968 in the treatment of 19 patients who underwent resection of aneurysms of the descending aorta or the repair of ruptured aortas.[8] A large-bore catheter is inserted into the inferior vena cava via the femoral vein, whence the blood is drained into a disposable bubble oxygenator and returned to the femoral artery (Fig. 20.4(b)). This allows a measured perfusion of the lower part of the body during aortic cross-clamping and decompresses the upper aortic segment. It has the additional advantage of removing cannulas and tubing from the operative field and avoids cannulation of the left atrium.

Although the use of this method does not seem to be widespread, it offers a great deal of control over the circulation above and below the aortic clamp but has the added complexity of requiring an oxygenator and full heparinization.

Ventriculo-aortic shunt

In 1970, Molloy reported the successful repair of ruptured thoracic aorta in three patients with the use of a left ventriculo-aortic shunt.[9] A plastic cannula was used, one end of which was inserted into the left ventricle at its apex and the other into the descending thoracic aorta below the site of trauma (Fig. 20.4(c)) The only complication reported was clotting of blood in the cannula on one occasion. Current practice is to use a heparin-bonded plastic shunt.[10]

The advantages of this method are the avoidance of heparinization on the one hand and the avoidance of elaborate bypass procedure on the other. It is relatively simple and it may well be that it will ultimately be favoured as the procedure of choice in the repair of traumatic rupture of the descending aorta. However, great care must be taken to ensure that the cannula does not pass back into the left atrium or flow will cease.

Aorto-aortic shunt

Khan[1] described the use of a similar type of temporary plastic shunt inserted at one end into the ascending aorta and at the other into the descending aorta (Fig. 20.4(d)) in operations to repair traumatic rupture of the aorta, but reported the occurrence of paraplegia in one patient which may have been due to too small a diameter of shunt.

Gott[10] described the use of a shunt from the left subclavian artery to the left femoral artery using a plastic tube lined with a non-thrombogenic substance.

At the present time most surgeons are veering away from complicated extracorporeal systems, utilizing left ventriculo-aortic bypass or subclavian-aortic bypass, with the Gott plastic shunt which is internally heparin-bonded and non-thrombogenic.

In those centres where extensive experience of descending aortic surgery has been obtained, some surgeons advocate operating without the use of left heart bypass or any form of shunting. It must be borne in mind that this small and select group of surgeons operates with extreme rapidity, thus avoiding prolonged periods of spinal cord ischaemia. Even so, their patients accept and sign a consent form which specifically names the complication of paraplegia. For the majority of surgeons, however, who have less experience but who from time to time necessarily undertake these operations, such surgery without bypass is reckless.

Moderate hypothermia

Moderate hypothermia at 30°C, which has now been superseded by bypass procedures, was used when surface cooling had an important place in cardiac and vascular surgery. Although several successful cases of suture of ruptured aorta and resection of thoracic aneurysm have been reported, the period of safe aortic occlusion in these conditions is so unreliable and variable, and the risk of ventricular fibrillation during the surface cooling of badly injured people is so high, that the use of this technique is no longer advised, unless supported by some form of bypass.

The monitoring of distal aortic pressures by electromanometric methods is clearly more sensitive and accurate than is the assessment by digital palpation alone. Although many experienced and distinguished surgeons would disagree with this last sentiment and claim that in their hands digital aortic palpation assessment of distal pressures has never been followed by paraplegia, it is likely that an uncomfortably large number of surgeons will have an operation complicated by paraplegia should they operate on a sufficient number of patients, whichever method of monitoring is used.

Cases are reported of paraplegia following short periods (under 20 minutes) of aortic cross-clamping, confirming the view that in a very small number of patients even short periods of aortic cross-clamping will not be tolerated—regardless of the skill and experience of the surgeon. It is advocated that sole reliance on estimation of aortic pressures by digital palpation should be abandoned and replaced in all cases by electromanometric measurement.

Although the use of somatosensory evoked-potential monitoring of the spinal cord is largely undeveloped in the UK, the work of Laschinger in the USA and Pollock in Glasgow shows clearly that this method has great potential. It is recommended that interested users, including thoracic surgeons, orthopaedic surgeons and neurophysiologists, collaborate and develop somatosensory evoked-potential monitoring in their own departments, in the expectation that they will eventually have at their disposal a comprehensive and reliable system of spinal cord monitoring.

Conclusions

I believe that the monitoring of spinal cord function by somatosensory evoked potentials may eventually be shown to be accurate and reliable, but this has not yet happened in the United Kingdom.

It is recommended that for the majority of surgeons some form of aortic bypass is used in descending aortic surgery when the pressure distal to the cross-clamp is inadequate by the criteria discussed.

References

1. Khan D.R. Discussion of: Crawford E.S., Fenstermacher J.M., Richardson W., et al., Reappraisal of adjuncts to avoid ischaemia in the treatment of thoracic aortic aneurysms. *Surgery.* 1970; **67:** 182–96.
2. Adamkiewicz A. (1882) Die Blutgefasse des Menschlichen Ruckenmarkes. I: Die Gefasse der Ruckenmarksubstanz. II: Die Gefasse der Ruckenmarkoberflache. *Sitz. Akad. Wiss. Wein. Math. Natur. Klass.* 1882; **84:** 469; **85:** 101.
3. Laschinger J.C., Cunningham J.N., Càtinella F.P., et al. Detection and prevention of intraoperative spinal cord ischaemia after cross-clamping of the thoracic aorta: use of somatosensory evoked potentials. *Surgery.* 1982; **92:** 1109–14.
4. Laschinger J.C., Cunningham J.N., Nathan I.M., Knop E.A., Cooper M.M., Spencer F.C. Experimental and clinical assessment of the adequacy of partial bypass in maintenance of spinal cord blood flow during operations on the thoracic aorta. *Ann. Thoracic Surg.* 1983; **36:** 417–26.
5. Pollock J.C., Jamieson M.P., McWilliam R. Somatosensory evoked potentials in the detection of spinal cord ischaemia in aortic coarctation repair. *Ann. Thoracic Surg.* 1986; **41:** 251–4.
6. Golden G.T., Sears H.F., Wellons H.A., Mueller W.A. Paraplegia complicating resection of aneurysms of the infrarenal abdominal aorta. *Surgery.* 1973; **73:** 91.

7. Keen G. Closed injuries of the thoracic aorta. *Ann. R. Coll. Surg. Engl.* 1972; **51:** 137–56.
8. Neville W.E., Cox W.D., Leininger B., *et al.* Resection of the descending thoracic aorta with femoral vein to femoral artery oxygenation perfusion. *J. Thoracic Cardiovasc. Surg.,* 1968; **56:** 39–42.
9. Molloy P.J. Repair of the ruptured thoracic aorta using left ventriculo-aortic support. *Thorax.* 1970; **25:** 213–22.
10. Gott V.L. Discussion of: Connolly J.E., Wakabayashi A., German J.C., *et al.* Clinical experience with pulsatile left heart bypass without anticoagulation for thoracic aneurysms. *J. Thoracic Cardiovasc. Surg.* 1971; **62:** 568–76.

21

The ureter

John P. Blandy, DM, MCh, FRCS, FACS

The ureter is so easily damaged in both endoscopic or open operations, and the complications and the consequences are so serious, that all surgeons of experience have learned to regard this little tube with profound respect.

A few years ago, operations in the pelvis—notably hysterectomy — were the principal cause of iatrogenic damage. Today, with the advent of the ureteroscope and the vogue for aggressive management of stones in the ureter, the urologist is now the principal perpetrator of iatrogenic trauma to the ureter.

Avoiding injury to the ureter

Endoscopic operations

Endoscopic injury to the ureter may be caused by operating on stones of less than 5 mm diameter. It has been known for many years[1,2] that these usually pass spontaneously without surgical interference. Removal of a small stone may be necessary, for example, when there is a combination of obstruction with infection in the urine, but impatience and the temptation to exercise a new instrument are not good indications. It is even worth questioning whether the ureteroscope should be discarded since the morbidity it engenders may far outweigh any possible benefit.[3–5] If we consider not only the urological literature, but the growing files of the medical defence societies, a randomized study comparing classical ureterolithotomy versus ureteroscopic extraction of stones is long overdue.

If the ureteroscope is to be used then three rules should *always* be applied:

1. Always pass a guide-wire first.
2. Make sure that the ureteric orifice and the ureter downstream of the stone are well-dilated. One may use graduated ureteric bougies or a balloon,[6] but best of all leave a double-J stent in position for four or five days before attempting to pass the ureteroscope.
3. Above all, it is essential never to use force in passing the ureteroscope.

Open operations

The best way to avoid injury to a precious structure in any surgical operation is to find it first. For the ureter this is not difficult except in just those cases where the ureter is most vulnerable, such as when there is fibrosis after irradiation, or inflammation, or when there have been several previous procedures. Here even the most experienced surgeon finds it difficult to identify a ureter when it is displaced from its expected position, dilated many times its normal size, and surrounded by hard fibrous tissue. *Any aid to the search will add to its safety.*

1. *Preoperative IVU.* It is very helpful to have had the forethought to obtain a urogram before embarking on an operation. This will reveal the rogue ureter with an unusual course, or one that is grossly dilated.

2. *Ureteric catheter.* The next manoeuvre is to pass a ureteric catheter. In identifying the ureter it is far more reassuring to feel a catheter inside it than to try to recognize it by its appearance, or to see it writhe when pinched with forceps. It only takes a few minutes—and no few minutes are more worthwhile—to rearrange the position of the patient and the operating drapes, to pass a cystoscope and to run catheters up the ureters and secure them to a small Foley catheter.

Most often the abdomen is already open when difficulty is encountered, but this should not exclude ureteric catheterization.

The search for the ureter should begin at least 5 cm higher than seems necessary, even if this means mobilizing the colon medially and dividing the splenic or hepatic flexure to expose the renal pelvis.

When the ureter has been found, the next step is to find the plane of cleavage between it and the adventitia. This plane is followed down the ureter using a right-angled forceps. The overriding tissue is divided with a knife (Fig. 21.1), taking extra care where the ureter is crossed by the gonadal and superior vesical vessels.

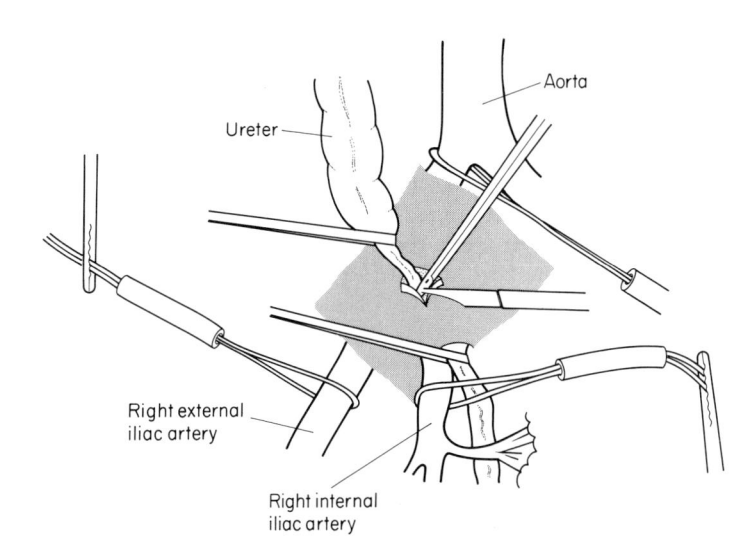

Fig. 21.1 When dissecting the ureter off the common iliac vessels to which it is often adherent, a tape should be placed around the vessels on either side of the fibrosis. A right-angled forceps is used to open up the plane of cleavage between ureter and surrounding fibrous tissue. (Reproduced from reference 12 by kind permission of Blackwell Scientific)

In retroperitoneal fibrosis and in node dissection for testicular cancer after chemotherapy, the ureter may be encased in a stiff mass of fibrous tissue stuck firmly to the aorta, cava, and common iliac vessels. The rules of vascular surgery are not abrogated merely because the structure one seeks is the ureter: before dissecting close to any great vessel one must have control on either side of the danger zone. Tapes, Rummel tourniquets and vascular clamps must be available. The ureter is often particularly adherent where it crosses the bifurcation of the common iliac artery. With control of the vessels, a hole in the common iliac artery is a trivial nuisance: without control it may be a life-threatening disaster.

The ureter injured at ureteroscopy

If a laceration in the wall of the ureter is seen through the ureteroscope it may be confirmed at once by injecting contrast and observing the extravasation on the fluoroscope. If a guide-wire is in position a double-J stent is easily passed and left *in situ*, and the patient may be safely observed; but any suggestion of a collection of urine in the retroperitoneal tissue demands prompt exploration and drainage, for infection in an undrained urinoma can lead to necrosis of several centimetres of ureter.

The ureter injured at open operation

Injury noticed at the time of operation

If the ureter has been crushed or caught up by mistake in a ligature, but not severed, it may recover merely by being splinted; so it is reasonable to undo the ligature, rearrange the drapes, reposition the patient, pass a cystoscope and run a guide-wire up the damaged ureter. Confirm that the wire has gone up into the renal pelvis, and then pass a double-J stent beyond the site of injury. Since young connective tissue continues to contract for up to six weeks, it is logical to leave the stent in for at least this period of time.

If the ureter has been cut right across and the ends are healthy and uncrushed, and if they can be brought together without tension, then they may be spatulated and anastomosed end-to-end using 4.0 or 5.0 absorbable catgut or collagen sutures. It may not be necessary to splint the anastomosis, but it is so easy nowadays to introduce a double-J stent and to remove it later with the flexible cystoscope[7] that it seems prudent to take this extra precaution.

More often when the ureter is accidentally cut it is not normal: it is unhealthy, inflamed, surrounded by scar tissue and its ends retract and do not come together without tension. In such cases, and in the lower ureter which is the usual site of injury, it is easier to reimplant it into the bladder with a Boari flap or a psoas hitch (see below) than attempt an end-to-end anastomosis.

Injury discovered at an interval after operation

After what was thought to have been a relatively straightforward pelvic operation the patient may still seem to be quite well, although with hindsight it is usually found that there has been some loin pain and fever.

Some five to seven days after the operation fluid is seen to seep from the vagina or the wound drain, or if a pack has been used the loss of fluid may be noticed only when this is removed. It is tempting for inexperienced staff to deceive themselves and the patient with the notion that the loss is no more than the expected exudation of lymph. To an experienced ward sister or charge nurse this seemingly innocuous loss of fluid brings a chill of recognition. *Two questions must be answered without delay*:

1. Is the fluid urine?
2. Where is it coming from?

Is the fluid urine?

Do not waste time by packing the vagina with tampons or injecting methylene blue. Fluid is easily shown to be urine by drawing up a few drops from the wound or the vagina with a syringe and having its creatinine or urea measured in the laboratory; if these are higher than the levels in the blood the fluid must be urine since no other body fluid can have an elevated level of creatinine or urea. A helpful laboratory will provide this information within the hour.

Where is it coming from?

To decide where the fluid is coming from, the next step is to obtain an IVU. This may show the track of the fistula: more often it does not, but when a ureter has been injured it is usually dilated. *The evidence of the IVU must always be verified by cystoscopy and ureterography.*

At cystoscopy a careful search is made for a fistula between bladder and vagina—for it is by no means unusual for a vesical and ureteric fistula to occur at the same time. Both these injuries can easily be repaired at the same operation so long as they have been detected; but if one has been overlooked, to repair it at a second procedure is exceedingly difficult.[8]

To obtain a ureterogram, a bulb-ended catheter is placed in the ureteric orifice and contrast medium injected while watching the fluoroscope. This usually does not show a leak, but it does show distortion and blockage of the ureter at the site of injury. An attempt may be made to pass a guide-wire up the ureter, and if successful this will allow a double-J stent to be inserted; but in practice this is rarely possible. Always check the other side since it is by no means rare for both ureters to be injured and, again, it is far more easy to repair them both at the first operation than to have to repair the other one at a second operation.

Bilateral injury obstructing both ureters

This is rare and difficult to diagnose. The patient may have undergone a difficult pelvic operation (e.g. removal of an extensive tumour or a Caesarian–hysterectomy), and the estimate of blood loss is likely to be inaccurate no matter how carefully swabs have been weighed. Hypovolaemic shock may well have led to acute tubular necrosis, and attemps to stop bleeding in the pelvis may well have obstructed both ureters.

In the recovery room it is soon found that no urine is being passed. Is this the result of bilateral ureteric obstruction or acute tubular necrosis? The patient going into acute tubular necrosis from shock does not develop anuria immediately: the onset is usually gradual, and at first a small volume of rather brownish urine (rich in granular casts) is passed before there is total anuria. Examination of this tiny volume of urine—if it has been collected—may be very helpful in making a diagnosis. In contrast, when both ureters have been ligated the catheter is dry from the outset.

If both ureters have been ligated, the upper tracts will be dilated and this will be detected with an ultrasound scan. If ultrasound is not available or is inconclusive, a large dose of contrast medium may be given and delayed films—12 to 24 hours later, with tomography—will show the dilated renal pelvis and ureter.

Today, the management of these patients has been revolutionized by percutaneous nephrostomy. This is done as soon as possible, and gives time for the patient to recover from the original operation.

Delayed treatment of the injured ureter

Either there and then, or more often a day or two later when the patient is better, it may be possible to negotiate a guide-wire through the nephrostomy down past the obstruction and relieve the condition with an angioplasty balloon catheter.[8]

Operative correction

When either or both ureters are obstructed, the percutaneous nephrostomy will buy enough time to allow the patient to recover from shock or septicaemia; but the sooner they are unblocked the better.

Where the problem is not so much obstruction but a urinary *fistula*, there has usually been several days delay before the fistula is diagnosed. There is still a widely-held opinion that one should defer intervention for six weeks in such cases to allow oedema and inflammation to settle down.[10] For the patient, this delay brings protracted misery, leakage of urine, soreness and stink. On readmission to hospital, the patient is demoralized, resentful, and understandably apt to litigate.[11]

This is a strange convention (for which there is no evidence), because early intervention is easy and successful: the tissues are not bound together with impenetrable scar tissue, and the results of early intervention show that the sooner the ureter is repaired the better.[8]

Choice of operation

The Boari flap (refer to Fig. 21.2)

Be ready to operate immediately after the diagnostic cystoscopy and ureterography.[12,13] Leave a catheter in the bladder connected to a bottle of normal saline, left shut off at this stage.

Unless the previous operation has been a vaginal hysterectomy, the old incision is reopened: it is no more difficult to repair the ureter through a

Delayed treatment of the injured ureter 275

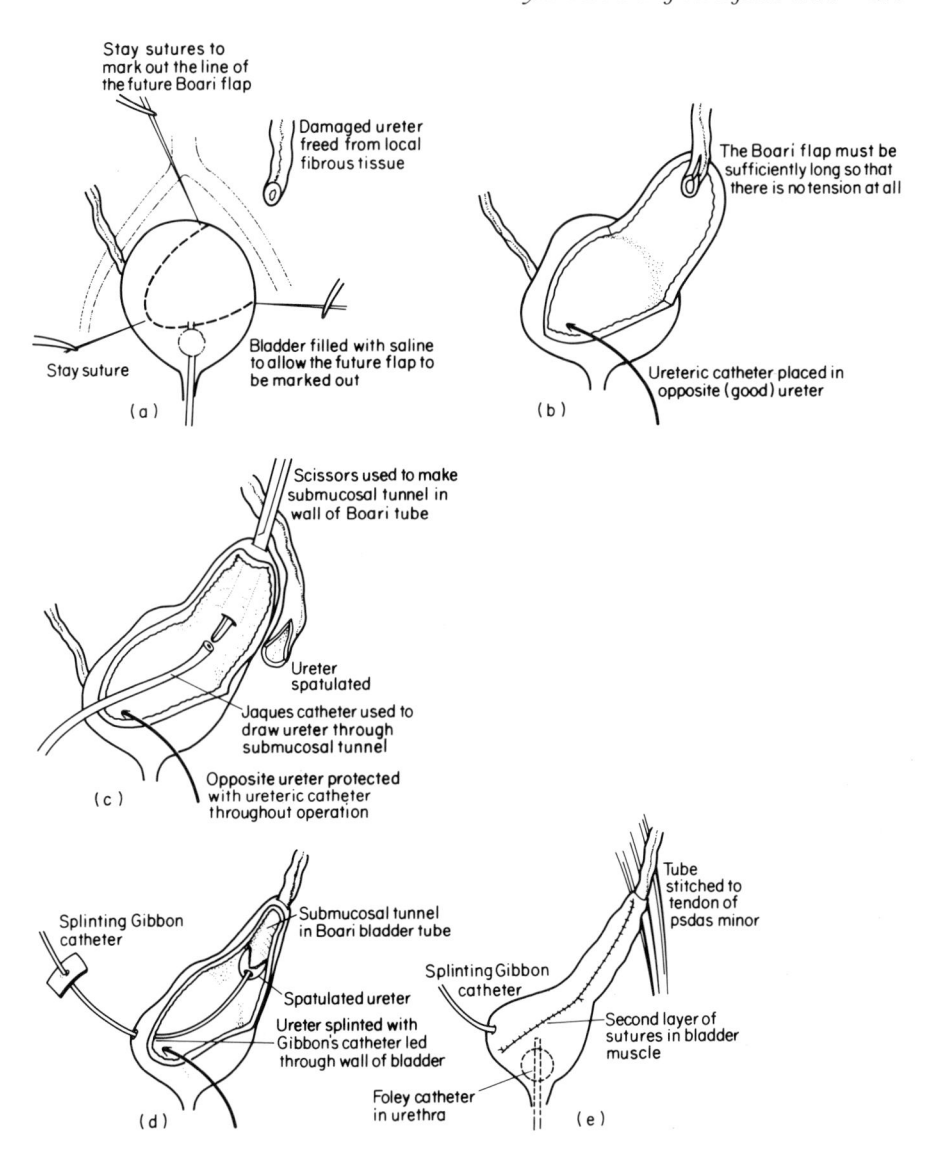

Fig. 21.2 (a) The Boari flap is marked with stay sutures. (b) The flap is mobilized, the damaged ureter mobilized, and the opposite ureter catheterized. (c) A tunnel is made with scissors and the ureter led through it. (d) The ureteric anastomosis complete, both ureters are splinted for safety. (e) The Boari flap is complete; if necessary, tension is relieved by suturing it to the tendon of psoas minor. (Adapted from reference 13 by kind permission of Churchill Livingstone)

Pfannenstiel than a midline incision. Adhesions will need care because the small bowel, sigmoid colon and ovaries are often stuck to the back of the bladder.

Find the ureter above the bifurcation of the common iliac artery and follow it down to where it disappears into granulation tissue. This becomes progressively more hard and difficult to dissect the longer the operation has been postponed. Seldom can one identify the offending ligature. When the damaged ureter has been dissected free it usually retracts, revealing a gap between ureter and bladder that is much longer than was envisaged at the beginning of the operation.

Saline is now run into the bladder to distend it so that the Boari flap may be planned and marked out with stay sutures, to provide a flap that will bridge the gap without any suggestion of tension. The bladder wall is then cut along the line bit by bit, taking time to pick up all its little arteries with suture-ligature rather than diathermy. A tunnel is made with scissors, through which the ureter is led. Spatulate it and sew it to the mucosa over a suitable splint catheter, and close the Boari in the form of a tube in two layers using continuous catgut. The wound should always be drained. The splinting catheter is left in position for three or four days (or until it blocks) and is then removed. The urethral catheter is removed at ten days.

An IVU is performed three months later, by which time it is usually difficult to tell which side has undergone the reimplantation.

The psoas hitch

An alternative technique[12] involves making a transverse incision in the wall of the bladder and closing it longitudinally: sometimes a short tunnel can be made for the ureter. The bladder has to be sutured to the tendon of psoas minor to relieve tension. Exponents of this operation claim results nearly as good as those of the Boari flap.[14]

Uretero-ureteric anastomosis

The injured ureter is cut off and anastomosed to the good one.[15] The danger is that the good ureter may suffer obstruction.[14] The procedure should be reserved for very selected cases.

Ureteric injury combined with vesicovaginal fistula

When injury to a ureter is found at the same time as vesicovaginal fistula, Walters' technique[12,16] is used to close the fistula, interposing omentum to bring healthy, well-vascularized tissue between the suture lines in the bladder and the vagina. This is a very reliable method for post-hysterectomy fistulae.[8] If, in addition, it is necessary to reimplant one or both ureters, Boari flaps can be fashioned out of the halves of the bladder, and the ureter implanted as described above.

Although two methods only have been mentioned, further illustrated text can be found in textbooks of operative urology.[12]

References

1. Badenoch A.W. *Manual of Urology.* 2nd ed. London: Heinemann, 1974: 613.
2. Kinder R.B., Osborn D.E., Flynn J.T., Smart J.G. Ureteroscopy and ureteric calculi: how useful? *Brit. J. Urol.* 1987; **60:** 506–8.

3. Carter S.StC., Cox R., Wickham J.E.A. Complications associated with ureteroscopy. *Brit. J. Urol.* 1986; **58:** 625–8.
4. Ford T.F., Payne S.R., Wickham J.E.A. The impact of transurethral ureteroscopy on the management of ureteric calculi. *Brit. J. Urol.* 1984; **56:** 602–8.
5. Chang R., Marshall F.F. Management of ureteroscopic injuries. *J. Urol.* 1987; **137:** 1132–5.
6. Schultz A., Krestensen J.K., Bilde T., Eldrup J. Ureteroscopy: results and complications. *J. Urol.* 1987; **137:** 865–6.
7. Blandy J.P., Fowler C.G. Lower tract endoscopy. *Brit. Med. Bull.* 1986; **42:** 280–3.
8. Badenoch D.F., Tiptaft R.C., Thakar D.R., Fowler C.G., Blandy J.P. Early repair of accidental injury to the ureter or bladder following gynaecological surgery. *Brit. J. Urol.* 1987; **59:** 516–18.
9. Glanz S., Gordon D.H., Butt K., Rubin B., Hong J., Sclafani S.J.A. Percutaneous transrenal balloon dilatation of the ureter. *Radiology.* 1983; **149:** 101–4.
10. Mattingly R.F., Thompson J.D. Vesico-vaginal fistulas. In: Mattingly R.F., Thompson J.D. (eds.): *Te Linde's Operative Urology.* 6th ed. Philadelphia: Lippincott, 1985: 613.
11. Flynn J.T., Tiptaft R.C., Woodhouse C.R.J., Paris A.M.I., Blandy J.P. The early and aggressive repair of iatrogenic ureteric injuries. *Brit. J. Urol.* 1979; **51:** 454–7.
12. Blandy J.P. *Operative Urology.* 2nd ed. Oxford: Blackwell, 1986: 89–114.
13. Bowsher w.G., Shah P.J.R., Costello A.J., Tiptaft R.C., Paris A.M.I., Blandy J.P. A critical appraisal of the Boari flap. *Brit. J. Urol.* 1982; **54:** 682–5.
14. Ehrlich R.M., Skinner D.G. Complications of transuretero-ureterostomy. *J. Urol.* 1975; **113:** 467–73.
15. Smith I.B., Smith J.C. Transureteroureterostomy: British experience. *Brit. J. Urol.* 1975; **47:** 519–00.
16. Walters W. Omental flap in the transperitoneal repair of recurring vesicovaginal fistulas. *Surg. Gynec. Obstet.* 1937; **64:** 74–00.

22

Injuries from bandages, splints, plasters and tourniquets

P.G. Stableforth, FRCS

Poorly applied tourniquets, splints, bandages or plasters continue to cause permanent limb damage with pain, functional disability and handicap. Claims for negligence in such circumstances are often successful.[1] Damage may be caused in three ways:

1. Any tightly and unevenly applied, or poorly padded, device may produce skin and subcutaneous necrosis over bone or tendon prominences.
2. Any encircling device may cause local pressure damage to underlying tissues.
3. Least commonly, more distal muscle and nerve ischaemia with fibrosis or necrosis may follow prolonged compression of the feeding vessels, or may arise within a closed fascial compartment from the soft tissue hyperaemia and swelling of tourniquet release.

In injured patients, soft tissue damage caused by trauma, whether caused externally by compression or internally by fracture or dislocation, may be increased by excessive local pressure or by inappropriate circumferential limb compression.[1,2]

Tourniquets

A properly applied and inflated tourniquet will stop blood from entering the limb through the vessels lying exposed within the soft tissue. If the band is applied to the proximal part of the limb, blood will still flow through interosseous vessels and through collaterals at the elbow or knee, and will slowly congest the distal part of the limb.

Whilst prolonged tourniquet ischaemia will cause distal deep tissue fibrosis or necrosis, most clinical problems are caused by local damage to the nerves and to other soft tissues under a cuff of inappropriate size, from its careless application, or from too high an inflation pressure.[3-7]

Physiological results of tourniquet ischaemia

Cellular swelling, metabolic acidosis, increased capillary permeability and a rise in interstitial fluid volume occur within 15 minutes. The changes become progressively more severe with time, but are full reversed in previously healthy tissues on tourniquet release after up to 150 minutes of total ischaemia. In ischaemia, nerve function is lost before muscle function but muscle necrosis precedes nerve death.

Venous congestion, tissue damage from trauma or previous tourniquet application, partial tissue ischaemia from previous trauma or radiotherapy, all increase susceptibility to ischaemia. Tissues in patients with atherosclerosis, diabetes or rheumatoid disease may be damaged more rapidly.[7] Tissues in a cooled limb can withstand longer periods of ischaemia before undergoing structural change.[8,9]

After tourniquet release there is a reactive hyperaemia with limb swelling which reaches a peak after 5 minutes. If the circulation is restored after 30 minutes the metabolic and structural changes are reversed in 5 minutes, after 90 minutes of ischaemia recovery may take up to 15 minutes, and after 240 minutes a full 40 minutes is required for recovery.[10-13]

The use of a tourniquet does not seem to alter the incidence of postoperative deep venous thrombosis.[14] In patients with sickle cell disease tourniquet ischaemia may provoke a haemolytic crisis.

Exsanguination

Simple elevation of the limb for two or three minutes will drain most of the venous blood, and cause arteriolar constriction.[15]

Exsanguination by an Esmarch bandage or Rhys Davis device causes systemic changes. In an adult the 500–750 ml of blood squeezed from the leg into the general circulation (some 8–10 per cent of the blood volume) produces a temporary rise in the central venous pressure, and in an emaciated patient or one with myocardial ischaemia or strain this may lead to heart failure.[16]

Fatal pulmonary embolism from dislodged venous thrombus has followed both limb exsanguination and tourniquet application in patients previously bed-fast or previously limb-immobilized in plaster.[17-19] Septicaemia or tumour embolism may follow exsanguination of an infected or tumour-bearing limb, and in these clinical situations the limb should be drained by elevation and not exsanguinated by pressure.

Correct tourniquet application

A pneumatic tourniquet[20] with a pressure monitor should be used to provide a 'bloodless' field for surgical or anaesthetic procedures on the limbs. A 'double cuff' tourniquet is available for regional intravenous blocks, allowing anaesthesia of tissues under the cuff and thus increasing patient comfort. There is a range of cuff widths and lengths.

The Esmarch rubber bandage is very rarely needed, and then only in an emergency to control life-threatening bleeding. *A patient with the device applied must never be left unattended.*

The cuff should only be applied snugly around the proximal part of the limb over a smooth layer of wood-wool or similar padding, and once secured should not then be 'adjusted' or twisted round the limb as the padding can become ridged or the underlying soft tissues stretched or distorted, increasing the chance of pressure damage.

Burns may follow the use of diathermy if the padding becomes wetted by an alcohol-containing skin preparation solution; they can usually be avoided with careful skin preparation and occlusion of the tourniquet and padding with waterproof strapping.

The cuff with its 'tail' should allow at least 12.5 cm overlap, and should ideally encircle the limb twice to prevent slippage after inflation. If slippage with premature tourniquet release would be dangerous (e.g. in regional IV anaesthesia or cytotoxin administration) the tail should be secured by a clip or Velcro fastener and further secured with adhesive strapping.

The broader the cuff the lower the inflation pressure needed to exclude blood from the limb. Many adult cuffs in general use are 9 or 9.5 cm wide and need to be inflated to at least 100 mmHg above systolic blood pressure, or more ideally 50 mmHg above systolic in the upper limb, and twice the systolic pressure in the lower limb.[21] With the wider 12.5 cm cuff inflation needs to be little above mean arterial pressure to prevent blood inflow, though an overpressure of 35 mmHg in the upper limb or 125 mmHg in the lower limb is advised for clinical use.[22,23] In thin limbs, overpressure can be reduced, and on the smaller limbs of children a 60 mm cuff is adequate.

As monitoring gauge faults are a frequently reported cause of cuff overinflation with soft tissue damage,[3,24–26] the gauge should be checked weekly for accuracy against a mercury manometer. Electronic sensors that warn of, or prevent, overinflation are now available with many systems.[27]

If a procedure has taken 60 minutes and a bloodless field is still required, surgery should be interrupted, the wound compressed with moist packs, the limb elevated and the cuff released for at least 10 minutes. The cuff is then re-inflated and the limb lowered and a further 60 minutes of limb ischaemia is safe. Experimental studies have shown that full recovery can follow four hours of tourniquet ischaemia.[10]

Digital tourniquets. A rubber band stretched firmly and secured around the base of the digit after digital nerve anaesthesia will provide a satisfactory field for short surgical procedures, although the band is usually tightened excessively.[28–30] The finger of a rubber glove, or a finger cot rolled up the digit, is an alternative, but must always be 'marked' with a clip so that it is not forgotten under a dressing. Total digital nerve block can be induced with 1.5–2 ml of 1% local anaesthetic. Large fluid volumes or adrenalin-containing solutions may cause digital gangrene and should never be used.

Tourniquet complications

Tourniquet 'palsy'

This variable mixture of motor-sensory and occasional autonomic dysfunction is reported to follow 1 in 8000 tourniquet applications.[31] The arm is more commonly affected (though this may merely reflect the more frequent use of the arm tourniquet). Fifty per cent of lesions affect all of the nerves of the limb; the radial nerve is the most frequently and the musculocutaneous nerve the most rarely damaged.[32] The motor component is the most important, the sensory disturbance is usually relatively minor, and autonomic damage with causalgia and disturbance of sweating are rare.

The clinical picture varies from a patchy and transient paralysis with full recovery over a few days, to an initially more complete motor loss and patchy sensory disturbance with full recovery over 3–9 months; clinically important permanent impairment is rare. Careful examination of patients in whom recovery seems to be complete may show residual oedema, minor colour change, patchy sensory disturbance, weakness and stiffness from muscle and nerve fibrosis.[33] Such a limb is more susceptible to compression and ischaemia from further tourniquet application or trauma.

Distal ischaemia

Prolonged tourniquet ischaemia may lead to gangrene. This occurs most commonly when a finger band is hidden under a dressing and forgotten, or may follow the use of an adrenalin-containing local anaesthetic solution for digital block.

Less severe ischaemia may affect the whole distal limb, or affect all the structures within a fascial compartment in the forearm or lower leg. There may be rest pain, with pain on passive stretching of all muscles within the space, and a more patchy distal paralysis with sensory disturbances from damage to any nerves that traverse the space.[2]

The symptoms and signs may be apparent early or the onset may be delayed for a few minutes to a few hours, as the reactive hyperaemia of tourniquet release causes circulation compromise from raised compartment pressure.

Management of complications

Tourniquet 'palsy'

There is no evidence that the speed or extent of recovery from tourniquet palsy can be altered by later local measures, though perhaps perineural neurolysis may prove to be valuable. Neuropraxia will recover within hours, axontmesis will recover following myelin degeneration and later axonal growth over many weeks, whilst any neural and perineural fibrosis from compression ischaemia will slow and may jeopardize full neurological recovery.

Insensible skin must be protected from cuts or blows, from burns and from pressure sores, and oedema avoided when possible by support bandaging and limb elevation. Splintage may prevent overstretching of affected joints, though they should ideally be put through a full range of movements at least twice a day to maintain mobility. Muscle atrophy is rapid, though arguably slowed by repeated galvanic stimulation; degeneration though inevitable is delayed if muscle stretch tears and soft tissue oedema are carefully avoided.

As recovery starts, range-of-movement and muscle-stretching and strengthening exercises are commenced.

Distal ischaemia

Limb gangrene is usually treated by amputation. Very rarely, sympathetic block or fasciotomy may limit tissue death, but these need to be performed very early to be of use.

Although there are differences between the closed compartment ischaemia seen after tourniquet mishap and Volkmann's contracture,[34] the principles of management are similar.

Open fasciotomy to decompress all involved compartments may avert or limit tissue damage; muscle rest pain, pain on passive muscle stretching, distal numbness or paraesthesia, or a compartment pressure over 50 mmH$_2$O and probably over 40 mmH$_2$O, should lead to open decompressive fasciotomy.[35]

At its mildest, established ischaemic fibrosis is limited to the deep flexor and intrinsic hand and foot muscles. Stretching by dynamic splintage and an exercise programme may suffice, though tighter contractures may require a musculotendinous lengthening or distal slide of the common muscle origins,[36] or an intrinsic release at their wing insertions into the extensor tendon. In a growing child such surgery may need to be repeated.[37]

With severe ischaemia both superficial and deep muscles are affected and nerve function is disturbed by neural and perineural fibrosis. Musculotendinous lengthening or distal slide may need to be combined with neurolysis, or where possible transfer of the nerve to a more vascular bed. Totally necrotic muscle should be excised to avoid irretrievable joint stiffness, and later tendon transfer may restore some function, though impaired sensation may limit useful recovery.[38]

Plaster of Paris and synthetic casts

Unprotected skin under a cast is always vulnerable to damage; anaesthetic, ischaemic or adherent skin is particularly at risk.

Pressure from a poorly placed cast edge may cause nerve damage (the radial and common peroneal nerves are the most commonly injured); inadequate padding or careless moulding of a cast may lead to skin marking or necrosis over the bony prominences (iliac crest, medial epicondyle and ulnar styloid, fibular head and lateral malleolus) or over the tendo-achillis or other unshielded tendon.

More general limb compression with vascular compromise may occur under a cast following reactionary swelling after fracture, or from the hyperaemia of tourniquet release, or may more rarely follow deep venous thrombosis. If a limb tourniquet has been applied for surgery it is advisable to delay plaster of Paris cast application for a full five minutes after tourniquet deflation to allow the hyperaemic swelling to develop.[39]

Any encircling cast, dressing or bandage applied to a limb shortly after injury, after closed manipulation or surgery, should be split end-to-end and down to skin to allow for reactionary swelling and thus avoid the need for urgent removal of a damp plaster encircling a swollen and painful limb.[40] A 'backslab' or incomplete cast secured with a firm bandage is of course just as likely to compress the limb, but is easier to release in an emergency.

Tissues under the newer, quick-setting resin casts need to be padded with even greater care as the casts are less easily moulded and their edges are rough and hard; direct contact by curing resin on the skin may occasionally cause redness or blistering.

Wherever possible, a cast should be split or removed whilst the patient is awake so that skin laceration by oscillating saw, scissors, shears or knife can be avoided. Particular care is needed if the cast has been applied over anaesthetic skin.

Splints and bandages

Any rigid, non-contoured splint or brace can cause pressure damage to unprotected and vulnerable skin, or damage the deep structures; whilst the newer heat-mouldable conforming materials are less dangerous than wood or metal, they are often non-porous and may produce troublesome skin maceration and soreness from sweat unless applied over a suitable pad or sock of absorbent material.

An inexpertly applied tight bandage may 'ridge' or press to cause skin and subcutaneous necrosis over a bone or tendinous prominence, though more commonly the bandage is applied too loosely and slips to impact further down the limb, compressing and partially strangulating the more distal structures.

It must be emphasized that a surgical wound or a reduced fracture does not produce rest pain; a patient with rest pain under any encircling device should never be given analgesics until the limb has been carefully examined for signs of ischaemia or local pressure. The safe limb has pink digits and a brisk capillary return after pressure, there is normal feeling, the muscles can be braced against resistance and passive stretching does not provoke muscle belly pain.[41] It should be possible to move an encircling cast gently on the limb without soreness over prominences.

Management of complications

Compression

If there is sluggish capillary return after pressure release, if there is distal swelling or congestion, the limb should be elevated above heart level for 15–30 minutes. If the swelling or congestion persists, or if there is muscle pain at rest or pain that is induced by passive muscle stretching, the cast, bandage, dressings and anything else encircling the part must be split immediately end-to-end, and down to the skin, to release compression.[40,42]

Should the symptoms and signs still persist, then an open fasciotomy to decompress the relevant compartment or compartments is needed urgently.[39] A compartment monitor probe will probably show a pressure in excess of 40 mmH$_2$O.

The wound is packed open and firmly dressed, bandaged and splinted as needed; the part is elevated. Although delayed primary suture is occasionally possible at 3–5 days, partial skin closure with split skin grafting of the remaining defect is more usually necessary.

Established muscle ischaemia is treated as described above.

Pressure necrosis

Localized pain under a cast, splint or bandage demands immediate inspection of the painful area.

Skin marking with local tenderness and hypersensitivity usually settles once pressure is relieved, and a new, carefully padded cast (etc.) can be applied.

A small area of skin and subcutaneous necrosis (less than 1 cm across) will usually demarcate, separate and heal under an occlusive dressing once pressure has been relieved, though separation may be speeded by regular moist dressings.

The separation and healing of larger superficial sloughs and those involving deeper structures may be very slow and may be complicated by secondary infection. Formal surgical excision of necrotic material will speed the process, and the defect can then be allowed to heal naturally, or can be closed by an immediate local rotation flap or by free skin grafting once granulation has occurred.

References

1. Eadie D.G.A. Post-traumatic ischaemia. *J. Bone Joint Surg.* 1979; **61B:** 265–6.
2. Sarokhan A., Eaton P.G. Volkmann's ischaemia. *J. Hand Surg.* 1983; **8:** 806–9.
3. Bruner J. Tourniquet time, pressure and temperature factors for safe surgery of the hand. *The Hand.* 1970; **2:** 32–42.
4. Ochoa J., Fowler T.J., Gilliat R.W. Anatomical changes in peripheral nerves compressed by a pneumatic tourniquet. *J. Anatomy.* 1972; **113:** 433–55.
5. Fowler T.J., Danta G., Gilliat R.W. Recovery of nerve conduction after a pneumatic tourniquet. *J. Neurol. Neurosurg. Psych.* 1972; **35:** 638–47.
6. Parkes A. Ischaemic effects of external and internal pressure of the upper limb. *The Hand.* 1973; **5:** 105–7.
7. Tubiana R. The use of the tourniquet. In: *The Hand*, vol. II. Philadelphia: W.B. Saunders, 1985: 31–7.
8. Paletta F.X., William V., Ship A.G. Prolonged tourniquet ischaemia in dogs: an experimental study. *J. Bone Joint Surg.* 1960; **42A:** 945–50.
9. Irving G.A., Noakes T.D. The protective role of local hypothermia in tourniquet-induced ischaemia of muscle. *J. Bone Joint Surg.* 1985; **67B:** 297–301.
10. Klenerman L., Biswas M., Hulands G.H., Rhodes A.M. Systemic and local effects of the application of a tourniquet. *J. Bone Joint Surg.* 1980; **62B:** 385–8.
11. Newman R.J. Metabolic changes in muscle due to tourniquet ischaemia. *J. Bone Joint Surg.* 1983; **65B:** 658.
12. Newman R.J. Metabolic effects of tourniquet ischaemia studied by nuclear magnetic resonance spectroscopy. *J. Bone Joint Surg.* 1984; **66B:** 434–40.
13. Sapega A.A., Heppenstall R.B., Chance B. Optimizing tourniquet application and release times in extremity surgery. *J. Bone Joint Surg.* 1985; **67A:** 303–14.
14. Angus P.D., Nakielny R., Goodrum D.T. The pneumatic tourniquet and deep venous thrombosis. *J. Bone Joint Surg.* 1983; **65B:** 336–9.
15. Lister J. *Collected Papers,* vol. 1. Oxford: Clarendon Press, 1909, 196.
16. Sanders R. The tourniquet: instrument or weapon. *The Hand.* 1973; **5:** 119.
17. Austin M. The Esmarch bandage and pulmonary embolism. *J. Bone Joint Surg.* 1963; **45B:** 384–5.
18. Pollard B.J., Lovelock H.A., Jones R.M. Fatal pulmonary embolism secondary to limb exsanguination. *Anaesthesiology.* 1983; **58:** 373–4.
19. Hoffman A.A., Wyatt R.W.B. Fatal pulmonary embolism following tourniquet inflation. *J. Bone Joint Surg.* 1985; **67A:** 633–4.
20. Cushing H. Pneumatic tourniquets: with special reference to its use in craniotomies. *Med. News* NY. 1904; **84:** 557–80.

21. Klenerman L. Tourniquet paralysis. *J. Bone Joint Surg.* 1983; **65B:** 374–5.
22. Newman R.J., Munhead A. A safe and effective low-pressure tourniquet. *J. Bone Joint Surg.* 1986; **68B:** 625–8.
23. Moore M., Garfin S.R., Hargens A.R. Wide tourniquets eliminate blood flow at lower inflation pressure. *J. Hand Surg.* 1987; **12A:** 1006–11.
24. Flatt A.E. Tourniquet time in hand surgery. *Arch. Surg.* 1972; **104:** 190–6.
25. Calderwood J.W., Dickie W.R. Tourniquet paresis complicating tendon grafting. *The Hand.* 1972; **4:** 53.
26. Durkin M.A.P., Crabtree S.D. Hazards of pneumatic tourniquet application. *Proc. R. Soc. Med.* 1982; **75:** 658–60.
27. Wheeler D.K., Lipscombe P.R. A safety device for a pneumatic tourniquet. *J. Bone Joint Surg.* 1964; **46A:** 870.
28. Salem M.Z. Simple finger tourniquet. *Brit. Med. J.* 1973; **1:** 779.
29. Lubahn J.D., Koenerman J., Kosar K. The digital tourniquet: how safe is it? *J. Hand Surg.* 1985; **10A:** 664–9.
30. Hixson F.P., Shafinoff B.B., Werner F.W., Palmer A.K. Digital tourniquets: a pressure study with clinical relevance. *J. Hand Surg.* 1986; **11A:** 865–8.
31. Middleton R.W., Vanian J.P. Tourniquet paralysis. *Aust. NZ J. Surg.* 1974; **44:** 124–8.
32. Sunderland S. *Nerves and Nerve Injuries.* Edinburgh: E.S. Livingstone, 1968.
33. Bruner J. Safety factors in the use of the pneumatic tourniquet for haemostasis in surgery of the hand. *J. Bone Joint Surg.* 1951; **33A:** 221–4.
34. Tsuge K. Treatment of established Volkmann's contracture. *J. Bone Joint Surg.* 1975; **57A:** 925–9.
35. Mubarak S.J., Owen S.J., Hargens A.R., Garretts L.P., Akeson W.H. Acute compartment syndromes diagnosis and treatment with the aid of a Wick catheter. *J. Bone Joint Surg.* 1978; **60A:** 1091–5.
36. Page C.M. Operation for the relief of flexion contracture in the forearm. *J. Bone Joint. Surg.* 1923; **5:** 233–4.
37. Tajima T. Post-traumatic hand contractures: Volkmann's contracture. *J. Hand Surg.* 1988; **13B:** 118.
38. Seddon H.J. Volkmann's contracture: treatment by excision of the infarct. *J. Bone Joint Surg.* 1956; **38B:** 152–74.
39. Ayoub M.H., Bennett G.C. A study of cutaneous and intracompartmental limb pressures associated with the combined use of tourniquets and plaster casts. *J. Bone Joint Surg.* 1986; **68B:** 497.
40. Bingold A.C. On splinting plasters. *J. Bone Joint Surg.* 1979; **61B:** 293–5.
41. Holden C.E.A. The pathology and prevention of Volkmann's ischaemic contracture. *J. Bone Joint Surg.* 1979; **61B:** 296–300.
42. Watson-Jones R. *Fractures and Joint Injuries.* Edinburgh: E.S. Livingstone, 1955.

23

The saphenofemoral junction: damage and bleeding

Georges Jantet, MB, FRCS

The saphenofemoral junction (SFJ) is the point where the long saphenous vein passes through the saphenous opening (fossa ovalis) in the groin and ends in the femoral vein.

As will be seen, two of the main causes of difficulties or accidents occurring during operations on the SFJ can be attributed to a wrongly sited incision (usually too low) or to a lack of appreciation of the normal anatomy and its variants. Anatomical considerations are therefore relevant.

Anatomy of the SFJ

Classically the SFJ is situated about 3 cm below the inguinal ligament.[1]

The *surface marking* of the centre of the saphenous opening is given as nearly 4 cm below and lateral to the pubic tubercle (pubic spine),[1] while the surface marking of the SFJ is given as 2.5–3.5 cm below and lateral to the pubic tubercle.[2] It must be remembered that the oblique skin crease at the groin, termed the inguinal fold, is not a reliable landmark as its position in relation to the inguinal ligament varies with the build of the patient. While it corresponds fairly accurately to the inguinal ligament in thin patients, it may lie as much as 5 cm below it in obese patients. Therefore it cannot be used as a landmark for all patients. In the thin or average patient lying flat on the operating table with a 10–20° head-down tilt and the legs abducted, the pulsating femoral artery is easily defined, the inguinal ligament can be traced (a line slightly curved downwards running from the anterior superior iliac spine to the pubic symphysis), and often it can be palpated. The femoral vein lies medial to the femoral artery and the SFJ 3 cm below the inguinal ligament along the femoral vein. There is nearly always a secondary skin crease just above that level along which an obliquely running incision, centred on the femoral vein, can be made.[3] This gives a better cosmetic end-result than a lower incision as it is in a skin crease and very often in the hair line. It is above the SFJ, but this presents no problem as with slight retraction (Travers self-retaining retractor and small Langenbeck's retractor held by an assistant), the wound can be 'moved' into different positions. It is much safer to site the incision slightly too high than too low in relation to the SFJ. This incision can easily be extended medially or laterally to improve access and still remain in a skin crease and can, of course, be extended medially and downwards in case of difficulties to convert it to a 'hockey-stick' incision.[2,4] If the patient is obese, or the femoral artery not palpable, an incision centred 2.5–3.0 cm below and lateral to the pubic tubercle and parallel to the inguinal ligament will expose the upper part of the SFJ very satisfactorily, but will result in a less cosmetically satisfactory scar.

The termination of the long saphenous vein, its tributaries and adjacent blood vessels

Correct identification of the anatomy is essential *before* any forceps or ligatures are applied or any vessel divided, to avoid any damage. Damage to, and bleeding from, any of the vessels mentioned below can occur.

The *long saphenous vein* runs vertically upwards, deep to the superficial fascia and enters the saphenous opening. It is encased in a thin prolongation of the femoral sheath which must be opened to define it and the SFJ clearly. In patients with marked saphenofemoral incompetence, the termination of the long saphenous vein can be very large but the vein itself remains straight and it can therefore be mistaken for the femoral vein; dissection may be difficult if it is the site, at its termination, of a saphena varix which may be very friable.

Classically there are six *tributaries* of the long saphenous vein at its termination, but it must be stressed that variants are frequent. *All the tributaries must be sought and divided or ligated in a properly conducted Trendelenburg operation.* A good description of the anatomy of the long saphenous vein termination and its variants is given by Furderer *et al*.[5]

1. The *anterolateral vein* runs obliquely upwards and medially in the subcutaneous tissues from the anterolateral surface of the thigh and joins the long saphenous vein at a variable point in its terminal few centimetres. It can be very tortuous and varicose.

2. The *posteromedial vein* runs obliquely upwards and laterally deep to the superficial fascia from the posteromedial surface of the thigh, and drains either in the terminal few centimetres of the long saphenous vein or at the SFJ, or, occasionally, into the medial aspect of the femoral vein at the level of the SFJ. It too can be very tortuous and varicose lower down the leg, but at its termination it is fairly straight and may be mistaken for the long saphenous vein.

3. The *superficial external pudendal vein* runs transversely in the subcutaneous tissues from the external genitalia and perineum to drain into the medial aspect of the long saphenous vein at its termination.

4. The *deep external pudendal vein* also runs transversely and medially, but in a deeper plane, and ends either just at the medial aspect of the SFJ or in the femoral vein itself deep in the saphenous opening. It must be deliberately sought and ligated by gentle lateral retraction of the SFJ and femoral vein to prevent persistent or recurrent varicosities of the external genitalia. It can be enlarged and very friable.

5. The *superficial epigastric vein* runs vertically downwards from the anterior abdominal wall in the subcutaneous tissues and drains into the termination of the long saphenous vein.

6. The *superficial circumflex iliac vein* runs obliquely downwards and medially just below the inguinal ligament and joins the termination of the long saphenous

vein close to the superficial epigastric vein or, sometimes, by a common trunk with it. It and the superficial epigastric vein run within the same fascial sheath as the long saphenous vein and may therefore be missed if not properly exposed as they lie 'plastered' on the termination of the long saphenous vein within the sheath. This is particularly liable to happen if the original incision is sited too low. As a consequence the ligature on the SFJ, instead of being flush on the femoral vein, is placed below these missed tributaries and persistent or recurrent varicose veins result.

Rarely, there may be a *duplication of the long saphenous vein* which can cause difficulties in identification and may be mistaken for the femoral vein or, more seriously, vice versa. However, it lies in a more superficial plane than the femoral vein although deep to the superficial fascia. Correct identification of all the vessels at the SFJ, before any damaging procedure is carried out, is the only way to prevent a serious accident.

The *femoral vein* runs vertically deep to the saphenous opening just medial to the femoral artery and encased in the femoral sheath. On the operating table it may be collapsed and mistaken for fibrous tissue. It is essential that it be unequivocally identified by exposing its anterior surface for 1 cm above and 1 cm below the SFJ, thereby confirming its identity, and also by exposing its medial and lateral aspects to secure any tributaries running into it at those sites.

Similarly, the *femoral artery* must be identified although it need not be exposed.

Unequivocal identification of the femoral vein and artery is the key to a safe flush saphenofemoral ligature and stripping or avulsion of the long saphenous vein or tributaries.

This is particularly important in thin patients in whom the femoral vessels may lie very superficially as they have been mistaken for the long saphenous vein with disastrous results.[6-8]

Rarely the *profunda femoris artery* arises high (just below the inguinal ligament) and may run downwards and medially across the femoral vein just above or below the SFJ, where it may cause confusion and may be injured.[1,2]

The *superficial and deep external pudendal arteries* are small arteries which arise from the medial aspect of the femoral artery and run medially across the femoral vein in the region of the SFJ. The *superficial* artery usually runs above the SFJ and is not encountered, but it can cross medially lower down, anterior to the long saphenous vein at its termination, and may be injured. The *deep* artery runs medially, posterior to the termination of the long saphenous vein, in the inferior border of the saphenous opening. The interest of these arteries is that they can be damaged and lead to mild arterial bleeding but, more importantly, the deep artery serves as a very helpful landmark to the SFJ as it is the only transversely running artery in that region and it runs most commonly behind, but sometimes in front of, the termination of the long saphenous vein. They should therefore be preserved as they may be particularly helpful landmarks if second operations have to be carried out on the SFJ for inadequate flush ligation, in which situation the operation may be difficult because of local recurrent friable varicose veins and scar tissue from the previous operation. Furthermore, cases have been reported of sexual impotence in the male following ligature of an external pudendal artery.[9]

Causes of damage and bleeding

Inexperience

With good basic surgical training, varicose vein surgery is usually fairly straightforward. However, errors can lead to serious trouble, and unfortunately this type of surgery is sometimes left in the hands of inexperienced surgeons who are unsupervised and left to their own resources.

An inexperienced operator may run into difficulties from simple lack of knowledge of local anatomy and its variants, from the failure to appreciate that an error has been committed, and from the failure of calling for assistance. Thus, an error, even a serious one, may occur, and the operator may not be aware of this; or perhaps this error is discovered only when it is too late for any effective corrective procedures to be carried out. On the other hand the error may be recognized, but the operator may attempt corrective surgery for which he or she does not have the necessary experience. With appropriate training, this type of surgery can perfectly legitimately be left in the hands of surgeons in training; but it must be emphasized to them that they must request assistance of someone competent to deal with the situation if there is any difficulty and not to attempt to repair any error, as the evidence is that it is at this stage that the real damage is done. It is therefore incumbent upon any surgeon delegating this type of surgery to ensure that the operator is properly trained in this type of surgery, knows when to call for help and knows where to obtain that help. Even a trained and experienced general surgeon may need the help of a vascular surgeon if inexperienced in the repair of damaged large vessels, remembering that the outcome of failure to prevent or correct an accident may be the loss of the limb.

Failure to appreciate the true state of local anatomy

Difficulties may also arise in patients with 'abnormal' anatomy, when sometimes serious errors in identification can be made. Sound knowledge of the normal anatomy and its variants is therefore essential.

Inadequate exposure

An incision which is too small or wrongly sited may lead to difficulties in dissecting out the anatomy and errors in identification. Forceful retraction may well lead to tearing of a major vessel or to serious bleeding.

Inadequate lighting

Surgery in the groin may be combined with further surgery down the leg and there may not be adequate lighting to cover both areas at the same time. It is a truism to state that proper lighting is essential.

Lack of assistance

It is difficult to carry out safe surgery in the SFJ region without some assistance for retraction, ligatures, etc. Assistance becomes mandatory if the operator runs into any difficulty.

Re-operations for recurrent or persistent saphenofemoral incompetence.

Re-operating in the groin in these conditions may be very difficult because of local recurrent varicose veins which are usually very friable and because of scar tissue from previous operations. Usually the original incision was wrongly sited and nearly always it was too low. The solution is to operate through previously uninvolved tissues away from all the scar tissue and recurrent varices. The best course is to approach the femoral vein from above and medially. This is obtained through a high incision above the original incision, running close to the inguinal ligament centred on the femoral vein and curved downwards at the medial end; that is, a high 'hockey-stick' incision.[2,4] Nevertheless these are difficult and time-consuming operations which may be associated with quite severe venous bleeding and with an increased likelihood of accidental damage to other blood vessels. It is not surgery to be entrusted to the inexperienced.

Damage and bleeding

Illustrative case

Before discussing damage and bleeding to specific structures in the SFJ region, the description of an illustrative case may be helpful. Experience from medico-legal cases suggests the following situation is fairly representative of the commonest accidents. A surgeon in training,† assisted by the scrub nurse, wishing to carry out a saphenofemoral ligature (Trendelenburg operation), is misled by the patient's inguinal fold and sites his incision lower than it should be; very often the incision is also too small. In an attempt to find the SFJ after some dissection, forceful retraction is carried out with resultant tearing of a vein and a sudden surge of venous blood. If the bleeding arises from a small venous tributary, the situation is usually easily corrected; but if there is damage to the femoral vein owing to a tributary, or the long saphenous vein itself, being torn off the femoral vein, a potentially more serious situation results. Serious trouble can occur if the operator blindly applies haemostats to the bleeding spot. At the best this will be on the femoral vein itself, which thus risks being crushed, ligated or transfixed in the subsequent ligature or suture. This usually fails to control the bleeding completely and a further haemostat is then applied more deeply.

†It must be emphasized that surgeons in training are not the only ones who run into difficulties. Some of the more spectacular accidents have occurred in experienced hands, but the common situation described here is usually linked with inexperience.

This may cause further damage to the femoral vein and may also inadvertently involve the femoral artery. The subsequent further transfixing suture is therefore very likely to include the femoral artery or to result in bleeding from the femoral artery when the haemostat is removed. Further haemorrhage is then unfortunately dealt with by deep sutures which may involve the femoral artery or vein partially or completely until the haemorrhage is 'controlled'. This will result in thrombosis in these vessels very rapidly or during the following hours. If, at this stage, the operator seeks further help the situation may still be relieved, but tragedy may occur if the situation is not recognized.

In the recorded or known cases of damage occurring during intervention at the SFJ, the two important structures endangered have been the femoral vein and the femoral artery. Damage can, of course, occur to venous tributaries or arterial branches of these vessels, but this is of much less serious consequence. The author is not aware, in this context, of any cases (reported or not) of damage to the femoral nerve which is more laterally situated. Such damage has been reported during other operations in the groin or on the hip and during angiography via the groin, but these are outside the scope of this chapter. The saphenous nerve which arises from the femoral nerve in the groin is more likely to be damaged below the knee during stripping of the long saphenous vein below the knee.

Damage to, and bleeding from, the femoral vessels can occur from haemostats, scissors, scalpel and retractors during dissection, from sutures and ligatures, or even from stripping. Thus they can be crushed, tied, torn or stripped. Inexperience, forceful retraction, rough dissection, fibrosis and recurrent varices, failure to recognize 'abnormal' anatomy, are the main causes.

Vessels 'crushed'

The femoral vein or artery may be partially or completely crushed by haemostats applied to control bleeding. Fine mosquito forceps applied to a small tear in these vessels may be perfectly safe, but the use of larger haemostats is inappropriate. Such haemostats applied blindly to control bleeding and inadvertently applied on to the femoral vein or artery may result in the subsequent thrombosis of the vein, depending on the amount of damage caused. Prophylactic postoperative anticoagulation may be indicated, or even a formal repair of the vein. A crushed femoral artery may result in intimal damage with subsequent occlusion of the artery and loss of pulsation. This situation may be mistaken for spasm of the artery and misguided attempts made to overcome this. Intimal damage requires urgent exploration of the artery through an arteriotomy with a repair of the damaged intima and possibly a venous angioplasty. A severely crushed femoral artery may require excision of the crushed segment and reconstruction with an interposition vein graft.

Vessels 'tied'

Partial or complete ligature of the femoral vein will probably lead to thrombosis of the femoral vein. If the accident is spotted immediately, before thrombosis has occurred, it is safe to remove the ligature; but if there is any thrombosis, the vessel should remain ligated because of the danger of pulmonary embolism. Similar damage to the femoral artery may produce acute ischaemia of the limb. If spotted immediately the ligature can be removed, but the state of the femoral and distal pulses should be checked immediately and regularly during the postoperative period. In many cases the fact that the femoral artery has been ligated is unsuspected until the pale appearance of the limb is noted during the postoperative period.[7] Reconstruction of the damaged artery may require preliminary angiography and resection of the damaged segment with grafting procedures.

Vessels 'torn'

Tearing of the femoral vein itself, by direct trauma or by avulsion of one of its tributaries, will result in copious venous bleeding obscuring the whole operative field. Serious venous bleeding has occurred when the long saphenous vein has been stripped either from above or from below before dividing the long saphenous vein, which has thus been torn off the femoral vein at the SFJ. In this situation the cause of the bleeding must be accurately located. This is obtained by packing the operative field and lowering the head of the table 20° if not already done. An inexperienced surgeon should limit his activities to that and do no more except request more experienced help. Adequate exposure must be ensured and, if necessary, the incision extended in curved fashion downwards and medially as described above. After packing for a few minutes the venous bleeding is usually sufficiently reduced to allow identification of the source. Local pressure on the torn area by means of a swab on a holder will produce a dry field and thus allow full exposure of the femoral vein above and below the damaged area. The pressure is then transferred to the exposed vein above and below the damaged area and the damaged vein can then be repaired, under direct vision, with a vascular suture—the key to carrying this out successfully is a dry field. On no account should haemostats be applied blindly or sutures inserted blindly.

Arterial bleeding from a tear in the femoral artery is easily recognized. Local swab or finger pressure produces temporary control while adequate help is obtained. The artery should be adequately exposed by dissection and the appropriate vascular haemostatic clamp applied. Repair may be limited to a simple suture, but more extensive damage will necessitate local resection and grafting or venous patching.

During dissection, the deep pudendal artery, skirting around the saphenous opening, can be damaged, but the resultant bleeding is usually slight and easily controlled.

Vessels 'transected'

The femoral vein or artery can be completely divided. This is the result of incorrect or inadequate identification of the anatomy and can occur particularly if the anatomy is 'abnormal'. This accident has been described as occurring even in experienced hands.[7,10]

In reported cases of this accident,[10] the femoral vein has been mistaken for the long saphenous vein, and the divided proximal end ligated thinking it was the saphenous stump while the distal end has been left open; bleeding from the open end has then been controlled by firm bandaging of the leg. In the reported cases, the accident was not discovered until the wound was re-explored because of continued postoperative bleeding. In experienced hands an attempt may be made to reconstruct the divided femoral vein.

The femoral artery may be partially or completely divided, and the diagnosis should be obvious from the character of the bleeding. Temporary control can be obtained by pressure proximal to the damaged area. Repair of this arterial injury will be by means of a venous patch, or end-to-end anastomosis or reconstruction via an interposed venous (or synthetic) graft, depending on whether the artery has been partially or completely divided, and whether the cut is clean or ragged. If the correct diagnosis is not made and the divided ends are simply ligated, acute ischaemia of the leg will result.

It is imperative that in any case of difficulty in the SFJ region the presence of the femoral and distal arterial pulses is confirmed at the end of the operation and regularly postoperatively. Difficulties may occur in older patients who may have some absent pulses. It is therefore good practice to record the state of all the leg pulses preoperatively.

To prevent these serious accidents, no vessel should be cut or divided until it has been positively identified.

Vessels 'stripped'

Inadvertent stripping of the femoral vein or artery is well-documented.[7,11,12]

The femoral vein, mistaken for the long saphenous vein, has been stripped. While simple ligation of the femoral vein may have surprisingly few postoperative sequelae, stripping of the vein will result in marked bleeding during the stripping, which can, however, be controlled by bandaging. Reconstruction is not possible and the leg will eventually show the same changes as after a deep vein thrombosis.

The remarkable feature of the cases where the femoral artery has been stripped is that in most of them there was surprisingly little, if any, bleeding at the time of the stripping. Thus the accident was not recognized at the time of the operation and, in the reported cases, the correct diagnosis was not established until several hours or even days later when obvious ischaemia had developed. It is therefore important to note that *lack of bleeding at the time of the operation does not necessarily exclude the possibility that the femoral artery may have been stripped.* Reconstruction following this injury will require complex grafting procedures depending on the length of artery stripped.

Prevention of these very serious accidents to the femoral vessels lies in not introducing any stripper in a vessel until it has been positively identified as the long saphenous vein and the SFJ clearly demonstrated.

Minor bleeding

Bleeding not arising from the femoral vessels themselves can usually be controlled by simple pressure, ligation or bandaging of the leg, but correct identification of the damaged vessel is imperative in order to avoid serious accidents.

During stripping of the long saphenous vein, some venous bleeding occurs from the tract, particularly if a mid-thigh (Hunterian) perforator is present. This can be kept to a minimum by elevating the limb during the stripping, stripping from below upwards, and bandaging from below upwards as the stripping is carried out.

Delayed bleeding

Bleeding from the wound postoperatively may indicate a slipped ligature or bleeding from the tract of the stripped vein. If the ligature on the long saphenous stump slips there may be marked bleeding or a large haematoma. This accident can be completely prevented by not only ligating the saphenous stump flush with the femoral vein at the SFJ, but also by transfixing the distal part of the stump.

Bleeding from the tract of the stripped long saphenous vein is controlled by proper bandaging of the leg.

If local pressure does not control the situation, exploration of the wound will be necessary, the cause of the bleeding accurately identified and dealt with appropriately.

Injection of sclerosant into femoral artery or vein

Some phlebologists advocate obliteration of an incompetent long saphenous vein by injecting sclerosant into the termination of the vein at the groin. This may be safe in experienced hands, but serious complications have been described following inadvertent injection into the femoral vein or into the femoral artery.[7] This technique is best not used except by very experienced phlebologists.

Medico-legal repercussions, and conclusions

Serious complications occurring after what should have been a straightforward operation can well lead to litigation and compensation. It is essential, therefore, to keep accurate records of the operation and of the complications and to discuss any complications frankly with the patient and the relatives.

Serious damage to the structures around the SFJ in the groin can occur from a variety of causes. In the context of the treatment of varicose veins and venous insufficiency, accidental damage is essentially preventable. Inexperience, inadequate surgical exposure and inadequate identification of the various structures are the commonest causes of these accidents. Correct identification of all structures will thus help prevent accidents.

Inexperienced surgeons should be supervised and not left on their own to operate on varicose veins until they can do so safely. In case of difficulties they should seek experienced help and not attempt to correct a situation which may be beyond their capabilities and competence.

A serious injury to the femoral artery does not necessarily lead to bleeding, and when any doubt exists the pulsations of the femoral and distal arteries should be checked.

References

1. Williams P.L., Warwick R.(eds.): *Gray's Anatomy*. London: Churchill Livingstone, 1980.
2. Dodd H., Cockett F.B. *The Pathology and Surgery of the Veins of the Lower Limb*. 2nd edn. London: Churchill Livingstone, 1976.
3. Brunner U. Esthétique en chirurgie des varices en particulier dans la région de l'aine. *Phlébologie*. 1985; **38:** 683–5.
4. Greany M.G., Makin G.S. Operation for saphenofemoral incompetence using medial approach to the saphenofemoral junction. *Brit. J. Surg*. 1985; **72:** 910–11.
5. Furderer C.R., Marescaux J., Pavis d'Escurac X., Stemmer R. Les crosses saphéniennes: anatomie et concepts thérapeutiques. *Phlébologie*. 1986; **39:** 3–14.
6. Natali J., Benhamon A.C. Iatrogenic vascular injuries: a review of 125 cases. *J. Cardiovasc. Surg*. 1979; **20:** 169–76.
7. Benhamon A.C., Natali J. Les accidents des traitements sclérosant et chirurgical des varices des membres inférieurs. *Phlébologie*. 1981; **34:** 41–51.
8. Cockett F.B. Arterial complications during surgery and sclerotherapy of varicose veins. *Phlebology*. 1986; **1:** 3–6.
9. Henriet J.-P. Le confluent veineux saphéno-fémoral et le réseau arteriel honteux externe: données anatomiques et statistiques nouvelles. *Phlébologie*. 1987; **40:** 711–35.
10. Welch G.H., Gilmour D.G., Pollock J.G. Femoral vein division during Trendelenburg operation. *J.R. Coll. Surg. Edinb*. 1985; **30:** 203–4.
11. Eger M., Goleman L., Torok G., Hirsch M. Inadvertent arterial stripping in the lower limb: problems of management. *Surgery*. 1973; **73:** 23–7.
12. Liddicoat J.E., Bekassy S.M., Daniell M.B., De Bakey M.E. Inadvertent femoral artery 'stripping': surgical management. *Surgery*. 1975; **77:** 318–20.

24

Anorectal stenosis

J.D. Hardcastle, MA, MChir, FRCS, FRCP

Anal stenosis following haemorrhoidectomy

This used to be a common problem following the Whitehead operation, in which the entire haemorrhoid-bearing area of the anal canal was excised and the lower edge of the rectal mucosa sutured circumferentially to the skin of the anal canal. In practice primary union was rarely achieved, and patients were left with a circular granulating wound which inevitably led to an anal stricture. As a result of these experiences the Whitehead operation has largely been abandoned in Great Britain.

In patients with multiple or circumferential haemorrhoids, if inadequate mucosal bridges are left between the excised haemorrhoids, subsequent healing of the large granulating wounds may also result in anal stenosis. The ligation excision procedure, the most commonly performed operation for haemorrhoids, has been shown to result in anal stenosis of sufficient degree to prevent the passage of a 2 cm proctoscope in 4 per cent of cases.[1] The submucosal haemorridectomy introduced by Parks[2] was designed to excise the underlying haemorrhoidal tissue but retain as much of the mucosal lining of the anal canal as possible so that no raw areas were left to produce fibrosis and stricture formation. However, Watts et al.[3] found that after submucosal excision the anal wounds invariably separated. The authors noted that the clamp and cautery method left the largest wounds in the anal canal, but in all the cases mucosa regenerated rapidly and healing was complete in six weeks.

In a comparison of the complications associated with a number of difficult types of haemorrhoidectomy, Watts et al.[3] found that 4 per cent developed sufficient narrowing to prevent the passage of an average sized proctoscope, and 8 per cent had palpable fibrosis which was unassociated with difficulty in passing the finger or proctoscope. Stenoses were least common after submucosal excision and most common after the clamp and cautery operation.

In patients with circumferential haemorrhoids it is possible to secure the haemorrhoid tissue from under the mucosal bridge, following which the mucosal flap can be sutured to the internal sphincter. In order to avoid anal stenosis the wounds in the anal canal should be as small as possible and adequate mucosal bridges should be left from which regeneration can take place. After haemorrhoidectomy it is important to assess the anal canal by digital examination in the postoperative period. If some degree of narrowing is found at follow-up examination, it seldom causes symptoms and can be treated by the use of a dilator. Sometimes it is necessary to make the first dilation under general anaesthetic.

Y–V advancement flaps may be used in the treatment of patients with severe mucocutaneous strictures. Gingold and Arvanitis[4] report on the use of this technique in 14 patients with anal stenosis, good results being obtained in all cases.

Anorectal stenosis following perianal sepsis

Patients with fistula-in-ano, particularly in those with a horseshoe abscess in the ischorectal fossa, may require treatment by an extensive laying open procedure. The healing of this wound by granulation tissue and fibrosis will inevitably lead to some degree of anorectal stenosis. This can usually be treated adequately by digital dilatation. Care should, however, be taken not to overdilate these patients as incontinence may result because of their sphincteric damage.

Large granulating wounds can be treated by secondary skin grafting which may expedite healing by three or four weeks and reduce the scarring and stenosis following the procedure. In severe cases new skin can be brought into the area by the use of full-thickness rotation flaps[5] or by a C anoplasty.[6]

Rectal stricture following pelvic irradiation

Following pelvic irradiation, rectal damage may result because of the associated vascular damage and endarteritis which leads to progressive ischaemia, resulting in deep ulceration and eventually fibrosis and stricture formation. The occurrence of radiation-induced stricture is related to the total dose of irradiation, the volume of tissue treated and the interval between fractions. It is most commonly seen in women treated for carcinoma of the cervix by intercavity and external irradiation, and has also been reported following treatment for bladder carcinoma.[7]

The interval between irradiation therapy and the onset of stenotic complications is very variable. A mean time of 60 months was noted by Anseline,[8] but it may occur many years later.

In most cases the degree of stenosis is insufficient to cause major symptoms. However, severe obstruction may occur and a colostomy may be necessary. If a colostomy is to be the final treatment it should be of an end type and situated in the left iliac fossa. If further direct surgical treatment of the stricture is indicated it is important that any anastomosis should be made in non-irradiated tissue.

A coloanal procedure described by Parks et al.[9] achieves these objectives and results in the anastomosis of normal descending colon to the anal canal. This operation is also indicated if the rectal stricture is associated with a rectovaginal fistula. In this operation the rectum is mobilized to the point of fixation to the vagina. No attempt is made to free the diseased bowel from the vagina. The descending colon is divided at a level above the field of radiation. The perineal approach is used to strip the mucosa from the anorectal junction and the colon anastomosed to the anal canal at the level of the dentate line.

A possible alternative to resection has been suggested by Bricker and

Johnston[10] in which the sigmoid colon is patched over a transversely open colotomy at the site of the stricture.

Rectal stricture following colorectal or ileorectal anastomosis

After anterior resection some degree of narrowing at the site of the anastomosis is very common, but the majority usually spontaneously improve from the dilating affect of bowel motions. A severe rectal stricture usually occurs in those patients who have had partial dehiscence of the anastomosis followed by pelvic sepsis. In these patients, especially if treated by a temporary colostomy, spontaneous improvement of the stricture may not occur.

An anastomosis made using a circular staple gun technique is occasionally followed by a stenosis, particularly if the small size cartridge is used and if a leak develops. Strictures following a hand-sutured anastomosis usually undergo spontaneous dilatation unless there has been almost complete breakdown of the anastomosis. Low strictures within reach of the finger may be treated by digital dilatation or by dilatation using Hegars dilators.

Following the successful use of balloon dilatation in the treatment of strictures in the upper gastrointestinal tract, this method has also been applied to rectal strictures.[11] Eleven colorectal strictures and one ileorectal stricture were dilated. The majority of the colorectal strictures followed anastomosis using the EEA staple gun. Balloon-tipped 15–20 mg Gruntzig catheters (microvasive) were used, the balloon being introduced with the aid of the finger when the anastomosis was low in the rectum or through a rigid sigmoidoscope or by means of a guide-wire introduced through a flexible sigmoidoscope. The majority of the strictures had a diameter of less than 5 mm. Successful dilatation was obtained in ten patients.

Balloon dilatation has several advantages over the use of rigid dilators; in particular, the balloon can be accurately placed through the stenosis, and the dilating force is radial, thus avoiding the pushing force of a rigid dilator. This technique is particularly useful when the stenosis is located high in the rectum where the passage of a rigid dilator may be difficult and only possible using a curved metal dilator.[12]

Before dilatation of a rectal stricture the patient should be given antibiotic prophylaxis, as a Gram-negative form of septicaemia has on occasions occurred following these procedures.

Strictures following the use of the EEA stapling gun may often present a diaphragm-like appearance. Two techniques have been described to treat this complication endoscopically. The stenotic ring may be cut in two or three places along its circumference using the papilotomy diathermy cutting wire.[13] Alternatively, if it is possible to dilate the stricture sufficiently to admit the head of a circular stapling gun, it may be possible to excise part of the stricture.[14] The head of the gun is passed through the stricture and gently withdrawn until it engages the stricture; the gun is then displaced laterally and the jaws of the stapler closed to include a portion of the stricture; the gun is fired and a segment of the diaphragm-like stricture is resected.

An anal stricture may also occur after a coloanal or ileal pouch anastomosis and can usually be treated by dilatation using the finger or Hegars dilators.

References

1. Bennett R.C., Friedman M.H.W., Goligher J.C. Late results of haemorrhoidectomy by ligature and excision. *Brit. Med. J.* 1963; **2:** 216–19.
2. Parks A.G. The surgical treatment of haemorrhoids. *Brit. J. Surg.* 1956; **43:** 337–51.
3. Watts J.McK., Bennett R.C., Duthie H.L., Goligher J.C. Healing and pain after haemorrhoidectomy. *Brit. J. Surg.* 1964; **51:** 808–17.
4. Gingold B.S., Arvanitis M. Y–V anoplasty for treatment of anal stricture. *Surg. Gyn. Ostet.* 1986; **162:** 241–2.
5. Corman M.L., Veidenheimer M.C., Coller J.A. Anoplasty for anal stricture. *Surg. Clin. N. Amer.* 1976; **56:** 727–31.
6. Oh C., Zinberg J. Anoplasty for anal stricture. *Dis. Colon. Rect.* 1982; Nov–Dec: 809–10.
7. Hillyard R.W., El-Mahdl A.M., Schellhammer P.F. Intestinal strictures complicating preoperative radiation therapy followed by radical cystectomy. *J. Urol.* 1986; **136:** 98–101.
8. Anseline P.F., Lavery I.C., Fazio V.W., Jagelman D.G., Weakley F.L. Radiation injury of the rectum: evaluation of surgical treatment. *Ann. Surg.* 1981; **194:** 716–24.
9. Parks A.G., Allen C.L., Frank J.D. A method of treating post-irradiation rectovaginal fistulae. *Brit. J. Surg.* 1978; **65:** 417–21.
10. Bricker E.M., Johnston W.D. Repair of postirradiation rectovaginal fistula and stricture. *Surg. Gyn. Obst.* 1979; **148:** 499–506.
11. Skreden K., Wiig J.N., Myrvold H.E. Balloon dilatation of rectal strictures. *Acta Chir. Scand.* 1987; **153:** 615–17.
12. Hood K., Lewis A. Dilator for high rectal strictures. *Brit. J. Surg.* 1986; **73:** 633.
13. Accordi F., Sogno O., Carniato S., Fabris G., Moschino P., Coan B., Carlon C.A. Endoscopic treatment of stenosis following stapler anastomosis. *Dis. Colon Rect.* 1987; **30:** 647–9.
14. Hinton C.P., Celestin L.R. A new technique for excision of recurrent anastomotic strictures of the rectum. *Ann. R. Coll. Surg. Eng.* 1986; **68:** 260–1.

Index

Aarons cone in hydatid disease surgery 153
Abdomen, tuberculosis affecting *see* Tuberculosis
Abduction, bilateral recurrent laryngeal nerve palsy/paralysis in 247-8
Abscesses
　amoebic, in liver 206-7
　para-/sub-areolar 215
Adduction, bilateral recurrent laryngeal nerve palsy/paralysis in 247
Adenomatous polyposis, familial *see* Polyposis
Adjuvant therapy in colorectal cancer 125
Administrative tribunals, medical defence and 225
Adrenaline, injected, with bleeding peptic ulcers 17, 30
Airway
　cancers obstructing, laser therapy with 27-8
　facial fracture-related management 57, 63
Albendazole therapy in hydatid disease 158-9, 159
Alveolar margins, cancers of 66-83
Amoebiasis in children in India 206-7
Amoeboma in children in India 206
Anal cancer 104-5
Anandron, orchiectomy with, in prostatic carcinoma 173
Anaplastic thyroid cancer 87, 94
　surgery 94
Anastomoses
　with bile duct damage 254-6, 258
　coloanal
　　for post-irradiation rectal strictures 297
　　in rectal cancer surgery 103
　colorectal
　　in colorectal cancer surgery 103, 124
　　rectal stricture following 298
　facial nerve 235
　ileorectal
　　colectomy with *see* Colectomy
　　rectal stricture following 298
　in infertility treatment 185, 186
　laser-effected 27
　phrenic nerve to recurrent laryngeal nerve 248
　uretero-ureteric 277
Androgen withdrawal/ablation therapy in prostatic carcinoma 167-73
　total 172-3
Aneurysm, descending thoracic aortic, surgery-related complications with 265
Angiodysplasia, laser therapy for 30
Angiography, pulmonary, in postoperative thromboembolic disease 47
Angioplasty
　balloon
　　laser-assisted 28-9
　　percutaneous transluminal 28, 29
　laser 28
Anorectal stenosis 296-8
Anterolateral vein 287
Antiandrogen drug therapy in prostatic carcinoma 172
Antibiotics
　with abdominal tuberculosis 201
　with breast abscesses 215
　with facial fractures 61
　with staphylococcal pneumonia 195-6

Antibodies to sperm, post-vasectomy 186
Anticoagulant therapy in postoperative thromboembolic disease 41, 42, 43–4, 47–8, 49–50
 long-term 49–50
 prophylactic 41, 42
Aorta
 coarctation 262
 descending, spinal cord damage associated with surgery of 260–268
Aortic bypass techniques 265–8
Aortic pressure monitoring during moderate hypothermia 267–8
Aorto-aortic shunt 267
Aortoiliac surgery, infertility associated with 180
Areolar abscesses, para-/sub- 215
Areolar incision, circum-, necrosis at edge of 210
Argon lasers 12
 applications 27–34 *passim*
 with bleeding peptic ulcers 12–16 *passim* 30
 characteristics 24
 costs 36
Arteries *see specific arteries*
Ascariasis in children in India 202–5
Aspiration, with breast cysts 209–10
Aspiration biopsy, fine needle *see* Fine needle aspiration biopsy
Assistance, lack of, saphenofemoral junction damage caused by 290
Atriofemoral bypass, left 265–6
Azoospermia 181, 182, 184, 185, 187

Balloon dilatation with lower gastrointestinal tract strictures 298
Bandages, injuries from 278, 283–4
 management 283–4
Berry's suspensory ligament 241, 244
Bile duct injuries 251–9
 aetiology 251
 perioperative recognition 254–6
 postoperative recognition, early 257–9
 prevention 253
 repair 254–6, 257–9 *passim*
Bile peritonitis 257–8
Biliary ascariasis 205
Biliary calculi, laser surgery with 31

Biliary fistula 258
Biliary obstruction 258–9
Biliary surgery 251–2
Biopsies
 with colorectal cancer 120–121
 with oral cavity cancers 69–70
 with thyroid nodules and thyroid cancer 88–9, 91–2
Black, Hatcher v. 226–7
Bladder cancer, laser surgery with 33–4
Bladder controller device, Finetech-Brindley 191
Bladder neck surgery
 antegrade ejaculation restored by 192
 retrograde ejaculation caused by 181
Bleeding *see* Haemorrhage; Rebleeding
Bleomycin therapy with oral cavity cancers 82
Blood transfusion in colorectal cancer surgery 121
Boari flap 274–6
Bodkin Adams (Dr.), Regina v. 224–5
Bolam case, the 227–8
Bone, in familial adenomatous polyposis 133
Bone hooks in facial fracture management 62
Bone scans in prostatic cancer 174, 175
Bowel/intestine
 large
  carcinoma 137, 140–141
  in familial adenomatous polyposis 130, 137–42
 obstruction 109–10
  ascarideal 202–5
 ostomies, avoidance 100–112
Brachytherapy with oral cavity cancers 80
Breast, benign disease 208–17
Brindley sperm reservoir 187, 187–8, 189
Bronchoscopy, laser treatment via 27–8

Calculi
 biliary, laser surgery with 31
 urinary, laser surgery with 31
Calot's triangle 253
Cancers *see also* Carcinogenicity; Premalignant conditions; Tumours

airway obstructing, laser therapy with 27–8
bladder, laser surgery with 33–4
colorectal *see* Colorectal cancer; Rectal cancer; Rectosigmoid cancer
oral cavity *see* Oral cavity
photodynamic (laser) therapy with 35
testicular 180–181, 184, 272
thyroid *see* Thyroid cancer
Carbon dioxide lasers
 applications 26–34 *passim*
 characteristics 24
 costs 36
 tissue interactions with light from 24–5
Carcinogenicity (malignancy transforming potential)
 of nitrosamines 66–7
 of photodynamic therapy 36
Carcinoma(s) *see specific sites/types*
Carcinoma-in-situ
 oral cavity 70
  surgery 72–3
 testis 184
Cardiac surgery, lasers in 28–9
Cardiopulmonary bypass, pulmonary embolectomy on 49
Cardiovascular complications of oestrogen therapy for prostatic cancer 171–2
Cast(s), plaster and synthetic, injuries from 282–3
Castration by orchiectomy in prostatic cancer, avoidance 171
Catheter, ureteric 271
Cavitron ultrasonic dissection device in hydatid disease 155–6
Central nervous system in familial adenomatous polyposis 133
Cerebrospinal fluid rhinorrhoea with facial fractures 57
Cervical intraepithelial neoplasia, laser therapy with 34
Cervical lymph node involvement with oral cavity cancers 77
Cheek cancers 66–83
Chemotherapy
 antibiotic *see* Antibiotics
 anti-cancer
  with anal cancer 105
  with oral cavity cancers 71–2, 82
Children in India, surgery 194–207

Cholangiopancreatography, endoscopic retrograde (ERCP), in hydatid disease 149, 151
Cholecystectomy, complications 251, 252, 253
Choledocholithotomy, complications 251
Choledochotomy, complications 253
Cisplatinum therapy with oral cavity cancers 82
Colectomy with ileorectal anastomosis
 in diffuse neoplastic disease/familial adenomatous polyposis 108, 137, 139–42
  follow up 141–2
  functional outcome 139–40
 in idopathic constipation 108
 in inflammatory bowel disease 105–6
 mortalities and morbidity 139
Colitis, gangrenous, in children in India, amoebiasis-associated 206
Coloanal procedures
 for post-irradiation rectal strictures 297
 for rectal cancer 103
Colonoscopy, laser therapy via 32
Colorectal anastomosis in rectal cancer surgery 103, 124
Colorectal cancer 113–26, 137, *see also* Rectal cancer
 management 121–6
 staging and operability 113–21
Colorectal surgery 103, 121–6, 137–42
 lasers in 32–3
Colostomy, avoidance 101–5
Compensation
 no-fault 229
 saphenofemoral junction damage and 294
Complications, surgery-related *see* Iatrogenic surgical disease
Compression injuries
 with plaster and synthetic casts 282
 with splints and bandages 283
Computed tomography
 with colorectal cancer 117, 118
 with hydatid disease 149
 with oral cavity cancers 69
Connective tissue in familial adenomatous polyposis 131–2
Consent, informed 226
Constipation, idiopathic, permanent stoma avoidance in 108

Continence following rectal cancer surgery 104, *see also* Incontinence
Continuous-wave lasers 21, 23, *see also specific types*
Coroners' courts, medical defence and the 225
Cosmetic results in breast surgery, poor 211–12
Courts
 coroners', medical defence and the 225
 criminal, medical defence and the 224–5
Crile's incision 75
Criminal courts, medical defence and the 224–5
Crohn's disease, permanent stoma avoidance in 108–9
Crushing of femoral vessels 291
Cyproterone acetate therapy in prostatic cancer 172
Cyst(s)
 breast 208–10
 epidermoid, in familial adenomatous polyposis 131
 hydatid *see* Hydatid cysts
Cystopericystectomy in hydatid disease 155
Cystoscopy with ureteric damage 273
Cytology
 with oral cavity cancers 69–70
 with thyroid cancers 91–2

Deaths *see* Mortalities
Defaecation (bowel movements) following colorectal surgery 104, 139
Deltapectoral flaps in oral cavity cancer reconstructive surgery 79
Dentition *see* Teeth
Desmoid disease in familial adenomatous polyposis 131–2
Diathermy, laryngeal nerve damage caused by 246
Diet, with facial fractures 63
Diethylstilbestrol therapy in prostatic cancer 167
Digital tourniquets 280
Division of vessels at saphenofemoral junction, accidental 292–3
DNA content
 in colorectal cancer 121
 in thyroid cancer 97

Double-J-stent with ureteric injuries 272
Duct(s)
 bile *see* Bile duct
 ejaculatory, obstruction, treatment 187
 mammary/lactiferous
  ectasia 213–14, 215, 216
  excision 210–212
Dye lasers 21, *see also specific types*
 applications 34
 characteristics 24
Dysphagia, malignant, laser therapy with 30

EAA stapling gun 298
Ear, nose and throat surgery, lasers in 26
Echinococcus 159
 granulosus 146, 147
 multilocularis 147
Ejaculation
 failure 191–2
 retrograde 181, 192
Ejaculatory duct obstruction, treatment 187
Electrode systems, with bleeding peptic ulcers 12, 12–17 *passim* 30
Embolectomy, pulmonary 48–9
Embolism, pulmonary *see* Pulmonary embolism
Empyema in staphylococcal pneumonia 195, 196–7
En-bloc composite resection with oral cavity cancers 75
Endoscopy
 in infertility assessment and diagnosis 184
 therapeutic
  for bleeding peptic ulcers 8–19
  for colorectal cancer 125–6
  in ejaculatory duct obstruction 187
 ureteric injury caused by 270, 272
Endosonography in colorectal cancer 115–17, 117–18
Endotracheal tubes in facial fracture-related airway management 56
Entamoeba histolytica in children in India 206
Epidermoid cysts in familial adenomatous polyposis 131
Epididymis, obstruction 184, 185–6

Epididymitis 179–80
Epididymovasostomy 185, 186
Epigastric vein, superficial 287, 288
Epistaxis with facial fractures 57
Epithelial thyroid tumours 86
Erection, penis, surgery correcting dysfunction in 191
Erythroplakia 67
Esmarch bandage 279
Estramustine phosphate therapy in prostatic cancer 172, 173
Evoked potentials, somatosensory, in spinal cord functional assessment 262, 264, 265, 268
Exsanguination with tourniquets 279
Extracranial surgical damage, facial palsy caused by 232–4
Eyes *see* Ophthalmology

Facial fractures 52–65
　classification 54–6
　diagnosis 58
　late complications 65
　management/treatment 61–4
　　early 56–7
　radiography 60–61
Facial nerves, iatrogenic surgical damage to 231–5
　no permanent 234
　permanent 234
　prevention 234
　repair 234–5
　unknown 232–3
Facial palsy, iatrogenic 230–235
Fasciotomy in distal tourniquet ischaemia 282
Femoral artery
　anatomy 288
　damage 291, 291–4
Femoral nerve, damage 291
Femoral vein
　anatomy 288
　damage 290–91, 291–4
　mistaken as long saphenous vein 292–3
Femoral venous-to-arterial oxygenation 266
Fertility in men *see also* Infertility surgery improving 188–90
Fibrinogen, radiolabelled, in deep vein thrombosis studies 41, 43
Fibromatosis in familial adenomatous polyposis 131–2

Fibrosis
　retroperitoneal 272
　submucosal 68
Fine needle aspiration biopsy/cytology
　with oral cavity cancers 69–70
　with thyroid nodules and thyroid cancer 88–9, 91–2, 97
Finetech-Brindley bladder controller device 191
Fistula
　biliary 258
　mammillary 212–13
　urinary 274
　vesicovaginal, ureteric injury combined with 276
Fixation
　extraoral 63
　intermaxillary 64
Flaps
　in anal stenosis surgery 297
　in oral cavity cancer reconstructive surgery 78–80
　in ureteric damage repair 274–6
5-Fluorouracil therapy
　with anal cancer 105
　with oral cavity cancers 82
Follicle stimulating hormone levels, sperm levels related to 181, 183
Forehead flaps in oral cavity cancer reconstructive surgery 79
Fractures, facial *see* Facial fractures
Free flaps in oral cavity cancer reconstructive surgery 80

Gangrene, tourniquet ischaemia leading to 281
Gangrenous colitis in children in India, amoebiasis-associated 206
Gas lasers 21, *see also specific types*
Gastric cardia carcinoma, laser surgery with 30
Gastrointestinal tract
　laser surgery 12–17, 18–19, 29–31
　lower, balloon dilatation with strictures of 298
　upper, in familial adenomatous polyposis 130–31, *see also specific parts of tract*
General hospitals, roles and responsibilities 5–7
General practitioners, surgical specialism and generalism concerning 3

Index

General surgeons, roles and responsibilities 3–7
Generalism in surgery, specialism and 1–7
Gillies' temporal approach 62
Glaucoma, lasers in treatment of 26
Goitre
  laryngeal nerve affected by 241
  surgery-related complications in 241–2, 244
Grafts, nerve 234, 235, see also Flaps
Graves' disease 241–2, 244
Gynaecology, laser surgery in 34

Haematoporphyrins in photodynamic therapy 35
Haemorrhage/bleeding see also Rebleeding
  at saphenofemoral junction, causes 289–95
  with facial fractures 57
  with peptic ulcers see Peptic ulcers
  stigmata of recent (with peptic ulcers) 9–11, 13–14
Haemorrhagic telangiectasia, hereditary, laser therapy for 30
Haemorrhoidectomy, anal stenosis following 296–7
Hamartomatous polyposis, types 128
Hatcher v. Black 226–7
Heart surgery, lasers in 28–9
Heater probes 12
  with bleeding peptic ulcers 12–17 *passim*, 30
Heparin therapy with postoperative thromboembolic disease 41, 42, 43–4, 45, 47–8
  long-term 50
  prophylactic 41, 42
Hepatic conditions/surgery see Liver
Hepatic ducts, injury to confluence of 257
Hepaticoduodenostomy 256
Hepaticojejunostomy 256
Hepatobiliary surgery, lasers in 31–2
Histopathology, with oral cavity cancers 68–9
Hormonal therapy in prostatic cancer 167–74
  choices 170–172
  side-effects 170
  timing 168–70
  treatment after relapse from 173–4

Hospitals, roles and responsibilities 3–7
Hydatid cysts, hepatic
  structure 147
  surgery 149–56
Hydatid disease, hepatic 146–59
  chance encounters with 156–7
  diagnosis 148–9
  future for 159
  medical therapy 158–9
  natural history 148
  surgery 149–56
    contraindications 158
    follow-up 158
Hyperplasia, verrucous, oral cavity 70
Hypertension, pulmonary, pulmonary embolic disease presenting with 50
Hyperthermia, interstitial laser 31–2
Hypothermia, moderate 267–8

Iatrogenic surgical disease 217–99
  infertility as 179–81
  introduction to 221–2
  laser-related 36
  thyroidectomy-related 94, 238, 239, 241–2, 242, 242–3, 249
Ileal reservoir, proctocolectomy with, in inflammatory bowel disease 106–8
Ileorectal anastomosis see Anastomoses
Ileostomy, permanent, avoidance 105–9
Iliac vein, superficial circumflex 287–8
Imaging in thyroid cancer 90–91, see also Radiography *and specific techniques*
Impotence, organic 191
Incontinence, Young-Dees operation for, modification of 192, see also Continence
India, paediatric surgery in 194–207
Inexperience, surgical, saphenofemoral junction damage caused by 289
Infarction, pulmonary, postoperative 44–5, 50
Infections with facial fractures 61
Inferior vena cava, operations to obstruct 50
Infertility in males, see also Fertility
  causes 179–81, 181, 183, 190
  diagnosis, surgery in the 181–4
  prevention, surgery in the 179–81

treatment, surgery in the 184–92
Inflammatory bowel disease, permanent stoma avoidance in 105–8
Inflammatory polyposis, types 128
Inguinal surgery 179
Intestine see Bowel
Intracranial surgical damage, facial palsy caused by 231–2
Iodine-125 therapy in prostatic cancer 166
Iodine-131 therapy in thyroid cancer 96
Ipsilateral gracilis muscle transfers in iatrogenic facial palsy treatment 235
Irradiation see Radiotherapy
Ischaemia, tourniquet-related
  distal 281, 281–2
    management 281–2
    physiological results 278–9
Isotope/radionuclide scanning (scintigraphy)
  in colorectal cancer 118
  in prostatic cancer 174, 175
  in thyroid cancer 90, 91

J-stent, double, with ureteric injuries 272
Johnsen technique of grading spermatogenesis 183–4
Jordan, Whitehouse v. 228

Kelami sperm reservoir 187–8, 188
Ketoconazole therapy in prostatic cancer 173

Lactiferous ducts see Ducts
Laparoscopy in abdominal tuberculosis 201
Laryngeal nerve(s) 237–49
  anatomy 237–8
  damage 239–49
    causes 239–46
    prevention 242–5
    treatment 246–7
  physiology and function 238–9
  recurrent see Laryngeal nerve, recurrent
  superior see Laryngeal nerve, superior
Laryngeal nerve, recurrent
  anatomy 237
  anomalous 242
  branches 237, 241
  damage 238, 239, 239–45
    causes 239–42
    prevention 242–5
    treatment 246–8
  divisions 241
  identification 243–4
  paralysis/palsy 246–8
Laryngeal nerve, superior
  anatomy 237–8
  damage 239, 245–6
    treatment 248
  external branch 238, 239, 245–6
  internal branch 239
  paralysis 248
Laryngoscopy in prevention of laryngeal nerve damage
  postoperative 245
  preoperative 244–5
Laser(s) (in surgery) 12, 21–36
  applications 25–35
    with bleeding peptic ulcers 12–17, 18–19
    in bowel/colorectal surgery 32–3, 109–10, 125
  cost-effectiveness 36
  fundamentals 21–2
  safety 36
  tissue interactions with light from 24–5
Laser knife 25
  in hepatic resection 31
Law, medical defence and the 226–9, see also Litigation
Le Fort's fractures 55, 58, 59
  level I 54, 55, 63
  level II 54, 55, 58, 62
  level III 54, 55, 58, 62, 63
  management 62, 63
Legal proceedings see Litigation
Leukoplakia 67
Ligation of femoral vessels, damage caused by 291–2
Lighting, inadequate, saphenofemoral junction damage caused by 289–90
Limb compression injuries
  with plaster and synthetic casts 282
  with splints and bandages 283
Lithotripsy
  extracorporeal shock-wave 34
  laser 34
Litigation 226–9

saphenofemoral junction damage
and 294
Liver *see also entries under* Liver
amoebic abscesses in, in children in
India 206–7
in familial adenomatous polyposis
134
hydatid disease of *see* Hydatid disease
metastases, with colorectal cancer
118–20
resection
complications 252
in hydatid disease 156
Lobectomy (thyroid gland) 244
in thyroid cancer 93
Lung scans, ventilation and perfusion, in
pulmonary infarction 45, *see also
entries under* Pulmonary
Luteinizing hormone-releasing hormone
analogue therapy in prostatic
cancer 172
Lymph gland tuberculosis 200
Lymph node involvement
in colorectal cancers 115, 117–18
surgery regarding 121–2
with oral cavity cancers 71, 77, 83
with thyroid cancers 94
Lymphoma, thyroid 88, 89, 96
surgery 96

McFee incision 75
Magnetic resonance imaging
with colorectal cancer 117, 118
with oral cavity cancers 69
Males, fertility and infertility in *see*
Fertility; Infertility
Malignancy *see* Cancer; Carcinogenicity
Mammaplasty 5
Mammary ducts *see* Ducts
Mammillary fistula 212–13
Mammography
with benign breast microlesions 215
with duct ectasia 213, 214
Mandible
anatomy, trauma-related 53
anterior arch reconstruction, following
oral cavity cancer surgery 79
fractures 55–6, 59
Mandibulectomy (for oral cavity cancers)
marginal 73
median, with mandibular swing
73–5

Maxillary sinus, packing the, in facial
fracture management 62
Medical and Dental Defence Union of
Scotland 224
Medical defence (medico-legal
matters) 223–9, 294
history 223–4
saphenofemoral junction damage
and 294
the State in relation to 224–5
Medical Defence Union 223–4
Medical Protection Society 224
Medico-legal matters *see* Medical defence
Medullary thyroid cancer 87, 95
surgery 95
Megestrol acetate therapy in prostatic
cancer 173
Men, fertility and infertility in *see*
Fertility; Infertility
Meningeal infection with facial
fractures 61
Menorrhagia, laser surgery in 34
Mesorectal excision in colorectal cancer,
complete/total 123, 124
Metastasis
colorectal cancer 102, 118–20
oral cavity cancers 70, 71, 77, 83
prostatic carcinoma 167–74
Methotrexate therapy with oral cavity
cancers 82
Microcysts, breast 210
Microlesions, benign breast 215
Microvascular muscle transfers in
iatrogenic facial palsy treatment
235
Mitomycin C therapy with anal cancer
105
Mortalities/deaths
with peptic ulcers 9, 10, 15, 16
in total colectomy with ileorectal
anastomosis 139
Muscle transfers, microvascular, in
iatrogenic facial palsy treatment
235, *see also* Myocutaneous flaps
Mycobacterium tuberculosis 197
Myocutaneous flaps in oral cavity cancer
reconstructive surgery 78, 79

National Health Service, medical defence
and the 225
Neck
dissection, with oral cavity cancers
77–8

modified 77–8
radical 77
supraomohyoid 78
fascial layers, right laryngeal nerve in relation to 240–241
Necrosis
at edge of circumareolar incision 210
nipple, partial 211
pressure, with splints and bandages 284
of skin edge (of breast) 210–211
Negligence 227–8
Neodymium-YAG dye eximer laser 24
Neodymium-YAG laser(s) 12
applications 26–34 *passim*
with bleeding peptic ulcers 12–16 *passim*, 19, 30
in colorectal surgery 32, 123
characteristics 24
costs 36
tissue interactions with light from 24–5
Neodymium-YAG Q-switched laser 24
Neoplastic disease, diffuse, permanent stoma avoidance in 108, *see also* Cancer; Tumours
Neoplastic polyposis, types 128
Nerves
grafts and anastomoses 234, 235
surgical damage 231–50, *see also specific nerves*
Neurological involvement in familial adenomatous polyposis 133
Neurosurgery, lasers in 26
Nipple
discharge 211
partial necrosis 211
Nitrosamines, oral cavity cancer caused by 67
Nodules, thyroid 88–9, 90
Nuclear magnetic resonance *see* Magnetic resonance imaging

Obstruction
airway, cancers causing, laser therapy 27–8
biliary 258–9
bowel/intestine *see* Bowel
sperm deficiencies and infertility caused by 183, 184, 184–7
treatment for 184–7
ureteric 274

Occlusion, dental, in facial fracture patients 59
Oesophageal carcinoma, laser surgery with 30
Oestrogen therapy in prostatic cancer 171–2, 173
Oligospermia 181, 182, 183
causes 181, 183
Ophthalmology
in facial fracture patients 59
in familial adenomatous polyposis 134
lasers in 25–6
Oral cavity
cancers 66–83
diagnostic procedures 68–71
geographic pathology and mechanism 66–7
prognostic factors 83
treatment 71–82
premalignant conditions 67–8
Oral hygiene with facial fractures 63–4
Orbital fissure syndrome, superior 53
Orbital floor fracture, management 62
Orchidopexy 179
Orchiectomy in prostatic cancer 171
with Anandron 173
Osteomyocutaneous flaps in oral cavity cancer reconstructive surgery 79
Otorhinolaryngology, lasers in 26
Oxygenation, femoral venous-to-arterial 266

Paediatric surgery in India 194–207
Pain
with facial fractures, management 61
in prostatic cancer 173–4
Palliative surgery in colorectal cancer 125–6
Palomo operation 190
Palsy *see also* Paralysis
facial, iatrogenic 230–235
laryngeal nerves 246–8
tourniquet 280–281, 281
management 281
vocal cord *see* Vocal cord paralysis/palsy
Pancreatic surgery, lasers in 31–2
Paralysis *see also* Palsy; Paraplegia
laryngeal nerves 246–8
vocal cord *see* Vocal cord paralysis
Paraplegia after aortic surgery 265, 268

Parotid tumours, iatrogenic surgical
    disease with 232–3
Parotidectomy 4
Pectoralis major myocutaneous flaps in
    oral cavity cancer reconstructive
    surgery 79
Pelvic radiotherapy, rectal stricture
    following 297–8
Pelvic surgery
  in colorectal cancer 123–4
  infertility associated with 180
Penis erection, surgery correcting
    dysfunction in 191
Peptic ulcers, bleeding, endoscopic
    therapy for 8–19, 29–30
  costs 17–19
  objectives 8–9
  prognosis 11
  targets 9–11
  trials 12–17
  weapons 12–17
Percutaneous transluminal balloon
    angioplasty 28–29
Perforation, ascarideal/roundworm
    205
Perfusion lung scans in pulmonary
    infarction 45
Perianal conditions, laser therapy with
    32–3
Perianal sepsis, anorectal stenosis
    following 297
Peritoneal abdominal tuberculosis 200
Peritonitis
  amoebic, in children in India 206
  bile 257–8
Phalloplasty 191
Phlebography in deep vein thrombosis
    42
Photoablation effects of lasers 25
  in menorrhagia 34
Photodynamic therapy with lasers 25,
    35
  risks with 36
Photomechanical reactions with lasers
    25
Photothermal reactions with lasers 25
Phrenic nerve to recurrent laryngeal
    nerve anastomosis 248
Pigment epithelium, retinal, in familial
    adenomatous polyposis 134
Plaster casts, injuries from 282–3
Plastic surgery 5
  lasers in 26

Pneumatoceles in staphylococcal
    pneumonia 195, 196
Pneumonia, staphylococcal, in children
    in India 195–7
Pneumothorax in staphylococcal
    pneumonia 195, 196
Polidocanol and adrenaline, injected,
    with bleeding peptic ulcers 17
Polyp(s) 129
Polyp cancer, colorectal 122
Polyposis 128–44
  familial adenomatous 128–44
    clinical features 129–35
    diagnosis 135–7
    differential diagnosis 136
    incidence 129
    inheritance 129
    management 137–42
    permanent stoma avoidance in
        108
    screening 136–7
  registry for 142–3
  types 128
Population inversion with lasers 22
Porphyrin compounds in photodynamic
    therapy 35
Port wine stain, laser surgery 26
Posteromedial vein 287
Pouchitis 108
Premalignant conditions in oral cavity
    67–8
Pressure necrosis 284
Proctocolectomy
  in familial adenomatous polyposis
    137
  restorative
    in diffuse neoplastic disease/
        familial adenomatous polyposis
        108, 137–8
    with ileal reservoir, in
        inflammatory bowel disease
        106–8
Profunda femoris artery 288
Progesterone and progestogen therapy in
    prostatic cancer 172, 173
Prostate-specific antigen 163–4
Prostatectomy, radical 165–6
Prostatic acid phosphatase 163
Prostatic carcinoma 162–74
  catastrophes avoided with 170
  diagnosis 163–5
  general ill-health 169
  local progression 169

natural history 163
quality of life 169
treatment 163–74
    in advanced (localized) stages 166–7
    in early (localized) stages 163–6
    hormonal *see* Hormonal therapy
Psoas hitch 276
Pudendal artery, external
    damage 292
    deep 288–9
    superficial 288–9
Pudendal vein, external
    deep 287
    superficial 287
Pulmonary angiography in postoperative thromboembolic disease 47
Pulmonary embolectomy 48–9
Pulmonary embolic disease, longstanding, management 50–51
Pulmonary embolism
    acute massive 45–7
        presentation 46
    perioperative 41–2
    postoperative 42, 43, 45–7
        management 48–9, 50–51
    recurrent 50–51
    tourniquet-related 279
Pulmonary hypertension, pulmonary embolic disease presenting with 50
Pulmonary infarction, postoperative 44–5, 50
Pulsed lasers 21, 23 *see also specific types*
Pyelopneumothorax in staphylococcal pneumonia 195, 197

Radiation
    ionizing, therapeutic *see* Radiotherapy
    stimulated emission of 21
        light amplification by (LASER) *see* Laser
Radiography/radiology *see also* Imaging *and specific techniques*
    with abdominal tuberculosis 201
    with colorectal cancer 115–17, 117–18
    with facial fractures 60–61
    with intestinal ascariasis 203
    with oral cavity cancers 68–9
Radio-iodine therapy in thyroid cancer 96

Radionuclide scanning *see* Isotope scanning
Radiotherapy
    with anal cancer 105
    with colorectal cancer 125
    infertility associated with 181
    with oral cavity cancers 80–81
        advantages and disadvantages 80
        complications 81
        postoperative 81
        preoperative 81
    pelvic, rectal stricture following 297–8
    with prostatic cancer 166, 167, 173–4
Rebleeding, with endoscopically treated peptic ulcers 14, 16
Reconstructive surgery with oral cavity cancer 78–80
Rectal cancer 101, 101–4, 103–4, 113–26, 121–6 *see also* Colectoral cancer; Rectosigmoid cancer
    distant metastases 102, 118–20
    local spread 101–2
    staging and operability 101–3, 113–21
    surgery for
        anterior resection in 101, 103–4, 124
        functional results following 103–4
        local excision in 105
        recurrence rates following 101–2, 103
        total rectal excision in 101, 105
    tumour level 101
Rectal carcinoma, incidence with familial adenomatous polyposis 140–141
Rectal excision
    for rectal cancer 101, 105, 141
    other reasons for 141
Rectal stricture
    following colorectal and ileorectal anastomoses 298
    following pelvic irradiation 297–8
Rectoscope, urological, in colorectal cancer palliation 126
Rectosigmoid cancers 122
    laser surgery with 32
Rectum, management following total colectomy with ileorectal anastomosis 141
5 α-Reductase inhibitor therapy in prostatic cancer 173

Retinal pigment epithelium in familial adenomatous polyposis   134
Retroperitoneal fibrosis   272
Retroperitoneal surgery, infertility associated with   180
Rhinorrhoea, cerebrospinal fluid, with facial fractures   57
Rhys Davis device   279
Roundworms in children in India   202–5

Saidi cone in hydatid disease surgery   153
Salazopyrine therapy, infertility associated with   180
Salivary gland tumours   4
Saphenofemoral incompetence, persistent or recurrent, re-operations for   290
Saphenofemoral junction   286–95
  anatomy   286–9
  damage and bleeding   289–95
Saphenous nerve, damage   291
Saphenous vein, long
  anatomy relating to   287–9
  duplication   288
  femoral vein mistaken for   292–3
  incompetent, obliteration of   294
  stripping   294
Scars, breast   210–211
Scintigraphy see Isotope scanning
Sclerosant injected into femoral artery or vein   294
Scolicidal agents in hydatid disease   151–3
Sepsis, perianal, anorectal stenosis following   297
Sidaway case, the   227
Sigmoid colon cancer see Rectosigmoid cancer
Sigmoidoscopy in familial adenomatous polyposis   137
Skin
  edge (of breast), necrosis   210–211
  in familial adenomatous polyposis   131
Skull, subdivisions   52–3
Solid state lasers   21, see also specific types
Somatosensory evoked potentials in spinal cord functional assessment   262, 264, 265, 268
Specialism/specialization in surgery   1–7
  advantages   2
  disadvantages   2
  generalism and   1–7
  trends towards   1–2
Sperm
  antibodies, post-vasectomy   186
  retrieval, operations facilitating   187–8, 189
Spermatogenesis, defects and deficiencies in   181–4
Spinal artery, anterior   260–261, 262
Spinal cord   260–268
  anatomy   260–262
  blood supply   260–261, 263
  damage associated with descending aorta surgery   260–268
  functional assessment   262
  monitoring   263–5
  protection in surgery   265–8
Splints, injuries from   278, 283–4
  management   283–4
Squamous cell carcinoma, oral cavity   70
Staphylococcal pneumonia in children in India   195–7
Stapling gun, EAA   298
State, medical defence in relation to the   224–5
Stoma construction, avoidance   100–112
Stones see Calculi
Streptokinase therapy with postoperative thromboembolic disease   48
Stripping
  of femoral vessels, inadvertent   293
  of saphenous vein   294
Strontium-89 injections in prostatic cancer   173–4
Students, medical, surgical specialism and generalism concerning   3
Submucosal fibrosis   68
Sulphomucin staining with colorectal cancer   121
Suspension wires, extraoral, with facial fractures   63

Taenia echinococcus   146, 159
Tearing of vessels at saphenofemoral junction   292
Technetium-99-labelled nanocolloid, bone scans with, in prostatic cancer   174, 175

Teeth
　in familial adenomatous polyposis
　　132
　occlusion in facial fracture patients
　　59
　septic/infected, radiation therapy
　　and　81
Telangiectasia, hereditary haemorrhagic,
　　laser therapy for　30
Testicles/testes
　exploration　181
　maldescent　179
　size　181, 183
　torsion　179–80
　transplantation　188
　tumours/cancers　180–181, 184, 272
Testosterone stimulation, blockage, in
　　prostatic cancer therapy　172
Thoracic surgery, lasers in　27–8
Thromboembolic disease,
　　postoperative　39–51
　prevention　39–42
Thrombolytic therapy with postoperative
　　thromboembolic disease　47–8
Thrombosis, venous
　deep
　　diagnosis　40–41, 42–4
　　management　50
　　responses to clinical suspicion of
　　　42–4
　tourniquet-related dislodgement　279
Thyroglobulin measurements in thyroid
　　cancer　96
Thyroid (gland)
　cancer see Thyroid cancer
　in familial adenomatous polyposis
　　133–4
　laryngeal nerve in relation to　241
Thyroid artery
　inferior, recurrent laryngeal nerve in
　　relation to　239–40, 242, 244
　superior, superior laryngeal nerve
　　external branch in relation to
　　245–6
Thyroid cancer　85–98
　classification　87–9
　　biopsy features related to　91
　epidemiology　85–6
　investigations　89–92
　management　93–6
　　complications/hazards　94, 96
　pathology and pathogenesis　85–6
　presentation　88–9

Thyroid cartilage, inferior cornu, as a
　　surgical landmark　244
Thyroid pedicle, ligation　244
Thyroidectomy　93–4
　complications　94, 238, 239, 241–2,
　　242, 242–3, 249
　safe, prerequisites　242–3
　in thyroid cancer　93–4
Tissues, laser light interactions with
　　24–5
TNM staging of oral cavity cancers
　　70–71
Tobacco chewers, oral cavity cancer in
　　66–7
Tongue cancers　66–83
Tourniquets　278–82
　correct application　279–80
　injuries and complications from　278,
　　278–82
　management　281–2
Tracheostomy in facial fracture-related
　　airway management　56
Tracheotomy with laryngeal nerve
　　surgical damage　247, 248
Transection of vessels at saphenofemoral
　　junction, accidental　292–3
Transosseous wiring in facial fracture
　　management　62
Transurethral resection (TUR)
　in bladder cancer, lasers compared
　　with　33–4
　in prostatic cancer　166, 167
Trendelenburg's operation　46, 291
Tribunals, administrative, medical
　　defence and　225
Tuberculosis, abdominal, in children in
　　India　197–202
　clinical picture　200–201
　epidemiology　197–200
　investigations　201
　management　201–2
　types　201
Tubulovasostomy　185, 186
Tumours see also specific sites/types of
　　tumours
　iatrogenic surgical disease with
　　232–3, 272
　laser therapy with　27–8, 30–31, 32
　malignant see Cancer
Tying of femoral vessels, damage caused
　　by　291–2

Ulcers, peptic see Peptic ulcers

Ultrasonic dissection device in hydatid disease 155–6
Ultrasonography *see also* Endosonography
 in colorectal cancer, for liver metastases 119
 in hydatid disease 149, 159
 in prostatic cancer, transrectal 163, 164
 in thyroid cancer 90–91
University hospitals, roles and responsibilities 3–5
Ureteric catheter 271
Ureteric injury 270–276
 at open operation 272–4
 at ureteroscopy 270, 272
 avoidance 270–272
 delayed treatment 274–6
 with vesicovaginal fistula 276
Ureteric obstruction 274
Ureterography with ureteric damage 273
Ureteroscopy, ureteric injury caused by 270, 272
Uretero-ureteric anastomosis 277
Urinary calculi, laser lithotripsy with 31
Urinary fistula 274
Urine loss/seepage with ureteric injury 273
Urography, intravenous 271, 273
Urology, laser surgery in 33–4

Vas (deferens), obstruction
 diagnosis 181–2
 treatment 186
Vascular surgery, lasers in 28–9
Vasectomy 180, 186
Vasography 181–2
Vasovasostomy 185, 186

Veins *see specific veins*
Vena cava, inferior, operations to obstruct 50
Venography
 with deep vein thrombosis 43, 44
 with pulmonary embolism 45
Venous thrombosis, deep *see* Thrombosis
Ventilation and perfusion lung scans in pulmonary infarction 45
Ventriculo-aortic shunt 267
Verrucous cancers, oral cavity 70
Verrucous hyperplasia, oral cavity 70
Vesicovaginal fistula, ureteric injury combined with 276
Veteran's Administration study of prostatic cancer 162, 165, 168, 169, 171
Visceral abdominal tuberculosis 200
Vocal cord paralysis/palsy 238, 246–9
 treatment 246–9
Vulvar intraepithelial neoplasia, laser therapy with 34

Warfarin therapy with postoperative thromboembolic disease 42, 44
Whitehouse v. Jordan 228
Wires, extraoral suspension, in facial fracture management 63
Wiring, transosseous, in facial fracture management 62

Y-V advancement flaps in anal stenosis 297
Young-Dees operation for incontinence, modification of 192
Young's syndrome 181

Zoladex therapy in prostatic cancer 172
Zygomatic arch fracture 58, 62
Zygomatic complex fracture 55, 58, 62